Social Wo   Care

A Handbook for Practice

About the Editors

Kay W. Davidson, DSW, is Associate Professor at Hunter College School of Social Work in New York City. She brings to her current teaching position many years of experience working in England and the United States as a practitioner and administrator in social work in health and mental health care. Dr. Davidson has published articles on social work issues in health care and social work education. She is an active member of the Society of Hospital Social Work Directors and the National Association of Social Workers.

Sylvia S. Clarke, MSc, is a nationally known leader in health care social work who has spent the major portion of her career as administrator of social work departments in two large, urban medical centers. She has also been active as a social work educator. The editor of the journal *Social Work in Health Care* (The Haworth Press, Inc.) since its inception in 1975, she has conducted numerous workshops and seminars in writing for professional publication.

Social Work in Health Care

A Handbook for Practice

Part II

Kay W. Davidson, DSW
Sylvia S. Clarke, MSc
Editors

The Haworth Press
New York • London

The Haworth Press, Inc., 10 Alice Street, Binghamton, NY 13904-1580
EUROSPAN/Haworth, 3 Henrietta Street, London WC2E 8LU England

Library of Congress Cataloging-in-Publication Data

A Handbook for practice.

Selected articles reprinted from Social work in health care. v.1-11, 1974-86.
Includes bibliographical references.
1. Medical social work. 2. Medical social work—United States. I. Davidson, Kay W. II. Clarke, Sylvia S. III. Social work in health care. [DNLM: 1. Delivery of Health Care. 2. Social work. W 322 H236]
HV687.H26   1990   362.1'0425   89-24535
ISBN 0-86656-846-8 (set)
ISBN 1-56024-025-3 (pt.I)
ISBN 1-56024-026-1 (pt.II)

ISBN 0-86656-907-3 (pbk.set)
ISBN 1-56024-005-9 (pt.I)
ISBN 1-56024-006-7 (pt.II)

CONTENTS

PART I

CONTENTS

PART II

PART 6: PROFESSIONAL AUTHORITY, AUTONOMY, AND ACCOUNTABILITY

PART 8: PREPARATION FOR SOCIAL WORK IN HEALTH CARE

PART 9: AN EXPANDED ROLE FOR SOCIAL WORK

PART 6
PROFESSIONAL AUTHORITY, AUTONOMY, AND ACCOUNTABILITY

Introduction

Clearer definitions of professional role and functions have helped social workers accrue greater autonomy and accountability in complex health care organizations. The articles included in this chapter examine this development; they illustrate the progression from services based on referrals by others toward broader, population-based approaches in which social workers themselves identify patients' psychosocial needs, initiate services, establish independent priorities, and develop social work management systems in response to calls for greater accountability in an era of increased fiscal and regulatory constraints.

DEVELOPMENT OF AUTHORITY AND AUTONOMY

The articles selected for this section demonstrate achievements in moving toward increased professional authority and autonomy in practice through development of systems for identifying appropriate recipients of service, for instituting case-finding mechanisms, and for defining professional roles and activities.

Berkman, Rehr, and Rosenberg's article illustrates how social workers in health care can initiate the development of professional criteria for identifying patients' needs for social work services. The authors demonstrate that when social workers cease to rely on the perspectives of others to define their role, their services may be outlined clearly and used effectively.

Boone, Coulton, and Keller report study findings that support the value of early and self-defined intervention. They demonstrate the benefits of research to test and confirm the effectiveness of autonomous social work practice in health care.

The conceptual framework for identifying patients at risk for medical and psychosocial complications that Sulman and Verhaeghe present in their article about social work with myocardial infarction patients supports autonomous decision making about timely and appropriate social work intervention and services.

The article by Pfouts and McDaniel examines persistent issues of autonomy, "handmaiden" status, and bureaucratic constraints on social workers in hospitals. It provides a challenging analysis of ways in which social workers define their roles and activities, illustrated by a study of social work services in the pediatric department of a teaching hospital.

MANAGEMENT AND ACCOUNTABILITY

Given the changing nature of social work practice, social work managers place emphasis on staff development programs that support, promote, and reward staff for the continuing accrual of a professional knowledge base which includes ideas adapted from other sources and tested for their applicability to health care social work. Although space did not permit their reproduction here, articles that offer reports of varying programs for staff supervision and development are suggested as additional readings.

The articles that are included here report innovative approaches to management and accountability. Many articles about these issues that appeared in the pages of the journal have by now been established as classics reprinted many times in a variety of professional publications (see, for example, Lurie and Rosenberg, 1984; Bracht, 1978). Rather than reproduce articles that are readily available elsewhere, we have selected for this chapter articles that, although less frequently cited and reprinted, make a valuable contribution to understanding management and accountability from the perspective of the social work practitioner.

These articles were selected because they expand the concept of accountability beyond that of responsibility to external authorities, such as funding sources, employing agencies, and regulatory bodies, to a broader one that considers responsibility to the recipient of services, the client, and seeks to answer the practitioner's question, "Is what I do helpful?"

The article by Ferguson et al. illustrates an early effort by practitioners to implement and evaluate a quality assurance program. The authors demonstrate the critical importance of peer review and staff participation in the accountability system. This innovative work forms an excellent base for comparison with reports of subsequent efforts by the same authors to refine this quality assurance program (see Ferguson et al., 1980).

Grob, Eisen, and Edinburg contribute an example of a client satisfaction study in a psychiatric hospital setting. Adolescent and young adult patients and their parents and social workers were interviewed to develop data about the adequacy of social work services to meet clients' needs. The report of the study's findings and discussion of its implications provide the basis for a widely replicable model.

Krell and Rosenberg's article on social work staffing furnishes a framework for studying and predicting patterns of social work staffing for hospital settings. The steps in the development of the proposed formula constitute a seminal effort to approach systematically a critical management issue of universal concern to social workers in health care.

Garber, Brenner, and Litwin's article reports on a client satisfaction study. Although some of the research assumptions need further exploration, the study, based on a survey, is clearly reported and replicable. It is of particular significance as an example of a research study and accountability program undertaken by practitioners.

A Social Work Department Develops and Tests a Screening Mechanism to Identify High Social Risk Situations

Barbara Berkman, DSW
Helen Rehr, DSW
Gary Rosenberg, PhD

SUMMARY. This paper described a model for developing and testing a screening mechanism to identify high psychosocial risk patient situations in need of early intervention by social workers. Although the criteria developed need further refinement, it was found that multiple criteria are significantly more predictive of high risk than single factors and that three variables, (1) severity of illness: life threatening, (2) severity of illness: physically dysfunctional; and (3) chronic illness, were good predictors of need for social work services. It is suggested that similar screening mechanisms be developed and utilized in hospitals throughout the country.

A major problem which has handicapped the delivery of comprehensive social work services in the hospital setting is the dysfunctional aspect of the traditional case finding system. In that system

At the time of writing Dr. Berkman was Adjunct Associate Professor of Community Medicine (Social Work) at the Mount Sinai School of Medicine of the City University of New York, and Research Associate at the Department of Social Work Services, Mount Sinai Hospital, One Gustave Levy Place, New York, NY 10020. Dr. Rehr was Edith J. Baerwald Professor of Community Medicine (Social Work) at the Mount Sinai School of Medicine. Dr. Rosenberg was Assistant Professor of Community Medicine (Social Work) at the Mount Sinai School of Medicine, and Director, Department of Social Work Services, Mount Sinai Hospital.

Reprinted from *Social Work in Health Care*, Volume 5(4), Summer 1980.

other health care professionals determine who is in need of social work services and when that help should be requested. Social workers in the health care system have not assumed consistent responsibility for finding those persons who could benefit from their services, except in a few social programs such as young unmarried pregnant girls, neonatal defects, drug addicted pregnant women, and those entering renal care programs.

Because persons outside social work perceive psychosocial need from their own professional view, and because they may not be familiar with the types of problems dealt with and the range of services offered by social workers, a referral-based system tends to lead to referrals of those clients with obvious, easily visible needs, but often fails to refer those patients and family members who could utilize help with the range of psychosocial stresses that accompany illness and hospitalization (Berkman and Rehr, 1973). When referrals *are* made, most of them come to the social work department late in the course of the patient's hospitalization, and thus limit the service the patient and family can receive by imposing a time constraint that can adversely influence the outcome of the situation (Berkman and Rehr, 1972).

Despite the existence of several vanguard programs where social work casefinding is institutionalized, this characteristic referral system has remained basically unchanged through the years and even appears to have been introduced into the newer "innovative" health settings, such as the neighborhood health center and the health maintenance organization (Berkman, 1977). Clarification of the role of the social worker and appropriate utilization of social work services will not be assured as long as social workers continue to rely on the perspectives of other professions to determine not only the timing of social work intervention but also the specification of the problems with which they can help.

In a move to grapple with the problem of late referrals of limited perspective, social workers at the Mount Sinai Medical Center, a 1,200 bed acute care hospital in New York City, have been developing a high social risk (HSR) screening procedure. The mechanism tries to identify those patients and their family members whose social situations, stress, or predicted social and physical problem resulting from the illness and hospitalization may interfere with their ability to make an optimum plan for the post-hospital period or to cope with daily life expectations. This paper presents the steps in developing and testing a screening mechanism with criteria relevant to the hospitalized population served in this medical center (Blumberg, 1957; Cochrane and Holland, 1971).

A MODEL FOR DEVELOPMENT
OF THE SCREENING MECHANISM

There were four phases in the development of the screening mechanism (Chart I): Phase I involved the development of the High Social Risk Indicators by the professional staff; Phase II involved a test utilization of the screening mechanism on all admissions with expected lengths of stay of 7 days or longer; Phase III utilized Master's degree level social workers to act as judges in the review of all patients scored as positive for High Social Risk by the screening device. In this process, they were expected to determine the validity of high social risk situations uncovered in the screening. During Phase IV those patients who were screened as non-high social risk were followed statistically through departmental records to assess the validity of that determination.

Phase I: Development of High Risk Indicators

The social work staff of the adult medical and surgical inpatient units met over a three month period to determine indicators of high social risk (HSR) for patients and families. From their knowledge of the impact of illness on social functioning, and their experience-based views of the relationship of illness and social problems, they worked to identify the characteristics of social work clients in this health setting. They then worked to translate the social factors into screening criteria that could uncover "at admission" those patient/family situations at presumptive high social risk who would then be followed with a psychosocial diagnostic assessment (Appendix A). The screening mechanism was designed so that the risk variables projected by professional social workers could be identified from data available on the patient's admission sheets by a trained non-professional screener at the time of the patient's admission.

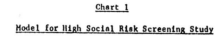

Chart 1

Model for High Social Risk Screening Study

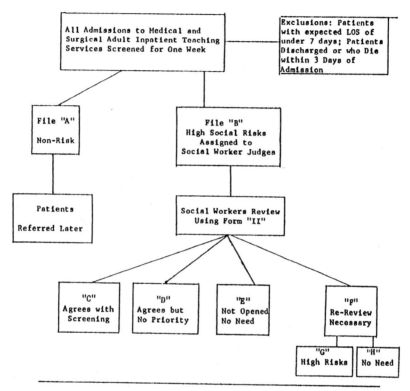

Group "A" is monitored statistically for two months to see what proportion of cases are referred to social workers after screening is completed. This will capture false-negatives which may occur in Group "A." In addition, a random sample of Group "A" should be interviewed during hospitalization as another way to determine whether screening represented a false-negative (i.e., screening mechanism found patient not potentially at risk but interview proved differently.) Also monitored are Groups "E" and "H" to be sure the judgments of the social workers were sound.

Phase II: Screening All Admissions

During six days in April 1978, a secretary trained in the screening procedures reviewed all daily admissions to the adult in-patient medical and surgical services of the hospital. Utilizing the eight criteria established by the social workers, she screened the daily admission sheets, pulling those which fell into a high social risk category. For this pilot study, those patients with expected lengths of stay of under seven days were excluded from review. This policy was based on past experience which demonstrated that long stay patients were the primary users of the service. This policy derived from the extent of social work services available rather than the judgment that short stay patients are without social problems. At the end of each day, admission which was designated high social risk was assigned to the social worker who covered the appropriate service area.

Phase III: Social Work Review

This phase checked on the validity of the positive screenings, i.e., those patients who were identified by criteria as High Risk through a review (Appendix B) within three days by one of fifteen staff social workers who acted as judges in determining the validity of the screening decision.

This study was designed purposely to fit the department's organizational structure wherein social workers cover designated service areas. It would have been better to distribute the screenings randomly among the fifteen MSW social worker judges, protecting us from possible sources of bias due to variations in workers' clinical experience. In addition, staff members covering services which had a larger number of high social risk admissions experienced a greater impact of review work. An alternate study approach which would have reduced the impact on those workers, would have been to select randomly from among the high risk screenings designated for their review. In future studies of this nature this procedure is suggested if randomization across all workers is not feasible.

The method of review was left to the discretion of each social worker-judge and could consist of an in-person intake interview, review of information available in the medical chart, discussion with the physicians and nurses, informal rounds, or through combinations of these approaches. Excluded from review were patients discharged or those who died within three days of admission. Following review there were three options for worker decision: (1) to consider the patient at High Social Risk and needing social work intervention; (2) to decide not to give service because of "no need"; (3) to defer decision at that time with a plan for a second review one week later. Those latter two options indicated possible errors in the High Social Risk screening mechanisms. "Too many" of these would be an indicator that the instrument was screening in too many "false positives."

Phase IV: Monitoring

This phase monitored through departmental records those patients who had been screened out as Non-High Social Risk. The question to be answered was whether they would be referred to the social work department at any time during the course of the patient's hospital stay. If a large number of these patients were subsequently referred to social workers, it would be an indication that the screening mechanism was not working adequately and was screening out too many "risk" cases. In addition, those HSR situations which the social workers reviewed in Phase III and determined there was "no" need for social work intervention, or which they "deferred," were also monitored at this time to insure the validity of the early judgments by checking whether they were not served later in the patient's hospitalization.

FINDINGS

In the six day period 613 adult patients admitted to the Medical and Surgical Services of the hospital with expected lengths of stay of seven days or more were screened. Three hundred ninety-four (67%) of the patients were screened as Non-High Social Risk "at admission." One hundred ninety-three patient situations (33%) were designated as potentially at High Social Risk and referred to social worker-judges for review. Twenty-six situations were excluded from the review: 22 patients who were discharged and four patients who died within 3 days of admission.

The High Risk Patients

The first question asked during analysis was which, if any, potential risk factors were prevalent in the admissions identified as High Social Risk. Would one or two factors, or combinations of factors, account for a major proportion of the admissions screened as high risks? It was found that two factors were present in 57% of all the screenings which designated patients as High Social Risk: (1) severity of illness: life threatening, occurred in 33% of the HSR cases and (2) severity of illness: physically dysfunctioning, occurred in another 34% of the HSR situations. Among the diagnoses included in these categories were those patients with metastatic or terminal cancer, those with blood dyscrasias, patients admitted to the various intensive care units, patients with organic and/or mental brain syndrome, and sight threatening conditions (Appendix A).

Of the 193 patients screened in as High Social Risk, the social worker-judges agreed that 68 situations (35%) were high risk and needed immediate intervention. Thirty-five (18%) were assessed "at possible risk" by the social workers but not considered of immediate priority when compared to other situations in which they were intervening. Thus, while they believed there was a "possible risk" they did not intervene "at admission." In an additional 42 cases the workers could not make an "at admission" decision because of limited information and re-reviewed those situations one week later when eight (4%) were confirmed as high risk. Thus the total number of situations validated as high risk (true positives) were 111 or 58% of the total screened "in" High Social Risk cases.

In 48 screenings (25%) the social worker-judges determined "no need" for intervention because their social assessments indicated there were adequate psychosocial supports in the family situation to allow the situations to be handled without social work intervention. Adding to this number the 34 deferred cases (17%) which were re-reviewed and then determined not in need of social work services brought the total of "false positive" screenings to eighty-two or 42%.

The issue which must still be determined is whether these "no need for intervention" situations, for whatever reasons posed, should be considered "false positive" screenings. It is important to note that the instrument utilized was intended for identification of high social risk from specified documented data available at the time of admission to the hospital. Information available either from professional in-person interviews with the patient-family system or from interactions with or materials derived from the provider system, following the admission, would need to be considered additive to early casefinding. Therefore these "no need" or "deferred" situations would need to be reviewed in the context of later referrals, if any. It would be helpful to learn more about these types of situations to see if other dimensions need to be deliberated for early casefinding.

Of the 193 patients screened as at high social risk, 120 (62%) had one risk factor present (Table 1). Seventy-three cases (38%) had multiple risk factors. Of the one risk factor screenings, 52% were true positives in the judgment of the social workers. Of the multiple factor cases significantly more, 67%, were judged true positives (X^2 = 3.82, df = 1, P *lth .05). Thus it would appear that the presence of more than one risk criterion is a better predictor of high social risk than a single risk criterion.

In continuing the comparative analysis of High Social Risk situations that were judged "true" positive or "false" positive, individual risk factors and combinations of factors were reviewed to determine which were predictive of high risk (Table 2). It became clear that neither of the age criteria alone were predictive of high risk, i.e., neither those patients in their eighties, nor those in their seventies and living alone, were judged at risk because of these factors

Table 1

Distribution of High Social Risk Screenings
by Number of Risk Factors Present and Validity Judgments

	Number of Risk Factors					
	One Risk Factor		Multiple Risk Factors		Total	
Validity Judgment of Social Workers						
	N	%	N	%	N	%
True Positive	62	52%	49	67%	111	58%
False Positive	58	48%	24	33%	82	42%
	120	100%	73	100%	193	100%
	(62%)		(38%)		(100%)	

X^2=3.82, df=1, P<.05

Table 2

Distribution of High Social Risk Screening by Risk Criteria Present and Validity Judgement

Validity Judgment of Social Workers	Single Criteria Present						Multiple Criteria Present			Total
	80 Years Old	70 Years Old	Emergency Admission	Severity Illness Life Threatening	Severity Illness Phys. Dysfunctional	Chronic Disease	Severity Illness Life Threatening Plus Other	Severity Illness Phys. Dysfunctional Plus Other	Other Multiples	
	N %	N %	N %	N %	N %	N %	N %	N %	N %	N %
True Positive	4 (44%)	3 (43%)	5 (33%)	23 (66%)	17 (44%)	10 (67%)	23 (64%)	22 (86%)	4 (36%)	111 (58%)
False Positive	5 (56%)	4 (57%)	10 (67%)	12 (34%)	22 (56%)	5 (33%)	13 (35%)	4 (14%)	7 (64%)	82 (42%)
TOTAL	9 100%	7 100%	15 100%	35 100%	39 100%	15 100%	36 100	26 100%	11 100%	193 100%

solely. Nor was an "emergency admission," as a single indicator, predictive of High Social Risk. However, severity of illness that was life-threatening, as a single criterion, and the presence of chronic disease, as a single criterion, were predictive of high risk in two out of three situations. Severity of illness that was physically dysfunctional was not predictive as a single criterion. In analyzing those situations with multiple risk criteria present, we find that severity of illness which is physically dysfunctional, in combination with one or more other factors, is predictive of high risk in four out of five instances. Severity of illness which was perceived as life-threatening, combined with one or more other criteria, was predictive in approximately two out of three situations.

The Non-High Social Risk Patients

Three hundred and ninety-four patients (67%) were screened as non-high social risk since there were no high risk screening criteria identified. To test the validity of the screening determination these patients were followed through departmental statistics for two months to determine whether these "non-risk" patients were referred to social service through traditional referral methods. Any of the "non-high risk" cases which were referred would be considered an error, a false negative, for the screening process. Only 11 cases (3%) were referred to social work services during the course of the patients' hospitalization, indicating the "screening-out" process may be working effectively. However, the ideal way to have carried out this study would have been to interview those patients who were screened out to see whether professional social workers would have agreed with the screening. It is our plan to repeat the study and interview patients who are screened out as non-high risk to further substantiate this observation.

DISCUSSION

The primary intent of a casefinding system is to identify individuals and their families with specifically defined problems that have placed them at high social risk and then to link them with the appropriate, available social work services. Identifying high social risk factors is not difficult for social workers. They work with those in social need and with social problems. Education and experience sharpen their perceptions. Case reviews, chart assessment, and medical social rounds are other effective means to cull out "risks" in those utilizing the setting.

In these early efforts to develop a casefinding instrument, the professional staff stated their preference to continue interviewing patients and family members to confirm need. They also indicated a preference for continued utilization of medical-social rounds for essential interprofessional collaboration. It was clarified that the benefits of interprofessional rounds as useful in collaborative decision making and communication would continue, however, the traditional means of uncovering patients at social risk through professional interview of each admitted individual or through medical social rounds were costly structures for casefinding. The introduction of a valid screening mechanism utilized by a non-professional may prove more cost effective than these other methods.

This study demonstrated that the high social risk screening mechanism could screen out patients not-at-risk as evidenced by the very small percentage of hospitalized patients who entered the service by other referral methods. However, this finding is considered tentative until restudied with direct interviews of patients screened as non-risk to substantiate the validity of the finding. In this experience the screening "out" of patients was easier to achieve than the valid screening "in." It had been anticipated that a small proportion of patients screened as High Social Risk would be judged by the social workers as not needing their intervention since many patients have strong family supportive help or adequate resources which cannot be identified by the data on an admission fact sheet. At this time, the high social risk screening instrument has been developed for early casefinding only, and not for uncovering the internal or external resources in the patient-family or provider systems to deal with those risks. But a finding of major consequence in this pilot study was the large number of cases screened "in" as high risk via the screening mechanism and subsequently determined by the social worker-judges to be "non-risk." Because only 58% of the high social risk cases screened were considered valid as to needing social work services by the reviewing judges, the major question raised was whether the screening net as designed was too broad.

The one hundred and eleven patients screened "in" as HSR represented 18% of the adult admissions. This percentage represents approximately the same number of adult inpatient medical and surgical cases which social workers reach through traditional referral methods. However, at this time we do not know if the instrument is identifying the same patients. This must be determined in future study. If they are the same patients who were formerly reached near the time of discharge or at point of crisis, then the screening mechanism is clearly preferable because it enables us to reach patients earlier and allows for the necessary processes in intervention. If they are different patients than those reached through traditional referrals, the fact that we screen in the same proportion of cases will raise the question of how the current departmental resources can absorb a larger number of patients in need of social work service than we are currently serving.

Earlier intervention obviously is the preferable professional expectation. It would allow more time to be spent on each situation and enable social workers to deal with problems they were able to identify but were not able to deal with under the constraints of brief, limited service. However, the administrative and professional significance of potentially added numbers of clients would need to be considered before implementing any new method of casefinding. The instrument must now be taken back to staff and refined based on the findings of the study. Further modification of the instrument is needed to increase the specificity of the screening process.

Implications

Can social work in health care develop reliable social risk screening instruments? The immediate response is "yes." They are already in development and are being demonstrated as valuable by those initiating their own casefinding systems. We have suggested that screening instruments should be valid and economical. The objectives of a department must be clearly determined, resources have to be available and ready for achieving these objectives, and the screening program must be planned and tested before implementation. The achievement of a departmental screening device requires professional commitment and the allocation of time, money, and resources. Training and refresher meetings for staff, which affect the cost of the program, are essential for sound implementation and maintenance of the system (Rehr et al., 1980).

It is envisioned that screening mechanisms such as the one described will be utilized in hospitals throughout the country within the near future (Massachusetts General Hospital, Department of Social Services and Johns Hopkins Medical Center, Department of Social Services are utilizing screening mechanisms of this nature). A major issue in the process of implementing screening approaches is the orientation of hospital administration and medical staff to the new system. In the present case, this was done at the Medical Board level to secure a hospital mandate and policy decision. In these discussions we identified social work's focus, its roles and functions. Independent screening clearly establishes social work as the profession to deal with psychosocial problems in the medical setting. In addition, the possibilities for cost containment through the early identification of patients "at risk" for discharge cannot be underestimated. Early casefinding can help deter delays in appropriate medically indicated discharge. Also, those service areas which have greater numbers of high social risk patients can be identified and appropriate deployment and/or redeployment of manpower planned. Once we can anticipate the number of people and types of problems to be dealt with, we can plan for the types of services needed. The benefits of early intervention to patients and their families are self-evident. Administrators, particularly in times of scarce resources, are asked to set priorities. High Social Risk screening mechanisms are one means offered to determine priorities in a rational and systematic manner. It is believed that the methodology used for developing and testing this screening mechanism may be useful to comparable departments in their efforts to develop screening procedures geared to potential users of social work service.

REFERENCES

Berkman, B. Innovations for social services in health care. In F. Sobey (Ed.), *Changing roles in social work practice.* Philadelphia: Temple, 1977.

Berkman, B. & Rehr, H. The 'sick role' cycle and the timing of social work intervention. *The Social Service Review*, 1972, *46*, 567-580.

Berkman, B. & Rehr, H. Early social service case-finding for hospitalized patients: an experiment. *The Social Service Review*, 1973, *47*, 256-265.

Blumberg, M. Evaluating health screening procedures. *Operations Research*, 1957, *5*, 351.

Cochrane, A. L., & Holland, W. W. Validation of screening procedures. *British Medical Bulletin*, 1971, *27*, 3-8.

Rehr, H., Berkman, B., & Rosenberg, G. High social risk screening principles and problems. *Social Work*, 1980.

Appendix A

HSR Screening Form A

Category I.   Automatic Social Work Assistant Review- high social risk identified as:

_____ 1. Over 70 years, living alone, with eye surgery projected

_____ 2. Institutional transfers into the hospital

Category II.   Social Worker Review- High Social Risk identified as:

_____ 1. 80 year old and over

_____ 2. 70 year old and over, living alone

_____ 3. Emergency admission

(except appendicitis, hernias, pneumonias)

_____ 4. Severity of illness- life threatening

(i.e. metastatic or terminal CA and blood dyscrasias, all admissions to ND, CICU, Ames, CT, RT)

_____ 5. Severity of illness- physical dysfunctioning

(i.e. organic and/or mental brain syndrome, encephalopathies; syrengo-myelia; CVA and stroke, aphasia, pathological fractures; carcinoma of the colon, rectum, pancreas, brain or masses leading to "ostomies;" any limb surgery leading to amputation; (due to diabetes, gangreno, circulatory diseases); carcinoma of the throat, vocal chord, larynx, tongue, airway obstructions leading to "ectomies;" renal diseases leading to dialysis and/or transplant; multiple fractures; eye disorders i.e. glaucoma, retinal detachment, conditions which are sight threatening.)

_____ 6. Chronic Diseases

(i.e. lupus, Hodgkins, myasthenia gravis, ulcerative colitis, multiple sclerosis, cerebral palsy, hemophilia, sickle cell, muscular dystrophy, rheumatoid arthritis, liver diseases.)

Research Assistant_____   Date_____

Patient Admission Date_____   Worker assigned review_____

Patient's Name _____

Appendix B
Patient-Family HSR Review Form B

I. Worker Review (check method 1 or 2)

____ 1. In-Person Intake Review

____ 2. Other Review Method(s)
(circle applicable method(s)

a) Chart   d) Rounds Discussion

b) Doctor Discussion   e) Other (explain) _____

c) Nurse Discussion   _____

II. After Review did you:

____ a) Open Case

____ b) Open/close (in same day) Give reasons: _____
_____
_____

____ c) Not open case (give reasons) _____
_____
_____

____ d) MSW refers to Assistant after review (give name of Assistant, give reasons)
_____

____ e) Assistant refers to MSW after review (give name of MSW, give reasons)
_____
_____

____ f) Temporarily Deferred Decision on opening, will review again (give reasons)
_____
_____

____ g) Case previously opened (give date of prior opening)
_____

Patient's Name _____   Unit Number _____
Reviewer _____   Date _____

The Impact of Early and Comprehensive Social Work Services on Length of Stay

Charlotte R. Boone, MSW, ACSW
Claudia J. Coulton, PhD, ACSW
Shirley M. Keller, MSSA

SUMMARY. The efficient use of health care resources requires that patients remain in in-patient facilities only as long as is necessary. High-quality patient care requires that patients are physically, socially, and psychologically prepared for leaving the hospital and that plans for their post-hospital care are adequate. The authors discuss a study of Orthopaedic patients which demonstrates that early and comprehensive social work intervention can reduce the length of time patients stay in the hospital. They also describe the effect of the study on expanding the role of social work within the acute care, general hospital.

INTRODUCTION

As the cost of health care rises, there is increasing interest in utilization of hospital services in a more effective and efficient manner. Since in-patient hospital care is the most expensive health care

At the time of writing Charlotte R. Boone was Director, Social Service Department, Akron City Hospital, 525 East Market Street, Akron, OH 44309. Claudia J. Coulton was Associate Professor, School of Applied Social Sciences, Case Western Reserve University, Cleveland. Shirley M. Keller was Assistant Director, Social Service Department, Akron City Hospital. The authors are indebted to the entire Social Service Department and especially to Laura Schrank for her participation in this study.
Reprinted from *Social Work in Health Care*, Volume 7(1), Fall 1981.

service today, attention has focused on decreasing the length of time patients stay in the hospital.

Comparisons showing substantial regional differences in average length of hospital stay per patient have supported the view that some patients may be staying in the hospital when an alternative arrangement would be acceptable given their physical condition (NCHS, 1979). Thus, various procedures have been instituted in hospitals with the goal of assuring that patients' stays in the hospital are only as long as is medically necessary (Health Care Financing Administration, 1979). Although social workers support the appropriate utilization of acute health care beds, they are well aware of the fact that the length of time a patient remains in the hospital depends on many factors. Length of stay is not only dependent on physical condition, but also on the patient's personal capacities and resources in the environment. This perception is supported by numerous research findings. Glass et al. (1977) found that 18% of the hospital days for patients they studied were due to social factors rather than medical factors. Zimmer (1974) found that 11.9% of hospital days could not be attributed to medical need. Mason et al. (1980) reported that, for 21% of patients admitted to a metropolitan hospital, social factors were very important in the admission decision. Boaz (1979) noted that for patients admitted to the hospital on an emergency basis, length of stay was strongly affected by social factors. This may reflect these emergency patients' lack of opportunities to prepare emotionally and realistically for their hospital admissions and discharges.

Although social workers have known that services directed toward alleviating social and psychological problems are a vital component of reducing length of stay, this has been difficult to demonstrate. There has long been concern about whether patients with social and psychological problems were actually receiving timely and appropriate social work assistance. For example, Berkman and Rehr (1972) found that patients tended to be seen by social workers relatively late in their hospitalizations. In addition, in hospitals where social workers depend largely on referrals to identify their clients, the evidence from one hospital suggests that many patients who could benefit will never be seen by a social worker (Berkman & Rehr, 1973).

This interest in timely and comprehensive social work intervention has been based on the knowledge that the stress of illness and hospitalization can create a high level of anxiety in the patient and family. Early intervention is seen as increasing the possibility that the patient will be helped to cope with illness and/or anxiety in a more realistic manner. The reduction of the patients' anxiety level, which can be related directly to the illness and/or social problems, is expected to lead to more effective total health care. It is essential that emotional, behavioral, and social factors be included in defining adequate care and rehabilitation plans in order to guarantee patients' right to achieve their maximum health potential (American Hospital Association, 1980).

This article will report on a study of the effect of early and comprehensive hospital social work services to a group of Orthopaedic patients. The purpose of the study was to determine whether the provision of early and comprehensive social work services would affect the number of days that patients spent in the hospital. The propositions underlying this study were the following:

1. In any patient group, some patients will face social and psychological barriers that prevent them from being discharged from the hospital as soon as their physical condition permits.
2. If these patients can be identified early and receive comprehensive social work services, these problems are more likely to be resolved so that timely discharge can occur.
3. If social work services result in appropriate post-hospital care plans, if patients and families are prepared to cope effectively with these plans, and if follow-up contact is provided, timely discharge will be beneficial to both patients and society.

This study provides a test of only the second proposition. The authors recognize that there may be debate about the veracity of the third proposition. Some may argue that certain patients need extra time in the hospital for psychosocial reasons regardless of the timing and effectiveness of social work intervention. Resolution of this question awaits additional research.

By involving the patient early in the hospital stay, one of the goals of this project was to increase the patients' participation in active decision-making (Janis & Mann, 1977). Early intervention could enable the social worker to assist the patient and family in exploring a full range of sound, comprehensive services resulting in a plan tailored to their needs and preferences. Not only would the patient receive benefits, but the hospital would also be benefitted by proper utilization of acute health care beds and resultant reduction in the length of stay. The hoped for result of early and comprehensive social work services would be increased effectiveness and efficiency in the delivery of health care. An additional result might be that unnecessary readmissions through the Emergency Room would be prevented.

METHODOLOGY

With increased emphasis on better utilization of health care facilities, Akron City Hospital became interested in studying the impact of early discharge planning upon length of stay. The Chairperson of the Orthopaedics Department at the hospital was particularly interested in participating in a research project to investigate the effect of early and comprehensive social work intervention on reducing the length of stay on the Orthopaedic units.

This study gradually evolved from a general question to a clearly defined research plan. In the preliminary stages, it was crucial to provide an orientation regarding the study to the various disciplines involved, which included the Orthopaedic physicians and nurses. Throughout the study, monthly progress meetings were held with the key participating physicians, nurses, and social work staff.

The sample for this study was limited to Orthopaedic patients on the two Orthopaedic units at the hospital admitted during a six-month period. The study only included Orthopaedic patients directly admitted to the Orthopaedic units and those transferred to the units within three working days of admission. Orthopaedic patients who were transferred to other floors were eliminated from the sample.

This study utilized an experimental design in which 371 Orthopaedic patients were randomly assigned to two groups. One group was the experimental group and the other was the control group. Random assignment was accomplished by use of the date, time of admission, and last digit of the patient's admission number. The patients with even numbers were assigned to the experimental group. The patients with odd numbers were assigned to the control group.

Every patient in the experimental group received early and comprehensive social work services from a social worker for whom this service was a full time responsibility. During this study period, a temporary full time social worker was hired to permit the assignment of this experienced social worker for full time participation in the experimental group. Approximately 15 experimental patients were hospitalized at all times during the study.

In the experimental group, the social worker made contact with the patient and/or family within three (3) working days of admission to the Orthopaedic units. She immediately began to evaluate the psychosocial needs of the patient and/or family. A thorough assessment was made of the patient's physical condition and medical disability, if any; limitations imposed by diagnosis; social situation; psychological, cultural, and financial factors. Then an individualized discharge plan was developed with the patient and/or family or significant other to meet the physical, social, and emotional needs. To assist in forming the most comprehensive discharge plan, the social worker reviewed the medical chart; collaborated with the medical staff/nursing staff and other involved professionals; and contacted appropriate community agencies. After these assessments were completed, a plan was formulated with the patient and family or significant others. Patients were strongly encouraged to involve themselves actively in this planning process. This plan not only included the actual discharge of the patient, but provided a linkage to community agencies for additional counseling and/or other appropriate services.

Patients in the control group were provided with routine hospital services. At the time of this study, Orthopaedic patients were receiving social work services only on the basis of physician referral. These referrals were usually initiated late in the patient's stay and only a small proportion of patients were referred. Further, the social worker responding to these referrals served patients in many parts of the hospital and was not an integral part of the Orthopaedic team. One limitation of the experimental design was that control group contamination could not be ruled out. In other words, since the many hospital personnel were aware that the study was underway, they may have been sensitized to the need for social work services. Thus, the control group possibly received more social work services than they would have prior to the study. If this were, indeed, the case, the result would be a smaller difference between the experimental and control groups than would have occurred in the absence of contamination. However, since this bias was against finding differences between the two groups, the internal validity of the study was not seriously jeopardized.

Social work intervention for both groups was documented in the standard department's Progress Notes. The documentation included initial assessment, on-going progress notes, post-hospital care plans, and discharge summaries. For all study patients, information regarding their age, sex, the nature of surgery or discharge diagnosis, dates of admission and discharge, source of payment, disposition, actual length of stay, and certified length of stay by diagnostic category were entered on a data collection form. The information was retrieved from the medical record, and this coding was checked for its reliability.

RESULTS

The patients included in this study had a mean age of 62.68 (SD = 18.52) with the distribution being slightly skewed toward the older end of the age continuum. The average length of stay in the hospital for all study patients was 12.50 days. Table 1 presents some relevant characteristics of the experimental and control patients. There were no significant differences between the two groups in age, sex, discharge destination, or source of payment for medical care. The table reveals that the majority of patients in both groups were covered by Medicare or private insurance and were being discharged to their own homes.

It will be recalled that the major study hypothesis was that patients receiving early and comprehensive discharge planning (i.e., experimental group) would remain in the hospital for fewer days than patients receiving routine hospital services (i.e., control group). Table 2 suggests that all the differences are in the expected direction. For all diagnostic categories, patients in the experimental

TABLE 1

Description of Sample

Variable	Experimental Group	Control Group
Mean Age	64.25	61.09
Sex:		
Male (%)	36.4%	40.2%
Female (%)	63.6%	59.8%
Discharge Destination:		
Home (%)	75.9%	72.8%
Long-Term Care Facility (%)	24.1%	27.2%
Primary Source of Payment:		
Medicare (%)	48.1%	46.8%
Medicaid (%)	2.7%	1.6%
Private Insurance (%)	28.3%	30.4%
Other (%)	4.3%	8.7%
Unknown	16.6%	12.5%
TOTAL N	187	184

group spent, on the average, fewer days in the hospital than did patients in the control group. Overall, experimental patients remained in the hospital an average of 1.25 fewer days than did control patients.

In order to test the significance of the above differences, a two-way analysis of covariance was performed. Age served as a covariate due to its strong correlation with length of stay. The results of this analysis are presented in Table 3. The difference between the experimental and control group on mean length of stay is significant at the .001 level ($F = 10.10$, df = 1,362). Diagnosis and age are also shown to have statistically significant effects on length of hospital stay. The Eta^2 of, .21 suggests that 21% of the variance in length of stay in this patient group can be explained by age, diagnosis, and discharge planning.

During the six-month period of the study, there was a total saving of 234 hospital days for the experimental group as compared with

TABLE 2

Means and Standard Deviations*
For Length of Stay (in days) By
Treatment Group and Diagnosis

Treatment Group

Diagnosis	Experimental	Control
Hip Replacement	M=14.74 SD= 6.47 (34)	M=15.79 SD= 5.47 (29)
Knee Replacement	M=13.00 SD= 2.69 (14)	M=16.64 SD= 6.59 (14)
Hip Fracture	M=15.50 SD= 5.43 (50)	M=17.34 SD= 5.83 (41)
Other Fractures	M= 8.58 SD= 4.78 (89)	M=10.14 SD= 7.21 (100)
All Diagnoses	M=11.88 SD= 6.07 (187)	M=13.13 SD= 7.36 (184)

* Numbers in parentheses represent cell frequencies.

the control group. This resulted in a savings of $53,762.50 in health care dollars.

CONCLUSIONS

In addition to reducing health care costs and providing better patient care, an exciting gain from this study was that the Social Work Department demonstrated to itself, as well as to the hospital administration, the effectiveness of research as a social work tool. It was a new format for the department, and it opened many doors which had remained closed for years. It became clear, as a result of our experience with this study, that the social work profession has never been in a better position to demonstrate the effectiveness of service. The mandated need to demonstrate quality assurance combined with the professional commitment to providing effective discharge planning provided a winning combination.

TABLE 3

Analysis of Covariance of Length of Stay
by Diagnosis and Treatment Group
with Age as a Covariate

Source	df	Sum of Squares	Mean Squares	F
Main Effects				
Treatment Group	1	331.027	331.027	10.10*
Diagnosis	3	1864.794	621.598	18.96*
Covariate				
Age	1	2874.115	2874.115	87.66*
Interaction	3	13.852	4.617	.14
Error	362	11868.743	32.787	
TOTAL	370	16898.749	45.672	

N = 371
*p $<$ .001
Eta^2 = .21

The findings of the study demonstrated the cost effectiveness of hiring a full time social worker to cover the Orthopaedic units. It was statistically shown that the experimental group remained in the hospital on an average of 1.25 fewer days than the control group. In terms of cost, the average savings for Medicare and other insurances was a little more than a day of hospitalization cost. With the present health care concern about better utilization of hospital beds and cost-containment, this finding has great importance.

Although the reported findings are limited to the studied Orthopaedic patients, the implications of the results probably have relevance for other hospitalized patients. The Social Service Department found that the research design could be used in the future in other areas of the hospital to demonstrate the need for additional staffing. With the success of the study, the Social Service Department has been able to increase its entire staff by four social workers in the past year. This increase was a result of the study as well as other research projects in which the department participated. A future publication by the authors will illustrate the steps taken to achieve the staff increase.

As a direct outgrowth of the Orthopaedic study, the Social Service Department continued to retain the privilege of intervention in all cases when the department felt services would be most effective. This is a professional privilege which has been difficult to achieve in some places, but one which might never have been obtained except through demonstrated measurable results.

Another important gain from the study has been increased interest in the social work role on the multi-disciplinary team. This has led to further development of the team approach to total patient care and increasing respect for the social worker's contribution to this approach.

It is recognized that there are many factors not examined in this study which can slow down the discharge planning process. Studies have shown some of these factors might be lack of nursing home beds, change in patient's physical condition, and the lengthy welfare process (Schrager et al., 1978). Even though these factors can impede the discharge planning process, the reported findings still suggest the importance of early and comprehensive discharge planning in reducing additional overstays. Because the Orthopaedic study was so successful and has demonstrated the effectiveness of timely social service intervention, future research to measure the quality of social service intervention is planned.

REFERENCES

American Hospital Association (Committee on Discharge Planning of the Society of Hospital Social Work Directors) "Discharge Planning," American Hospital Association, Chicago, Illinois (1980).

Berkman, B. G. and Rehr. H. The Sick Role Cycle and the Timing of Social Work Intervention, *Social Service Review, 46*: 567-580, 1972.

Berkman, B. G. and Rehr, H. Early Social Service Case Finding for Hospitalized Patients: An Experiment, *Social Service Review, 47*: 256-265, 1973.

Boaz, R. F. Utilization Review and Containment of Hospital Utilization, *Medical Care, 17*:315-330, 1979.

Glass, R. I.; Mulvihill, M. N.; Smith, H.; Peto, R.; Bucheister, P.; and Stoll, B. J. The Four Score: An Index for Predicting a Patient's Non-Medical Hospital Days, *American Journal of Public Health, 67*: 751-755, 1977.

Health Care Financing Administration, *1979 PSRO Program Evaluation* (Washington D.C.: Health Care Financing Administration, 1979).

Janis, I. and Mann, L. *Decision-Making*, New York: The Free Press, 1977.

Mason, B.; Bedwell, C. L.; Zwagg, R. V.; Runyan, J. W. Why People Are Hospitalized, *Medical Care, 18*: 147-163, 1980.

National Center for Health Statistics. *Utilization of Short Stay Hospitals* (PHS 79-1557). (Washington D.C.: Department of Health, Education and Welfare, 1979).

Schrager, J.; Halman, M.; Myers, D.; Nichols, R. and Rosenblum, L. Impediments to the Course and Effectiveness of Discharge Planning, *Social Work in Health Care*, Vol. 4 (Fall 1978).

Zimmer, J. G. Length of Stay and Hospital Bed Misutilization. *Medical Care, 12*: 453-462, 1974.

Myocardial Infarction Patients in the Acute Care Hospital: A Conceptual Framework for Social Work Intervention

Joanne Sulman, MSW, CSW
Goldie Verhaeghe, MSW, CSW

SUMMARY. This paper describes a conceptual framework for identifying myocardial infarction patients in the acute care hospital who are at risk for medical and psychosocial complications that may impede recovery. Because of their precarious medical status, these patients present special issues for social work practice. Psychosocial factors affecting outcomes are reviewed and interventive strategies are outlined. The crucial role of adaptive denial in recovery is highlighted.

INTRODUCTION

A successful outcome for myocardial infarction patients is usually defined as physical survival and the resumption of a productive lifestyle. As with other seriously ill patients, a major goal of social work intervention is participation in the treatment plan to promote successful outcome. For myocardial infarction (M.I.) patients the interplay of medical vulnerability, psychological response and social characteristics calls for a unique practice approach.

At the time of writing Joanne Sulman was a Supervisor and Goldie Verhaeghe was a Clinical Social Worker at Mount Sinai Hospital, 600 University Avenue, Toronto, Ontario, Canada, M5G 1X5. The authors thank Verna Chandler, MSW, CSW, Renata Block, MSW, CSW and Gordon Dickinson, MD, FRCP(C) for their help.
Reprinted from *Social Work in Health Care*, Volume 11(1), Fall 1985.

The paper reviews a selection of the literature addressing psychological, social and demographic factors that influence outcome. Using these data, we propose a conceptual framework to identify patients who are at risk for medical and psychosocial complications that interfere with optimal rehabilitation. The implications for social work practice are discussed.

PSYCHOLOGICAL FACTORS

The meaning ascribed to the heart in human terms encompasses sympathy, courage, affection and survival itself. When one's heart is threatened with crushing pain, the dread evoked is overwhelming. Human beings react with shock, denial, massive anxiety and depression to this event which can radically alter or eliminate their future. These same emotions, although normal, can be major components in poor prognosis and death.

During the past fifteen years, researchers have investigated the links between these psychological responses and recovery from M.I. Most attention has been focused on denial, anxiety and depression. Other psychologically related factors that have been studied are control and predictability, behavioral adjustment and the effectiveness of psychotherapy.

Denial

Denial can have a positive or a negative effect on outcome depending upon its intensity and time of occurrence. Hackett and Cassem (1982) define denial as the repudiation of part or all of the total available meaning of an event in order to minimize or reduce anxiety. In their early work, as part of consultation-liaison in a large general hospital, Hackett, Cassem and Wishnie (1968) studied 50 patients in the Coronary Care Unit (C.C.U.) and found initial evidence that denial may have a positive influence on survival. In further work, Hackett and Cassem (1971, 1979, 1982) noted that denial can also be maladaptive if it causes critical delay in the recognition of cardiac symptoms or non-compliance with treatment. Croog, Shapiro and Levine (1971) and Garrity, McGill, Becker and

Blanchard (1976) also found that denial can produce a lack of compliance with rehabilitation measures.

Anxiety

The mobilization of denial may be viewed as an initial defense against the overwhelming, realistic anxiety that accompanies an encounter with one's mortality. Some patients experience this anxiety to a marked degree and a number of reports point to this having an adverse influence on both psychosocial (Cay, 1982; Winefield & Martin, 1981) and physical dimensions of recovery (Thomas, Lynch & Mills, 1975; Minckley, Burrows, Ehrat, Harper, Jenkin, Minckley, Page, Schramm, & Wood, 1979; Taggart & Carruthers, 1981).

Depression

Denial not only defends against anxiety but also acts as a mechanism to avoid acknowledging the physical, psychological and social role losses that can result from M.I. When denial of loss is no longer tenable, depression may ensue (Billings, 1980). Initial depression in the C.C.U. does not appear to be related to outcome. However, in a 2-1/2 year study patients who did not survive had displayed significantly more pessimism and depression at 3, 6 and 12 months post infarct (Obier, MacPherson & Haywood, 1977). This finding is in accord with the early work of Engel and Schmale (1967) who described the "giving-up, given-up" state of helplessness and hopelessness in illness behavior, and of Kimball (1969) who found the greatest incidence of death following open-heart surgery in depressed patients.

Control and Predictability

Control and predictability may also be related to positive outcome for M.I. patients. "The greater perceived controllability of a stressor, the less harmful are its effects on the organism" (Krantz, 1980). Similarly, Buell and Eliot (1980) provide strong support for the negative impact of unpredictability. In reviewing animal experimentation they found that heightened sympathetic arousal, hopelessness and helplessness were strongly linked to sudden death.

Behavioral Distress

In an interesting study that took a more global look at behavioral distress in the C.C.U., Garrity and Klein (1975) differentiated 48 M.I. patients as adjustors and non-adjustors when assessed for the presence of emotional/behavioral disturbance using a 21-point scale. The scale consisted of 18 items that described behavioral disturbance such as anxiety, hostility, and depression, and 3 items, calmness, cheerfulness and friendliness, that described positive behavior. Observations were made during the first five days of hospitalization following M.I. Patients were judged to be non-adjustors if they showed greater behavioral disturbance and little positive behavior over the five days, or if they showed increasing behavioral disturbance and decreasing positive behavior. Despite the preponderance of scale items relating to behavioral disturbance and non-adjustment, as many adjustors as non-adjustors were found in the sample. When these patients were followed for 6 months after discharge, Garrity and Klein discovered that 41% of the non-adjustors had died versus 8% of the adjustors. The relationship between behavior and mortality held even when the severity of the attack and the presence of prior heart disease were statistically controlled. To account for this finding, they suggest that chronic psychophysiological arousal, especially in subjects with already impaired hearts, will lead to greater risk of reinfarction and death.

Byrne, Whyte and Lance (1979) further analyzed behavioral responses of post-infarct patients and organized their data into four response clusters ranging from highly emotional reactions such as anxiety and depression to denial of illness and its consequences. The authors noted the hazards of both extremes. They state that anxiety has biochemical concomitants noxious to a vulnerable myocardium in the first few days after M.I., whereas denial, though initially protective, can become maladaptive if rehabilitation regimens are ignored. In a later prospective study, patients with poor cardiological outcomes at eight months were more likely than others to have reported a history of life stress prior to the M.I. and concern about somatic functioning following the infarct (Byrne, White & Butler, 1981). In the same study, patients who still had not returned to work at eight months were those who had accepted the sick role and who reported subjective feelings of tension.

Effectiveness of Psychotherapy

In an effort to deal with the negative impact of psychological reactions to M.I., the effectiveness of psychotherapy has been examined. Cassem and Hackett (1971) found a significant reduction in the mortality rate of patients provided with help for anxiety, depression and behavior disturbances in the C.C.U. Gruen (1975) randomly divided 70 patients between the ages of 40 and 69 with first M.I.'s into a treatment and a control group. The treatment group was provided with brief cognitively focused psychotherapy. The control group received no special psychotherapeutic intervention. Gruen found that the treated patients had shorter stays in hospital, were less likely to develop medical complications in the form of arrhythmias and congestive heart failure, showed fewer manifestations of depression or anxiety and were able to return to normal activities at four months follow-up.

However, adaptive denial that defends against disruptive anxiety and allows patients to participate in treatment should not be challenged. Gentry and Haney (1975) report on Foster's 1971 unpublished study where psychotherapy was provided to M.I. patients in the C.C.U. These patients were given the opportunity to ventilate feelings and thoughts about their illness and were offered realistic information and implications for the future. The intervention was found to be harmful to those patients who employed denial because they responded with greater anxiety following the treatment. Gentry and Haney conclude that psychosocial intervention should be directed only at patients experiencing emotional stress and not at patients for whom denial is an adaptive coping mechanism.

These results suggest that certain forms of psychological intervention can have a beneficial impact on the M.I. patient's emotional adjustment and physical recovery. Factors addressed in such intervention include excessive anxiety, depression, pessimism, non-compliance, somatization, and feelings of lack of control. Psychological factors, however, comprise only one area for exploration.

SOCIAL AND DEMOGRAPHIC FACTORS

Age

Age, sex and social class appear to exert a significant effect on outcome after M.I. Age-related indices suggest that older patients are better able to cope with social stress, pain and anxiety. Billing, Lindell, Sederholm and Theorell (1980) found that both older men and women reported less social stress, that older men required fewer analgesics and older women reported less anxiety than their younger counterparts.

Sex

The Framingham Study correlated the incidence and prognosis of M.I. with the sex of the patient (Kannel, Sorlie, & McNamara, 1979). That 20-year follow-up of 5,127 men and women initially free of coronary heart disease reported that although men were three times more likely to sustain an M.I., the prognosis was distinctly worse in women. Women had a 27% early mortality rate versus 16% in men, and a 40% reinfarction rate versus 13% in men. Other studies report that female M.I. patients are more likely to come from the lower social strata (Kottke, Young, & McCall, 1980) and are more likely to display anxiety than men (Byrne, 1980-81; Billing, Lindell, Sederholm, & Theorell, 1980).

Socio-economic Class

Outcome varies directly with socio-economic class. Blue collar workers are at greater risk for being non-compliers and dropouts from cardiac rehabilitation programs, especially if they smoke, do light work as opposed to hard work, and are inactive during leisure time (Oldridge, 1979). Kottke, Young and McCall (1980) used the five social strata developed by Hollingshead (1957) and found that only 35% of the lowest socio-economic class (Class 5) patients returned to work or to major activities, while almost 90% of Class 1 patients resumed these activities. Their findings indicate a direct relationship between socio-economic class and return to work or to major activities. The authors comment that when all cardiac events (death and reinfarction) are treated together, the lower socio-economic class patient apparently suffers from an excess burden of disease. These patients are exposed to multiple risk factors such as uncertain work opportunities, fragmented social supports, economic hardships, and reduced access to information (Ruberman, Weinblatt, Goldberg, & Chaudhary, 1984). Such risk factors may produce a lack of compliance with medication regimens and with necessary changes in lifestyle that adversely affect cardiac outcomes.

Life Events

Another measure of risk factors is seen in life events signifying change or distress prior to M.I. Obier Ell, de Guzman and Haywood (1983) support the contention that high risk is conferred by social stress. They found that the higher the pre-onset stress as measured by life change scores, the poorer the level of recovery. Byrne and Whyte (1980) found that M.I. patients reported more upset, depression and helplessness in response to life events than non-M.I. hospital patients, although the sums of life change scores showed no significant difference. They suggest that it is the meaning of the event to the M.I. patient rather than the event itself that is significant. Berkman (1982) proposed that the lack of social networks can increase the negative impact of life events.

RISK FACTORS AND OUTCOME

Given the profusion of variables related to survival and quality of life, we need to differentiate the positive and neutral factors from the negative. Some reactions such as denial have been shown to have both positive and negative characteristics. Others, like depression, are neutral if experienced in a limited way, but negative if protracted. It is important to note that positive or negative impact on outcome has little to do with the normalcy of a given behavior. When one is threatened with death, profound anxiety is a normal response; however, its effect on the M.I. patient is clearly negative.

Positive factors for survival and recovery include moderate denial of anxiety and loss, a sense of control and predictability, optimism, and compliance with treatment.

Negative factors include excessive denial that delays initial treatment or gives rise to non-compliance with treatment and rehabilitation; anxiety; prolonged depression; younger age on some indices; being female; being from a lower socio-economic class, and high levels of social stress and life change.

CONCEPTUAL FRAMEWORK
FOR IDENTIFYING HIGH-RISK PATIENTS

Although we have identified some primary psychosocial risk factors associated with outcome following M.I., this information is of limited help unless it can be structured into a clear conceptual framework. By this we mean that it must be available for use in identifying patients most in need of social work service and for informing our assessments and interventions.

M.I. patients who are high-risk for medical and psychosocial complications may be identified early in the C.C.U. or later, after they are transferred to a regular care floor. In some settings, all cardiac patients in the C.C.U. are reviewed by the social worker. In other settings, social work referrals are determined by the application of a high-risk screening tool (Obier Ell, de Guzman, & Haywood, 1983). In our setting, both in the C.C.U. and on the regular, cardiac care floor, we accept referrals from patients, families, medical, nursing and other patient care staff. In addition, we review all patients on the cardiac care floor on a weekly basis during multidisciplinary rounds.

We developed our conceptual framework as part of a multidisciplinary rehabilitation program for M.I. patients in our acute care hospital. The framework was designed as a screening and intervention guide for social workers, and is also taught to nursing, medical and other patient care staff on the cardiac care floor and in the C.C.U. in order to help them identify M.I. patients requiring social work intervention.

The framework combines four clusters of risk factors with outcome. The key concepts determining outcome are maladaptive versus adaptive responses paired with compliance or non-compliance with treatment and rehabilitation (see Table 1).

Group I consists of patients who are at risk for recurrence and

IDENTIFIABLE GROUPS	I	II	III	IV
RISK FACTORS	Maladaptive Anxiety or Depression Excessive Dependence Non-compliance	Anxiety Depression Dependence Compliance	Adaptive Denial Independence Compliance	Maladaptive Denial Excessive Independence Non-compliance
OUTCOMES	Risk of Recurrence Cardiac invalidism	Rehabilitation Potential	Best Rehab Potential	Increased Risk of Complications/ Recurrence

cardiac invalidism owing to their incapacitating anxiety or depression. Through their maladaptive attempts to cope with the crisis of their illness, they become pathologically dependent and non-compliant with rehabilitation measures.

Group II patients are moderately anxious or depressed but comply with treatment. They are dependent, but not excessively so, and have rehabilitation potential. However, their ability to participate in their recovery is tenuous because they have difficulty denying distressing affect.

Group III patients are characterized by the adaptive use of denial to ward off anxiety and depression (Billings, 1980). They appear optimistic and independent and participate in treatment.

They employ isolation of affect as a defense mechanism which allows them to acknowledge their illness without the intrusion of significant emotion. This group displays the greatest rehabilitation potential (Wrzesniewski, 1980; Garrity & Klein, 1975; Byrne, Whyte & Lance, 1979).

Group IV comprises patients who react to M.I. with maladaptive denial. Some refuse to acknowledge that they have had a heart attack and most deny that it will have much impact on their lives. They may speak as if fate alone rather than their own behavior will determine outcome. Excessively independent, they are notoriously non-compliant with rehabilitation efforts and therefore run a greater risk of complications and recurrence. In Byrne, Whyte and Lance's study (1979) this type of patient numbered half the sample.

INTERVENTION STRATEGIES WITH PATIENTS

For the social worker on the cardiac service, the assessment of the patient's response to M.I. should point to distinct strategies of intervention. Approaches that may be effective with one group of cardiac patients can be contraindicated for another.

Group I Patients

Patients in Group I require urgent intervention. They are unable to defend against the feelings associated with real losses of health and security, and therefore experience disabling anxiety and/or depression. Their feelings are so severe and prolonged as to render them incapable of actively participating in their treatment. Fears of inducing further damage and pessimism about the future pose barriers to recovery that, left untended, lead to cardiac invalidism. Patients in this group need help to manage their anxiety and depression more effectively so that they can comply with treatment.

Methods which have been proven effective include empathic listening combined with information and reassurance; prescription of anxiolytic medication, and the use of relaxation therapy (Billings, 1980; Hackett & Cassem, 1982). Relaxation techniques not only aid in reducing anxiety but also act against depression by promoting a sense of mastery.

A time of particular risk for this group of patients is the transfer from C.C.U. to a regular care floor. While the reduction of medical surveillance has positive connotations for staff, these changes tend to be perceived negatively by patients. Preparation for anticipated change can reduce the resulting anxiety.

Mr. B., a 65-year-old married librarian, suffered an M.I. shortly after retirement. Instead of slowly increasing his activity level, the patient was apprehensive about any physical self-care task, and unless prodded, would spend all his time in bed. He brooded about the future, was acutely sensitive to any bodily change, and was preoccupied with death. Mrs. B. mirrored her husband's feelings and thus increased the patient's sense of doom and hopelessness. Both husband and wife rejected support from family and friends, and became increasingly dependent upon professional staff.

Social work intervention consisted of regular meetings with the couple, individually and conjointly, to listen to their concerns, to identify areas requiring medical clarification, and to help the patient and his wife acknowledge progress. The social worker also maintained a close liaison with the cardiologist and nursing staff in order to ensure a consistent approach to information and support. Anti-anxiety medication prescribed by the cardiologist, combined with a co-ordinated team approach, helped Mr. B. to overcome enough of his misgivings to begin to participate in treatment. The social worker arranged discharge plans with maximum community support for the patient and his wife, and continued contact until Mr. B. was well-established in an out-patient cardiac rehabilitation program.

Group II Patients

Patients in Group II comply with treatment despite their anxiety and depression. Unlike patients in Group I who clearly signal their need for intervention, patients in Group II are deceptive. They are easily perceived as "good patients" because they make benign requests for encouragement and readily acknowledge apprehension and sadness. When their compliance with treatment is credited to the expression of these feelings, staff fail to identify the risk for these patients and are apt to encourage further exploration of anxiety and depression. Since these affects can have negative physiological consequences, Group II patients require preventive intervention that supportively acknowledges their participation in treatment regimens. Their consequent sense of mastery reinforces ego-strengths and promotes adaptive denial. Strategies suggested for Group I are equally effective with Group II and provide these patients with some armor once they are outside the hospital's protective cocoon.

Miss H., a 58-year-old unmarried secretary, in hospital for her first M.I., was referred to social work by her cardiologist. In spite of the patient's compliance with treatment, her anxiety appeared to be interfering with optimal recovery. Prior to her illness, Miss H. had experienced her job as demanding and had devoted all her time and energy to it. She had no social network apart from her job and no recreational outlets.

The social worker helped Miss H. to re-evaluate her priorities and also provided much-needed emotional support. In addition, the worker introduced the patient to relaxation tapes so that she might gain a sense of control over her anxiety. These interventions helped to relieve Miss H.'s apprehension, but her anxiety resurfaced prior to discharge. Careful discharge planning, including referral to a women's support group and an out-patient cardiac rehabilitation program, helped to reduce Hiss H.'s fears and ease her transition to a new lifestyle.

Group III Patients

Patients in Group III may be described as adaptive deniers. Their optimistic attitude and compliance with rehabilitation measures bode well for a successful outcome. Research provides evidence that their denial should be encouraged and supported, not challenged. When medical and nursing staff refer a Group III patient to social work, the request frequently reflects staff anxiety rather than patient need. Patients in Group III and their families generally cope well with the emotional and practical consequences of illness; so well, in fact, that staff may feel that affective issues are not being addressed. However, as long as the patient participates in treatment and rehabilitation, optimism need not be tempered with pessimistic versions of potential reality. When denial is more tenuous, and anxious or depressive feelings break through, staff should listen empathically and then actively point out positive aspects of the patient's progress and prognosis. The social worker's primary role with Group III is to alert staff to the need to support these patients in their successful adaptation.

Mr. L., a married 58-year-old man, suffered his first M.I. while he was in town attending a sales convention. Instead of the anxiety that one might anticipate in a patient who becomes seriously ill in a strange city, Mr. L. was jovial, outgoing and optimistic. Nursing staff referred him to social work because they felt that he wasn't taking their teaching efforts seriously. They were distressed that the patient responded with humor and mild sexual innuendo, instead of dealing with his feelings about the M.I. The social worker asked staff whether the patient was complying with treatment, and whether his family, who had flown in to be with him, were supportive of rehabilitation efforts. Nursing staff replied, "Oh yes. There's no problem there." The social worker then suggested that the nurses should join Mr. L. in his lighthearted approach, and support his adaptive denial. When staff followed this plan, their concerns about the patient disappeared.

Group IV Patients

Group IV patients, however, require specific intervention strategies aimed at altering their maladaptive coping methods. These are the patients whose denial prevents them from co-operating with treatment and rehabilitation. Members of this group are more likely to be men and frequently, though by no means exclusively, from lower socio-economic strata. Women are seldom found in this group because they are socialized to express feelings and are psychologically less likely to utilize the defense mechanism of denial.

In hospital, these patients may request special privileges to work from their bedside and are eager for discharge. Some have difficulty absorbing information because of their need to deny reality. For others, denial is compounded with faulty communication from caregivers. Once out of the hospital, Group IV patients refuse to pace their activity levels, discontinue medication without consultation, resume smoking, fail to recognize physical symptoms and drop out of cardiac rehabilitation programs. Their denial is clearly maladaptive.

Maladaptive denial ensues when reality and its consequences are perceived as overwhelming. Such patients employ excessive denial to defend against the anxiety aroused by a loss of control over destiny. The goal of intervention is to reconnect these patients with reality while bolstering their sense of mastery. This is done by providing patients with clear information regarding the rationale for medical protocols and then including them in making decisions about the rehabilitation process. Early involvement in physical rehabilitation is a powerful method for increasing the patient's sense of competence. Membership in a peer support group can also help to consolidate the rationale for compliance (Boyce, 1981). By reducing feelings of isolation and disability, the peer group encourages patients to participate in rehabilitation and to adopt a more constructive means of re-establishing control.

Mr. K., a 65-year-old married businessman, led an intensely active lifestyle prior to M.I. He took great pride in his success and the luxuries that accompanied it. Because his self-esteem was closely tied to his accomplishment, he was extremely resistant to treatment recommendations that appeared to limit his pace and undermine his sense of control. He bullied his somewhat passive wife into bringing him food that contravened his anti-hypertensive diet. He refused to learn about medication, stating that he never took pills. Predictably, he agitated for an early discharge.

The social worker assessed the patient as one who employed maladaptive denial to defend against anxiety and loss. Her efforts to provide Mr. K. with realistic information about the need for co-operation in treatment met with little success. She believed, however, that in a climate of peer support, Mr. K. might begin to participate in his treatment and rehabilitation. She therefore suggested that the cardiologist refer Mr. K. to a prestigious cardiac rehabilitation program in the city, and that the doctor emphasize the fact that many successful businessmen and professionals attended the program. The worker then met with the patient's wife to clarify rehabilitation goals and to enlist her help. To ensure that Mr. K. became connected to the rehabilitation program, the worker spoke to staff at the center and asked them to make special efforts to introduce Mr. K. to patients similar to himself. On follow-up, Mr. K. had not reduced his pace of activity, but was complying with medication, diet and exercise regimens.

INTERVENTION WITH FAMILIES

The preceding intervention strategies can only be effective if families and other social support networks are perceived as crucial to the patient's recovery (Mailick, 1979). The crisis of M.I. causes a major upset in the stability of the family system. Initial reactions of shock and disbelief can reinforce the patient's denial and delay treatment. Once the event is acknowledged, anxiety about the patient's survival prevails throughout the C.C.U. period.

The common practice of centering all attention on the patient and ignoring the family's need for information and support exacerbates this anxiety (Speedling, 1980). Rarely are provisions made for the family to meet regularly with physicians and nurses to ask questions and receive information about the patient's medical progress. When families are viewed by the medical team as passive outsiders, they tend to relate to the patient on the basis of their anxious misconceptions. This creates a barrier between family and patient that can turn visits into a source of stress rather than comfort. Instead of accepting this exclusion, the social worker should ensure that the family's unique knowledge of the patient and genuine desire to be helpful are harnessed to the common goals of recovery. This task is accomplished by facilitating the information flow between hospital staff and the patient's family. Greater input from the family not only enhances the care of the patient but also gives family members an opportunity to share their own feelings and regain a sense of control.

> Mr. E., a 65-year-old employed man, reacted to his first M.I. with denial about the severity of his illness, and displacement of his anxiety onto his job. In fact, his job was not in jeopardy. Nevertheless, C.C.U. staff were worried that he might sign himself out of hospital. The patient's wife responded to staff's concern by criticizing her husband for not realizing how sick he was. Her reaction forced Mr. E. into a more extreme form of denial and he demanded a phone by his C.C.U. bed so that he could call his customers. The social worker learned from the patient's family that Mr. E. was unable to tolerate inaction and tended to cope with problems by accelerating his pace of activity. In order to help Mr. E. reestablish a sense of control over some events in his life, the social worker conveyed the family's perceptions to staff and asked them to allow the patient some limited access to the telephone. She then counselled Mrs. E. to reassure her husband that he was improving and would soon be moved to a floor where he could gradually increase his activity. This intervention reduced the maladaptive responses of patient and family, and demonstrated to staff that the patient's co-operation with treatment could be improved when family perceptions were included in the treatment approach.

The family's participation is vital throughout the recovery period. As the patient improves, the family needs specific information about levels of activity, the purpose and effects of medication, recommended changes in diet and smoking habits, methods of reducing stress and resumption of sexual relations. This information can reduce the impact of new anxieties as the family shifts its focus from survival of the patient to long-range adaptation. Part of the social worker's role with the family is to help members obtain and clarify information and deal with necessary adjustments in their lifestyle.

Assuming that information needs are being met, the family still must contend with other feelings such as guilt, anger and depression that can impede adaptation. If family members feel that they precipitated the patient's M.I., their guilt feelings may prevent them from providing optimal support. Spouses may feel that they should have urged the patient more vigorously to slow down, change eating habits or exercise. Since M.I.'s are associated with business worries and are not uncommon following arguments (Kavanagh & Shephard, 1973; Greene, Goldstein & Moss, 1972), families may feel that they should have done more to protect the patient from life stresses. When these guilt feelings are not dealt with directly, they express themselves as over-protection of the patient and in demanding behavior towards staff. Families need help to examine the realistic basis for their feelings, not only what they have a right to feel guilty about, but also what they have taken unwarranted responsibility for. Family members need to be helped to understand that the patient's vulnerable physical condition was such that the M.I. could have occurred at any time – if not this stress, then the next. Their realistic guilt feelings can be further reduced by encouraging them to become positive participants in the patient's rehabilitation.

Mrs. S., an active professional woman in her mid-fifties, suffered a severe first M.I. following a stressful period of family contention. She responded with anxiety, demanding behavior and feelings of helplessness, and this was compounded by her family's over-protectiveness. Because her husband and her son felt guilty about the events in the family, they consequently complained to staff about inadequate care. In addition, they refused to allow Mrs. S. to do anything for herself, even when self-care activities were prescribed by the physician.

568 SOCIAL WORK IN HEALTH CARE: A HANDBOOK FOR PRACTICE

The social worker met with the patient's family and explored their feelings of responsibility. She praised their care and concern for Mrs. S., and pointed out that all families have stressful periods. She then helped them to meet with the physician to clarify that they could best help the patient by encouraging her in a graduated activity program and by reinforcing progress. Once the family was able to reframe its helping efforts in a way that was consistent with rehabilitation goals, Mrs. S. began to participate in her care.

Anger in families can occur as a mask for guilt feelings but also arises in response to the growing awareness of the disruptions that the M.I. brings to the family's former equilibrium. Family members are understandably reluctant to express their negative feelings towards the cardiac patient for fear of making things worse. Since this concern is a valid one, the social worker can help family members share and understand their feelings and prevent them from going underground or being acted out in a disruptive way towards staff. Families may, however, experience anger about genuine problems with the caregiving system. It is important to identify these problems and to act as an advocate in order to prevent the escalation of these feelings.

Mr. P. was a 47-year-old married businessman in hospital following a first M.I. His course in C.C.U. was uneventful and he presented an impatient but cheerful demeanor to staff after transfer to the regular cardiac care floor. The patient's wife made a complaint that her husband was not happy with his meals because they differed from what he had selected. Unfortunately no action was taken on the complaint, and two days later Mrs. P. again took her grievance to the nursing staff in a more heated fashion. At this time the nurse referred the patient to the nutritionist and his wife to the social worker for assessment. In rounds, other staff commented that the patient and his wife were not dealing with their feelings about the illness and were complaining about the food instead. The social worker assessed the patient and his wife and observed that they understood most of the treatment requirements, were optimistic about the future, but annoyed with the care in the hospital. The social worker contacted the nutritionist and asked her to explain the reasons for Mr. P's diet to both the patient and his wife. She then shared with the nursing staff her perception of the patient as one who used adaptive denial to cope with his M.I. She also suggested that if there had been an earlier consultation from the nutritionist, Mrs. P. might not have moved from complaint to anger.

Depression, sadness and grief are a response to the loss of what was. Hopes for the future are jeopardized. Along with health and financial stability, the integrity of the family is at issue (Dhooper, 1983). Feelings of anxiety and depression are especially prevalent at the time of discharge, a time when most families expect to be elated. It is as if the grim reality has set in and the change in health of the patient is most evident. To be prepared for this reaction can help family members reduce its impact. They need to know that this response is normal and common during the process of recovery. Reassurance consisting of realistic optimism and ready access to information can help patient and family master this phase.

Mrs. A., a 54-year-old self-employed married M.I. patient, was referred to social work because his depression was preventing him from increasing his activity level and delaying his discharge from hospital. He believed that he had lost his capacity to work and to lead a normal life. His wife shared his sadness and openly worried about being left a widow. The social worker assessed that the couple's information needs were not being met and so she intervened to increase communication by involving medical staff in regular joint meetings with the couple. The meetings reviewed the patient's progress, offered encouragement and helped to prepare for discharge. By treating this couple as a unit and offering them generous access to accurate information and support, their adaptation to the M.I. was infused with a sense of optimism.

A major support to families of M.I. victims can be provided through links with community services following discharges. Cardiac rehabilitation programs, public health nursing, and family counselling agencies are underutilized resources that can make an enormous difference to patients and families (Dhooper, 1983). One goal of social work follow-up is to identify and refer families that can benefit from these sources of help. Because high-risk patients are more likely to drop out of rehabilitation programs, continuing support may be required to maintain the connection.

DISCUSSION

During the past two years, social workers in our acute care hospital have been using the framework as a guide for their assessments and interventions with M.I. patients. They report that the framework has significantly altered their perceptions and practice with this patient population. Even those workers who have infrequent contact with cardiac patients note that the framework has helped them to focus their assessments and clarify goals for intervention.

The framework seems to be especially suited to social work's value base because it helps to identify and support the strengths and adaptive coping mechanisms of M.I. patients and their families. The approach also highlights the crucial role of patient and family as participants in the treatment and rehabilitation process.

In order to use the framework effectively, social workers need to differentiate those M.I. patients who can benefit from a rehabilitation approach from cardiac patients whose circumstances require palliation. The former include M.I. patients who have a reasonable hope of returning to an active lifestyle; the latter include patients with severe cardiomyopathy and other forms of end-stage heart disease.

If the social worker assigned to the C.C.U. or cardiac care floor does not personally assess every M.I. patient, then nursing, medical and other patient care staff need to be trained so that they can use the framework to identify patients for referral to social work. In our setting, as part of our cardiac rehabilitation program, we have discussed the framework with cardiologists and have participated in formal in-service training sessions with staff from nursing, physiotherapy, nutrition and pharmacy. This process has enhanced communication among team members, has improved the quality of referrals, and has promoted a more consistent approach to patients.

Although our evaluation of the effectiveness of the framework is anecdotal, the high-risk patients identified through its use and provided with appropriate intervention seem to have more success in linking up with out-patient cardiac rehabilitation programs, staying on medication regimens, and returning to an active lifestyle. We are in the process of designing a systematic evaluation of outcomes to examine these impressions.

SUMMARY

Social work practice with M.I. patients differs from approaches to other patients seen in the acute hospital setting. Many patients referred to social work require concerted exploration of anxiety and depression or confrontation of denial in order for them to benefit from treatment. When M.I. patients experience excessive anxiety, depression, denial or social stress, they are also at risk for psychosocial and physical complications. However, methods which are helpful to M.I. patients are markedly different. Strategies are indicated which support adaptive denial and increase compliance with treatment and rehabilitation measures. Families can also be a positive or negative force for recovery and call for careful attention to their own needs for information and support. The framework outlined in this article enables social workers to differentiate between adaptive and maladaptive responses to M.I., to meet the needs of patients and families more effectively and to avoid unproductive interventions.

REFERENCES

Berkman, L.F. Social network analysis and coronary heart disease. *Advances in Cardiology*, 1982, *29*, 37-49.

Billing, E., Lindell, B., Sederholm, M. & Theorell, T. Denial, anxiety and depression following myocardial infarction. *Psychosomatics*, August, 1980, *21*(8), 639-645.

Billings, C.K. Management of psychologic responses to myocardial infarction. *Southern Medical Journal*, 1980, *73*(10).

Boyce, M. Borgess hospital has outstanding example of cardiac rehabilitation program. *Michigan Medicine*, April 1981, 185-186.

Buell, J.C. & Eliot, R.S. Fundamentals of clinical cardiology: Psychosocial and behavioral influences in the pathogenesis of acquired cardiovascular disease. *American Heart Journal*, November, 1980, *100*(5), 723-740.

Byrne, D.G. Effects of social context on psychosocial responses to survived myocardial infarction. *International Journal of Psychiatry in Medicine*, 1980-81, *10*(1), 23-31.

Byrne, D.G., & White, H.M. Life events and myocardial infarction: the role of measures of individual impact. *Psychosomatic Medicine*, January, 1980, *42*(1), 1-10.

Byrne, D.G., White, H.M. & Butler, K.L. Illness behaviour and outcome following survived myocardial infarction: a prospective study. *Journal of Psychosomatic Research*, 1981, *25*(2), 97-107.

Byrne, D.G., White, H.M. & Lance, G.H. A typology of responses to illness in survivors of myocardial infarction. *International Journal of Psychiatry in Medicine*, 1978-79, *9*(2), 135-144.

Cassem, N.H. & Hackett, T.P. Psychiatric consultation in coronary care unit. *Annals of Internal Medicine*, 1971, *75*, 9-14.

Cay, E.L. Psychological problems in patients after a myocardial infarction. *Advances in Cardiology*, 1982, *29*, 108-112.

Croog, S.H., Shapiro, O.S. & Levine, S. Denial among male heart attack patients. *Psychosomatic Medicine*, 1971, *33*, 385-397.

Dhooper, S.S. Family coping with the crisis of heart attack. *Social Work in Health Care*, Fall, 1983, *9*(1), 15-31.

Engel, G.L. & Schmale, A.H., Jr. Psychoanalytic theory of somatic disorder: conversion, specificity and the disease onset situation. *Journal of the American Psychoanalytic Association*, 1967, *15*, 344-365.

Foster, S.B. Effects of interpersonal communication on urinary sodium-potassium ratio (a stress indicator). Unpublished Master's thesis, Washington, D.C., Catholic University of America, 1971. Cited in Gentry, W.D. & Haney, I. Emotional behavioral reaction to acute myocardial infarction. *Heart and Lung*, September-October, 1975, *4*(5), 738-745.

Garrity, T.F., & Klein, R.F. Emotional response and clinical severity as early determinants of six-month mortality after myocardial infarction. *Heart and Lung*, September-October, 1975, *4*(5), 730-737.

Garrity, T.F., McGill, A., Becker, M. & Blanchard, E. Report of the task group on cardiac rehabilitation. In Weiss, S.M. (Editor), *Proceedings of the National Heart and Lung Institute Working Conference on Health Behavior.* Department of Health, Education and Welfare, Publication No. 76-868, 1976.

Gentry, W.D. & Haney, T. Emotional and behavioral reaction to acute myocardial infarction. *Heart and Lung*, September-October, 1975, *4*(5), 738-745.

Greene, W.A., Goldstein, S. & Moss, A.J., Psychosocial aspects of sudden death. *Archives of Internal Medicine*, May 1972, *129*, 725-731.

Gruen, W. Effects of brief psychotherapy during the hospitalization period on the recovery process in heart attacks. *Journal of Consultation in Clinical Psychology*, 1975, *43*, 223-232.

Hackett, T.P. & Cassem, N.H. Coping with cardiac disease. *Advances in Cardiology*, 1982, *31*, 212-217.

Hackett, T.P. & Cassem, N.H. Psychological aspects of rehabilitation after myocardial infarction. In N. Wenger & H.K. Hellerstein, (Eds.), *Rehabilitation of the Patient after Myocardial Infarction*. Chichester: Wiley & Sons, 1979.

Hackett, T.P., Cassem, N.H., & Wishnie, H.A. The coronary-care unit — an appraisal of its psychological hazards. *New England Journal of Medicine*, December, 1968, *279*(25), 1365-1379.

Hollingshead, A.B. Two-factor index of social position. Mimeographed, 1957. Cited in Kottke, T.E., Young, D.T. and McCall, M.M. Effect of social class on recovery from myocardial infarction. *Minnesota Medicine*, August, 1980, 590-597. See also Hollingshead, A.B. and Redlich, F.C. *Social Class and Mental Illness*. New York: John Wiley & Sons, 1958.

Kannel, W.B., Sorlie, P. & McNamara, P.M. Prognosis after initial myocardial infarction: The Framingham Study. *American Journal of Cardiology*, July, 1979, *44*, 53-59.

Kavanagh, T. & Shephard, R.J. The immediate antecedents of myocardial infarction in active men. *Canadian Medical Association Journal*, July, 1973, *109*, 19-22.

Kimball, C.P. Psychological responses to open-heart surgery. *American Journal of Psychiatry*, September, 1969, *126*, 348-359.

Kottke, T.E., Young, D.T. & McCall, M.M. Effect of social class on recovery from myocardial infarction. *Minnesota Medicine*, August, 1980, 590-597.

Krantz, D.S. Cognitive processes and recovery from heart attack: a review and theoretical analysis. *Journal of Human Stress*, September, 1980, 27-38.

Mailick, M. The impact of severe illness on the individual and family: an overview. *Social Work in Health Care*, Winter, 1979, *5*(2), 117-28.

Minckley, B.B., Burrows, D., Ehrat, K., Harper, I., Jenkin, S.A., Minckley, W.F., Page, B., Schramm, D.E. & Wood, C. Myocardial infarct stress-of-transfer inventory: development of a research tool. *Nursing Research*, January-February, 1979, *28*(1), 4-10.

Obier, K., MacPherson, M. & Haywood, J.R. Predictive value of psychosocial profiles following acute myocardial infarction. *Journal of National Medical Association*, 1977, *69*, 59-61.

Obier Ell, K., de Guzman, M. & Haywood, L.J. Stressful life events: a predictor in recovery from heart attacks. *Health and Social Work*, Spring, 1983, *8*(2), 133-142.

Oldridge, N.B. Compliance with exercise programs. In M.L. Pollock and D.H. Schmidt (Eds.). *Heart Disease and Rehabilitation*. Boston: Houghton Mifflin Professional Publishers, 1979.

Ruberman, W., Weinblatt, E., Goldberg, J.D. & Chaudhary, B.S. Psychosocial influences on mortality after myocardial infarction. *The New England Journal of Medicine*, August, 1984, *311*(9), 552-559.

Speedling, E.J. Social structure and social behavior in an intensive care unit:

patient-family perspectives. *Social Work in Health Care*, Winter, 1980, *6*(2), 1-22.

Taggart, P. & Carruthers, M. Behaviour patterns and emotional stress in the etiology of coronary heart disease: cardiological and biochemical correlates. In D. Wheatley, (Ed.). *Stress and the Heart*, New York: Raven Press, 1981.

Thomas, S.A., Lynch, J.J. & Mills, M.E. Psychosocial influences on heart rhythm in the coronary-care unit. *Heart and Lung*, September-October, 1975, *4*(5), 746-751.

Winefield, H.R. & Martin, C.J. Measurement and prediction of recovery after myocardial infarction. *International Journal of Psychiatry in Medicine*, 1981-82, *11*(2), 145-154.

Wrzesniewski, K. The development of a scale for assessing attitudes toward illness in patients experiencing a myocardial infarction. *Social Science and Medicine*, 1980, *14A*, 127-132.

Medical Handmaidens or Professional Colleagues: A Survey of Social Work Practice in the Pediatrics Departments of Twenty-Eight Teaching Hospitals

Jane H. Pfouts, PhD
Brandon McDaniel, MS

SUMMARY. This paper, based on questionnaire data gathered in the summer of 1975, analyzes the ways in which social workers in the pediatrics departments of twenty-eight teaching hospitals define their roles and describe their activities. Data on overall social work coverage in these hospitals is briefly described, with emphasis on hospital size, professional preparation of staff, academic rank, and staffing patterns. Within this context, data analysis focuses on the extent to which pediatric social workers exercise autonomy in direct service, teaching, and research. Areas on the pediatric service which are examined include worker-bed ratios, direct practice coverage, and participation in grand rounds, medical rounds, policy-level committees, teaching, and research. Social work role priorities and obstacles to quality role performance are also discussed.

Autonomy has been called the hallmark of the professional practitioner. According to Carr-Saunders,[1] social workers lack profes-

At the time of writing Dr. Pfouts was Associate Professor, School of Social Work, University of North Carolina at Chapel Hill, 223 East Franklin Street, Chapel Hill, NC 27514; and Ms. McDaniel was Chief Social Worker, Pediatrics Department, Duke Hospital, Durham, NC.

An earlier version of this paper was presented at the Annual Forum of the National Conference on Social Welfare, Washington, D.C., June, 1976.

Reprinted from *Social Work in Health Care*, Volume 2(3), Spring 1977.

sional autonomy because the employer lays down the limits to the service and, to some extent, determines its kind and quality. Using this standard, Carr-Saunders would probably rate hospital social work as particularly vulnerable to the "handmaiden" label because of the formidable set of organizational pressures and constraints under which it operates. However, we believe that role definition is a fluid, interactive process between social work and its host institution. Even in the most difficult settings, social work is always involved, either actively or passively, in shaping its own destiny. Social workers are not the only professional group who must cope with the dilemmas of institutional adaptation. Increasingly, all professions have members who are salaried staff personnel in host agencies. Yet, with similar institutional constraints, autonomy varies among ancillary groups. Therefore, we suggest that the autonomy problem of hospital social workers involves more than constraints imposed by doctors and administrators. It also involves the way hospital social workers define themselves. Hallowitz[2] asserts that, in his experience as a social work director at a number of hospitals, "social workers do little more than complain bitterly to each other or to the administrator about their low level work and their treatment as physicians' handmaidens rather than as professional colleagues." Hallowitz pensively asks, "Do they really expect the administrator to call the physicians together, chastise them, and persuade them to treat social workers as professionals?" Hallowitz glumly opines that "these low status conditions have long persisted and the social workers, not the physicians, perpetuate the system." Most of us who have worked in hospitals would consider this to be an exaggerated and one-sided explanation of what actually goes on, but we would also have to admit that hospital-based social workers cannot escape some measure of responsibility for unsatisfactory as well as satisfactory role definitions.

This paper looks at the current role performance of social workers in twenty-eight teaching hospitals, based on information supplied by the social workers themselves. In the summer of 1975, social workers in the pediatrics departments of fifty-four teaching hospitals were asked to respond to a questionnaire, and thirty-four (63%) did so. Eight of these responses were later discarded because of incomplete data, leaving a total of twenty-eight questionnaires on which this analysis is based. A comparison between the twenty non-responding and the thirty-four responding institutions revealed no significant differences between the two groups in size or type.

Part I of the paper describes characteristics of the teaching hospitals and their social work departments. Part II analyzes some of the ways pediatric social workers in these hospitals define their roles and describe their activities. Data analysis focuses on the extent to which professional autonomy is presently exercised by pediatric social workers in the areas of direct service, teaching, and research.

I. CHARACTERISTICS OF THE TWENTY-EIGHT TEACHING HOSPITALS AND THEIR SOCIAL SERVICE DEPARTMENTS

Hospital Size

The twenty-eight hospitals in our survey are, in the main, large, complex teaching hospitals attached to prestigious university medical schools. Approximately one-half of these institutions have from 600 to over 1000 beds; one-fourth have 300 to 600 beds, and one-fourth are small, pediatric teaching hospitals with 100 to 300 beds. In all but two of these hospitals, the medical social workers are members of a centralized social service department.

Professional Training of Total Social Work Staff

Seventy-eight percent of staff members in our sample are master's level social workers, and 22% are BAs, BSWs, non-social work MAs, and others. In all cases, staffs include both MSW and non-MSW workers, but in only one instance are MSWs in the minority. The universal pattern is one in which the MSWs serve as administrators, supervisors, and case workers, and non-MSWs as case aides working under MSW supervision. Clearly, in this sample, MSW social workers continue to dominate the social work departments in teaching hospitals, and there is no evidence of a trend toward lower educational requirements for professional staff positions.

Academic Rank of Hospital Social Workers Exclusive of Psychiatry

The extent to which social workers on medical services, outside psychiatry, hold academic rank in these hospitals varies widely. In 29% of the cases, no medical social workers have an academic appointment, in 35% the only medical social worker holding rank is the departmental director, and in 36% other medical social workers also have faculty status. In only one department do all medical social workers also have faculty status. In only one department do all medical social workers with the MSW hold academic rank. These findings can be contrasted with those from a 1971 study by Large and Robinson of social workers in seventy-seven academic departments of psychiatry.[3] This study found that in 29% of the psychiatric departments surveyed, all social work clinicians with the MSW held academic rank, in 61% some of the workers held rank, and in only 10% did none have appointments. Clearly, for whatever reason, social work roles are more likely to be viewed as meriting academic status in psychiatry than in the medical services. We can also contrast our data with the Large and Robinson study on source of academic rank. In the case of psychiatry, over 90% of the appointments were in the psychiatric department or elsewhere in the medical school. On the medical side, in our study, roughly two-thirds of the appointments are also of this type, while one-third involve no medical school appointments at all, where only the director of social work holds academic rank, and that usually from a school of social work.

In our study, the rank held is mainly that of clinical instructor, with a minority of assistant professors and only two associate professors. There are no comparable data from the Large and Robinson study, but it is probable that tenured professorships are the exception in psychiatry as well. It appears clear that although many social workers in teaching hospitals can legitimately point with pride to their faculty status, it is important to remember that there are obvious autonomy problems for any group whose members are almost entirely confined to the untenured junior faculty ranks in an academic setting.

Staffing Patterns

Although, admittedly, worker-bed ratio is only one of several factors involved in staffing pattern decisions, this measure gives a rough estimate of staffing uniformity among hospitals. The average ratio of medical social workers to hospital beds in our survey is one to thirty, and the average number of medical social work staff is twenty-three. However, there is great variation among institutions, and there appears to be no generally accepted ratio of social work staff to hospital size. For example, the six hospitals in our sample with from twenty to thirty workers range in size from 250 to 1200 beds. Or, conversely, the seven huge medical centers in our sample with at least 1000 beds have medical social work staffs which vary between seventeen and fifty-five workers. A landmark 1954-55 survey of the social work departments of twelve hundred general and TB hospitals by the American Hospital Association, the Medical Social Work Section of NASW, and the United States Public Health Service[4] found the same disturbing lack of staffing uniformity and urgently recommended that social work develop criteria to establish professionally acceptable staffing patterns for hospitals by type and size. A 1969 survey of 359 hospitals (275 of which were teaching institutions) conducted by the American Society of Hospital Social Service Directors[5] had similar findings, and the researchers commented on the disappointing evidence of the lack of clear trends which might suggest some consensus on standards.[6] Recently, Abraham Lurie has argued in this journal that social work in health care agencies needs to reexamine its unsolved staffing problems now because of funding pressures, third-party payments, and administrative demands for explicit definition and measurement.[7]

Our limited data on staffing patterns suggests that not much has changed in twenty years. Social workers have still not carried out the recommendations of the 1957 American Hospital Association report which urged that studies be conducted to determine the need for social work by inpatients and outpatients, the nature and extent of services needed, and the number of social workers required to provide these services.[8] In the absence of empirical data, arbitrary standard setting is meaningless.

II. PEDIATRIC SOCIAL WORK ACTIVITIES

In our questionnaire, we inquired about pediatric staffing patterns, referral sources, case loads, roles, participation in medical rounds, teaching, and research.

Staffing Patterns

Not surprisingly, in view of the special needs of ill children, the average worker-bed ratio of pediatric social workers in our sample is one to twenty-four, in contrast to an average of one to thirty for total hospital beds. Our sample also shows that the average worker-bed ratio in the eight small pediatric hospitals (one to seventeen) is much more favorable than that of the twenty pediatric departments in general hospitals (one to twenty-six).

The average number of pediatric social workers in the twenty-eight hospitals in the sample is eight. The average in the eight pediatric hospitals is thirteen and in the twenty pediatric departments of general hospitals is six.

The proportion of total social work staff which is assigned to pediatrics in general hospitals suggests that both pediatricians and social workers set a high value on social work with sick children and their families. The even greater use of social workers by pediatricians in their own hospitals indicates that, given the administrative power to increase social work staff, pediatricians do exactly that.

Referral Sources

As Helen Rehr and her colleagues have documented,[9] the traditional system of case referral determines in advance the kinds of clients medical social workers see and do not see. Gorden and Rehr assert that, by not defining its own case-finding system, social work relinquishes the right to set its own priorities.[10] According to Weiner,[11] pediatric social workers have time and personnel to serve only 10% to 15% of the total pediatric population. In our study, an average of 11% of all pediatric patients is seen by social workers. Client needs will always outrun worker resources; therefore, it is essential that we give priority to the fraction of cases that need us most. To do so, we must control our case assignments. In order to assess the extent to which our sample displayed autonomous behavior in choosing clients, the pediatric social work respondents were asked to list referral sources in order of frequency. Social services case-finding ranks third, behind referrals from physicians and nurses, but ahead of patient and family, other hospital personnel, and outside agencies. The relatively high case-finding activity among our sample suggests a trend toward greater professional autonomy, and an important step away from the handmaiden role.

Pediatric Caseloads and Coverage

Our pediatrics sample differs widely in estimated average case load for workers. The reported range among departments of from twenty-five to one hundred twenty-five cases per month suggests that case loads are determined more on the basis of external pressures than on professional criteria.

The question of how social work priorities are set can also be approached by looking at which services are chosen to receive 100% coverage. Almost all the pediatric social work staffs in the study give total coverage to one or more specific patient groups, but the basis for choice is not apparent. Every conceivable pediatric problem group is given priority by somebody, but there appears to be little professional consensus among pediatric social workers about which groups are likely to profit most from intensive social work intervention. It is true that 100% coverage is most often given in the intensive care nursery and in areas of abuse and neglect, hematology, birth defects, and cystic fibrosis. However, differences in 100% coverage are far more evident than similarities, which suggests that service priorities are determined more by idiosyncratic factors within each department than by any widely held social work consensus concerning our professional mandate, knowledge, and skills.

Participation in Rounds

The strong interdisciplinary emphasis in the direct service activities of the pediatric social workers can be inferred from the data concerning their participation in rounds. Ninety-three percent of the respondents or their colleagues are routinely involved in pediatric medical rounds, and 75% have participated in grand rounds case presentations. Unfortunately, we did not request data about social work rounds, but a number of respondents mention the utility and success of this type of interdisciplinary case conference in their departments. It is easy to forget that not long ago social work participation in rounds was an issue, not an accomplished fact. The importance of our gains in this area cannot be overestimated because rounds offer opportunities for early case-finding and coordinated case management, in addition to serving as vehicles for social work teaching and consultation.

Teaching and Consultation

In our sample, the teaching of medical students and house staff, nursing students, social work students, and other trainees in the medical center is given high priority by the pediatric social workers. Ninety-three percent of the respondents report they are engaged in formal and informal teaching activities. Unstructured, informal teaching involving clinical demonstration and consultation about specific cases is frequently mentioned, but an impressive amount of formal teaching also takes place. There is widespread use of pediatric social workers as guest lecturers in courses taught by other faculty members, and a sizeable minority carry responsibility for conducting seminars, modules of courses, or elective courses for a wide variety of professional and paraprofessional groups. Subjects frequently covered in formal presentations include normal growth and development, interviewing, psychosocial components of health and illness, family dynamics, child abuse and neglect, and parent-child interaction.

Undoubtedly, much of the teaching activity of social workers in hospitals, particularly in case demonstration and consultation, is hidden from official scrutiny and is not labeled as such by others. Nevertheless, our data indicate that pediatric social workers are recognized throughout the hospital structure as authorities on the social components of health care. In some instances official recognition takes the form of academic rank, and in almost all instances unofficial recognition is evident through the widespread demands for social workers as formal and informal educators.

Research

William Gordon has characterized social workers in health care as the least theoretically and most realistically oriented of all social workers.[12] In our sample, 43% of the respondents report no research activity at all among their pediatric social work colleagues, 29% have members serving on medical research teams, 27% list involvement in both medical and social work research, and one person reports involvement in social work research only. Our questionnaire did not include an exploration of the extent or type of research activity involved, but our scanty data do suggest that where research activity exists there is a strong likelihood it will be on a medical team. Yet, Gordon has warned hospital social workers of the limited professional value to social work of involvement in medical research: "These studies conducted by someone else and to which you contribute are fine; but unless they provide for your testing and extending your own knowledge they contribute only to your appreciation and not to the growth of your professional base."[13]

The claim to autonomy of any profession rests, in large part, on the fund of knowledge which it creates and validates. Harriett Bartlett argues that by clarifying social work knowledge in the health field, social workers would be better able to specify the times and places at which intervention would be most fruitful, would be less dependent on referrals and guidance from physicians, and would have more to contribute to interdisciplinary practice and education.[14]

Because teaching hospitals are research institutions, all professionals, including social workers, are encouraged to conduct investigations in their areas of competence. Therefore, it is not lack of autonomy or institutional resources, but rather the lack of commitment of social workers themselves (and the schools of social work which trained them) to the research role that is the impediment.

Role Priorities of Pediatric Social Workers

Respondents were asked to state their most important social work roles in the pediatrics departments of the twenty-eight teaching hospitals in order to assess the relative emphasis given to direct service, consultation and teaching, research, and systems change. There is almost complete agreement (93%) that demonstration through direct service is the central social work role. Teaching and consultation activities also receive high priority. Nobody mentions research as an important role, and only one person lists program planning.

In general, our data are in agreement with findings of the 1971 study by Ullmann et al.,[15] which compares the professional activities of over 600 NASW hospital-based social workers and nearly 500 NASW social workers functioning in non-hospital settings. The Ullmann study concludes that

> even though there are some variations according to rank, the hospital is distinctive in its configurations of activities and interactions. Compared with non-hospital social work roles, it places more emphasis on direct service to clients as well as on interdisciplinary practice and teaching medical students, less emphasis on research and administrative program planning and roughly equal emphasis on collaboration with community agencies, consultation on community health needs, teaching social work students, participation in administrative staff conferences, and record keeping.[16]

CONCLUSION

Handmaidens or colleagues? As is the case with most social work questions, there is no clear-cut answer. In this paper, we have attempted to show that, in some aspects of their practice, hospital social workers are more autonomous than myth would have it, but that in others the opportunities to achieve greater autonomy are not grasped. The findings support our contention that it is not institutional forces alone, but the interaction of social workers and institution which determine the professional status of social work in the teaching hospital.

REFERENCES

1. Alexander M. Carr-Saunders, "Metropolitan Conditions and Traditional Professional Relationships," in *The Metropolis in Modern Life*, ed. Robert M. Fisher (Garden City, N.Y.: Doubleday, 1955), p. 283.

2. Emanuel Hallowitz, "Innovations in Hospital Social Work," *Social Work 17* (July 1972): 89-97.

3. Dorothy Large and Marie Robinson, "Social Workers in Academic Departments of Psychiatry," *Social Service Review 47* (December 1973): 613-615.

4. American Hospital Association, National Association of Social Workers—Medical Social Work Section, and United States Public Health Service, *Social Work in Hospitals: A study of social service departments in general and tuberculosis hospitals in the United States, 1954-55*, U.S.P.H.S. Publication 519 (Washington, D.C.: U.S. Government Printing Office, 1957), p. 117.

5. Report circulated to members of the American Society of Hospital Social Work Directors on questionnaire responses from 359 members concerning hospital programs and staffing, Leone Renn, chairman, December 1969.

6. Ibid, p. 2.

7. Abraham Lurie, "Staffing Patterns: Issues and Program Implications for Health Care Agencies," *Social Work in Health Care 2*, no. 1 (Fall 1976): 85-94.

8. *Social Work in Hospitals*, p. 84.

9. See Barbara Berkman and Helen Rehr, "Unanticipated Consequences of the Casefinding System in Hospital Social Work," *Social Work 15* (April 1970): 63-68; Barbara Berkman and Helen Rehr, "Early Social Service Casefinding for Hospitalized Patients: An Experiment," in *Social Service Review 47* (June 1973): 256-265; Barbara Gorden and Helen Rehr, "Selectivity Biases in Delivery of Hospital Social Services," *Social Service Review 43* (March 1969): 35-41.

10. Gorden and Rehr, "Selectivity Biases in Delivery of Hospital Social Services," p. 41.

11. Hyman J. Weiner, "The Workshop on Administration," in *Social Services in Pediatric Hospitals*, ed. Mary M. Lewis (Indianapolis, Ind.: The James Whitcomb Riley Hospital for Children; and Rockville, Md.: Maternal and Child Health Services, Public Health Service, Department of Health, Education and Welfare, 1972).

12. William E. Gordon, "The Challenge of Research to Today's Medical Social Worker," *Social Worker 1* (January 1956): 81-87.

13. Ibid., p. 85.

14. Harriett Bartlett, "Frontiers of Medical Social Work," *Social Work 7* (April 1962): 75-83.

15. Alice Ullmann, Mary M. Goss, Milton S. Davis, and Margaret Mushinski, "Activities, Satisfaction, and Problems of Social Workers in Hospital Settings," *Social Service Review 45* (March 1971): 17-29.

16. Ibid., p. 27.

Initiation of a Quality Assurance Program for Social Work Practice in a Teaching Hospital

Kris Ferguson, ACSW
M. Leora Bowden, ACSW
Donna Lachniet, ACSW
Anne Malcolm, BA
Gladys Morgan, MSW

SUMMARY. This first-stage paper describes the steps taken in implementing a quality assurance program. The rationale for writing social work protocols based on medical diagnosis or tasks rather than on psychosocial diagnosis is explained in detail. Protocols for adult rheumatoid arthritis, pediatric cancer, adult discharge planning, and adult nursing home placement are included to demonstrate the result of the medical diagnosis/task approach.

One critical issue in the field of social work is accountability. This issue has become particularly relevant because Professional Standards Review Organization (PSRO) legislation has raised difficult questions, such as to whom and for what social workers will be held accountable. These need to be addressed.

Although much has been written about the general issues related to peer review, such as the nature of the legislation and the impact of medical PSROs on hospital practice,[1] the profession of social work is just beginning the process of implementing peer review.

At the time of writing the authors were employed in the Social Work Department of the University of Michigan Medical Center.

Reprinted from *Social Work in Health Care*, Volume 2(2), Winter 1976-77.

Chernesky and Lurie[2] describe one aspect of quality assurance, assessing time spent in direct client versus nonclient activity.

A description of one phase of peer review, that of establishing standards to define quality social work practice, is the focus of this first-stage paper. A follow-up paper on the results of this type of program will be presented 1 year following its implementation.

THE SETTING

The Department of Social Work of the University of Michigan Medical Center employs 66 social workers in its various clinical units. The medical social work division, from which the current materials have generated, consists of 24 master's degree level and 5 bachelor's degree level staff. Staff assignments are made according to medical service and/or geographic units within the hospital and may involve both inpatient and outpatient responsibilities.

The initial work in the Quality Assurance Program was coordinated by a five-member committee comprised of one chief social worker, one bachelor's degree level social worker, and three master's degree level social workers. The committee's tasks included assuming a primary role in establishing a quality assurance program, obtaining input from all staff members regarding the essential components of such a program, and serving for 1 year as the coordinators of review activities.

PURPOSE AND PHILOSOPHY

The primary purpose of a quality assurance program is to devise the means for monitoring the quality and consistency of social work services in a way that demonstrates to any reviewer the effective delivery of service.

In the process of designing such a program, several serendipitous outcomes of quality assurance were discovered. In addition to monitoring delivery of service, quality assurance can also include: collecting information about staff development needs and recommending programs for meeting those needs; compiling detailed written descriptions of social work activity in various medical services for students and new workers; and using written material to describe social work practice to physicians and other allied health professionals.

Once the objectives for quality assurance have been established, the next step is identifying a system that can provide the information necessary to measure achievement of objectives. The decision to establish standards by medical diagnosis and tasks was made for several reasons. First, social work standards could then parallel programs being established by the medical profession in this center as well as in other medical settings. Second, specificity and uniformity are more attainable when medical diagnosis or actual task is used. Third, standards for practice should reflect the uniqueness of social work practice in hospitals. And finally, the staffing pattern of the department facilitated the medical diagnosis/task approach.

Parallel Medical Review

Since the medical profession is establishing its standards based on medical diagnosis, and because the future goal of PSRO legislation is for medicine and allied health professionals to conduct interdisciplinary reviews, it follows that social work should anticipate merging with medical reviews and establish standards that will facilitate that process. For example, a medical protocol for breast cancer might include referral to social work as one component of service delivery for quality care. If specific social work standards for care of patients with breast cancer are already established, information for an interdisciplinary review can be easily retrieved and understood by disciplines other than social work.

Specificity of Diagnosis Approach

The more specific protocols are, the easier it is to achieve consistency in practice. The committee decided it was possible to be more specific in using diagnostic and task-centered categories than psychosocial diagnostic categories that might cross multiple medical diagnoses.

For example, if a diagnosis such as "adjustment to illness and disability"[3] is established, the intervention of a social worker dealing with the family of a child with cancer would differ significantly from the intervention of a social worker dealing with an adult with rheumatoid arthritis. Operating from the diagnostic perspective, workers at this center were able to be very specific about what information needed to be obtained and what behaviors the individual or family engaged in that would indicate "adjustment to illness and disability," thus outlining specific measurable behaviors and eliminating some of the subjectivity inherent in assessing adjustment to illness or disability.

Uniqueness of Social Work in Hospitals

By defining standards according to medical diagnosis, recognition is given to the unique requirements of individuals affected by illness or injury. This then legitimizes the specialization of social work in medical settings and emphasizes the special knowledge required in dealing with patients and families around the stress or crisis precipitated by medical problems, injury, or disease.

In her description of crisis theory Rappaport[4] has indicated the need to identify specific events that a person or family needs to master in order to deal with stressful events successfully. The crisis event of a premature birth and the steps necessary to deal with it are described in detail by Kaplan.[5]

Since social workers who work with specific disease categories are usually aware of what the patient and family need to master in order to deal successfully with the illness or injury, the logical next step in quality assurance is to identify social work tasks that facilitate mastery of illness or injury and to set standards accordingly.

Staffing Pattern

Consideration of the setting also contributed to the decision to establish standards by diagnosis or task. Workers are assigned to medical services and work with patients and families that have a range of diagnoses within that medical specialty or subspecialty. Since each worker was asked to establish standards for his or her own practice, and since most activity is centered around a diagnosis or specific task, establishing standards on that basis seemed reasonable.

Task Protocols

While the disease/disability categories worked best for most services, there were certain situations in which this system was not appropriate, specifically when activity was primarily task oriented. For example, assisting with discharge planning and nursing home placement is consistent regardless of the patient's diagnosis or medical service.[6] In those circumstances, then, protocols were established according to the task rather than by diagnosis.

Although task protocols apply more to bachelor's degree level workers than MSW personnel, all protocols are intended to be used by staff at both levels. For example, nursing home placements should be done consistently throughout the department.

IMPLEMENTATION

In order to implement the program, full participation of social work staff was essential. Throughout the process staff input has been requested and incorporated into the program.

Once the committee presented and discussed the proposal of diagnosis and task protocols, individual workers were asked to write a protocol describing quality practice for the diagnosis or task they encountered most frequently. Since the intent of peer review is to assure the *overall* quality of service, initially it is necessary to establish standards only for the most common social work activities. The written protocols were then reviewed by the Quality Assurance Committee, and recommendations were made for revisions.

Based on the information obtained by reviewing these initial protocols, a standard format for outlining necessary information, the process for gathering information, and the process of service delivery was established. Information to be included was to be organized as follows: (a) criteria for referral to social work; (b) protocol for social work intervention (subheadings of assessment, goal setting, implementation of plan, recording); (c) unexpected complications; and (d) criteria for termination. As mentioned earlier, different diagnoses necessitate different types and levels of assessment. Specifying this information sets objective criteria that help determine the validity and comprehensiveness of social work objectives.

The decision to omit outcome criteria as part of the initial protocols was made primarily because including them made the task too overwhelming. As Levy[7] points out, there are many extraneous variables that limit social work's ability to predict consistent outcome accurately. It also may be possible to obtain more meaningful data for outcome criteria through the initial review process rather than in advance, so inclusion of outcome criteria has been postponed.

As a final step in establishing a quality assurance program, the committee has completed reviewing the final drafts of most protocols. Those that have been reviewed by the committee, with the author present, and submitted to social work administration include: breast cancer, suspected child abuse, childhood seizure disorder, failure to thrive, respiratory distress, obesity, adult nursing home placement, pediatric nursing home placement, adult discharge planning, childhood cancer, adult rheumatoid arthritis, juvenile rheumatoid arthritis, cystic fibrosis, migraine headaches, leukemia, and terminal cancer in adults. Four examples appear as appendices. Those yet to be reviewed include: adolescent pregnancy, burns, renal disease, and quadriplegia.

REVIEW PROCESS

Although the final audit procedure has not yet been determined, actual review will involve all members of the department at some time during the year. As mentioned earlier, because of the specificity of protocols, each worker should be able to review any other worker, regardless of educational background or experience.

In the actual review, the Quality Assurance Committee will set up task forces comprised of three or four social workers. In keeping with the interdisciplinary intent of the PSRO law, representatives from other allied health disciplines may be invited to participate. For example, if the physician, physical therapist, occupational therapist, and social worker all work closely together with spinal cord patients, then it would be appropriate for all of them to conduct an interdisciplinary review of that diagnosis. If physicians will be expected to have allied health personnel included in their PSROs, then allied health personnel will be expected to cooperate with physicians and each other in monitoring overall quality of health care.

Once each task force appointed by the committee has completed review of one diagnosis or task, it will disband. Each year new groups will be established to equalize the responsibility for review activities.

The committee has elected to have social workers do the initial reviews, rather than Medical Records personnel, because we believe the process itself will have educational value. Medical Records personnel will be involved in obtaining records and consulting about process, but will not be responsible for actual reviews. In the future, after the reviews have been done several times, it may be possible to have Medical Records personnel pull charts and quantify discrepancies which the Social Work Department could then review. At the present time, the system has not been refined enough to permit delegation of that responsibility, nor is such delegation required.

FEEDBACK

Once cases for review have been retrieved by Medical Records, each task force will take the protocol assigned and compare it to social work recording on the charts. Discrepancies will then be summarized and shared with the worker whose charts are being reviewed. After review by social work administration, recommendations for change in the protocol or in actual social work activity will be made. At the conclusion of that review we will have a better idea of how the system works and what its value is to the department.

EVALUATION

Because the concepts of quality assurance as described are as yet untested, there is no way to predict how this system will work in this particular setting or in any other institution. The entire process thus far has been a learning experience. The members of our department have learned new practice techniques as a result of discovering what other staff members are doing. We have also found that it is possible to describe our practice in terms of stated objectives and achievement of those objectives, and that by doing so practice can be improved.

The purpose of this paper has been to share the thinking that went into one way of establishing a quality assurance program. Its success in the setting described and its applicability to other settings have yet to be tested. It may be that what works in a large referral center cannot work in a small community hospital, but it is also possible that the principle of combining diagnostic categories could be relevant in institutions in which strokes, mastectomies, and nursing home placements are more common than childhood cancer or rheumatoid arthritis.

CONCLUSION

The University of Michigan Medical Center Social Work Department is in the process of establishing a quality assurance program based on actual *quality* of service delivered to complement existing administrative review. The system utilizes both diagnostic categories and task categories, since using one or the other does not adequately cover all activities of the department.

The entire Social Work Department will be involved in establishing standards for practice. The format for establishing protocols is the same throughout the department and specificity in assessment and goal setting has been requested. Standards will be applied to only those cases opened after standards have been approved.

The intent of review is to give peers responsibility for assessing their own practice. Social workers can no longer argue about the merits of peer review but should begin to develop objective measures of quality practice. This is a challenge but the potential rewards are great. Instead of being told by others what social work in hospitals should be, the profession can demonstrate in a positive way the value of social work intervention.

REFERENCES

1. Newman, Edward, and Turem, Jerry. "The Crisis of Accountability." *Social Work 19* (1974):5-16.
2. Chernesky, Roslyn H., and Lurie, Abraham. "The Functional Analysis Study: A First Step in Quality Assurance." *Social Work in Health Care 1* (1975-76):213-23.
3. Meites, Mable E. "One Adaptation of Social Work to A Peer Review Sys-

tem." PSRO Workshop Papers, E. W. Sparrow Hospital, Lansing, Michigan, February 1976.

4. Rappaport, Lydia. "Crisis Intervention as a Mode of Brief Treatment." In *Theories of Social Casework*, edited by Robert W. Roberts and Robert H. Nee. Chicago: University of Chicago Press, 1969.

5. Kaplan, David M. "Problem Conception and Planned Intervention." In *Health and Disability Concepts in Social Work Education*. Minneapolis: Vocational Rehabilitation Administration of the Department of Health, Education, and Welfare, 1964.

6. Kerstein, Jerrold. *Research Studies I through V and Narrative Article*. PSRO Publication, National Association of Social Workers, August 1975.

7. Levy, Charles S. "Inputs versus Outputs as Criteria of Competence." *Social Casework* 55 (1974):375-80.

APPENDIX A
Protocol for Adult Rheumatoid Arthritis

I. Criteria for referral to social worker (one of the following is sufficient justification for referral)
   A. Patient in need of additional community resources, including medical assistance, financial assistance, follow-up counseling
   B. Patient and/or family having difficulty understanding disease and treatment, with resultant lack of adherence to treatment program
   C. Patient and/or family requests contact with social worker
   D. Patient having personal or interpersonal problems that interfere with treatment of disease
   E. Patient having difficulty adjusting to disease symptomatology, including pain, fatigue, decreasing mobility
   F. Patient having functional pain
II. Protocol
   A. Assessment
      1. Description of patient, disease, length of time patient has had disease, general condition, prognosis, other illnesses
      2. Patient's general attitude about and adjustment to disease, that is, denying, accepting, depressed
      3. Patient's family composition, response to disease, employment status of household members, health of family members, financial constraints, division of labor at home

    4. Patient's employment status, potential for employability, and desire to work

    5. Patient and family's usual response to pain and stress

  B. Goal setting

    1. List of problems as seen by patient, family, physician, and other staff

    2. Goals established with patient and relevant staff

  C. Implementation of plan

    1. Make recommendations to patient regarding appropriate community resources

    2. Reinforce medical information and need for particular treatment with follow-up on questions. Refer to other medical personnel when appropriate

    3. Provide counseling to patient and/or family members or refer to community agency when family lives too far away or clinic visits are infrequent

  D. Recording

    1. Summary of assessment and treatment plan in chart

    2. Progress toward goals noted in chart

    3. Documentation of recommendations to patient regarding community resources in chart

III. Unexpected complications

  A. Patient's refusal of service

  B. Patient discharged prior to being seen by social worker

IV. Criteria for termination

  A. Cases will be terminated when goals have been reached or

  B. When it appears that goals cannot be achieved

APPENDIX B
Protocol for Pediatric Cancer

I. Criteria for referral to social worker (one of the following is sufficient justification for referral)

  A. Parental interest expressed in extended discussions on how to cope with their child's illness

  B. Problems in the family's social or economic situation requiring special planning (examples: parents not being United States citizens, patient being court ward, another handicapped child in the family, extended unemployment of breadwinners)

C. Unusual and unabating expressions of anxiety, depression, or fear on the part of either parent or the child that may show themselves in behavior disruptive to patient unit

D. Conflict between parents regarding illness (example: what to tell patient or significant others about the illness)

E. Parental delay or reluctance in accepting medical treatment program for child that extends beyond 1 week after presentation of a treatment plan

F. Social isolation of family — that is, no close relatives, neighbors, friends, or church contacts

G. Preexisting mental illness, substance abuse, or chronic illness in any of the child's caretakers

H. Lack of adherence to recommended treatment, including pattern of missed appointments, suspicion that drugs are not given as prescribed despite adequate education

I. Pattern of minimal visiting by family of inpatient (once a week or less with children 12 and under) or prolonged absence of either parent if still part of nuclear family

J. Parents are increasing child's anxiety by inappropriate information sharing or their own maladaptive behavior

II. Protocol for social work intervention

A. Assessment

  1. Process

    a) Review medical chart

    b) Clarify extent of parental information and stage of medical planning through discussion with house staff and appropriate specialty service (pediatric hematology, neurosurgery, orthopedic surgery, thoracic surgery, etc.)

    c) Initiate contact with at least one parent/caretaker of the child to establish mutual problem definition and contract

  2. Information to be obtained about

    a) Adequacy of family's medical information

    b) Adequacy of resources, both financial and emotional

  c) Adjustment to diagnosis and treatment up until time of social work assessment

  d) Previous adjustment to stresses

  e) Child's role within the family before illness

  f) Level of social and emotional functioning prior to diagnosis including marital relationship, family composition, life-style, level of physical activity of patient

  g) Extended family's and community's response to the diagnosis

  h) Parent's attitudes toward physicians and "experimental" treatment for terminal illness

B. Goal setting

  1. Define initial goals with caretakers, staff, and social worker within 1 week of receiving referral

  2. Redefine goals as problems are resolved and new critical events present themselves (such as relapse, tumor recurrence, recall for additional therapy, unexpected complications from treatment, impending death)

C. Implementation of plan

  1. Engage in brief intermittent or ongoing treatment with family members needing assistance

  2. Identify appropriate community agency when local intervention is required (obtaining releases for information sharing)

  3. Inform appropriate local agencies (including school, DSS, LMD) of availability for ongoing consultation when patient is followed jointly

  4. Arrange and lead team discussions with appropriate hospital staff when medical record is insufficient for information sharing and good parent/family care

D. Recording

  1. Summary of assessment and treatment plan in medical chart

  2. Progress toward goals or resolution of major problem noted in medical chart

  3. Documentation of recommendations made to patient regarding community resources (including names of agencies, name of contact person, address, phone numbers)

III. Unexpected complications
    A. Parent's refusal of service
    B. Patient withdrawn from medical treatment
    C. Family crisis occurs (another serious illness, divorce, death, layoff)
    D. Lack of community resources
IV. Criteria for termination
    A. Medical treatment transferred elsewhere
    B. Parents refuse social work service
    C. Goals achieved and family appears stable with coping skills intact
    D. Patient is in long-term remission
    E. Goals cannot be achieved
    F. Above recording is complete

APPENDIX C
Protocol for Adult Discharge Planning*

I. Criteria for referral
    A. Patient or family unable to state or complete feasible discharge plans
    B. Significant personal care or nursing care needs identified that require investigation prior to discharge
    C. Patient's behavior or care at home prior to admission causally related to medical problems or need for admission
    D. Patient's mental limitations preclude his planning living arrangements after discharge
    E. Patient or family identifies problems to hospital staff regarding patient's return to community, such as housing, finances, care arrangements, and social isolation, which cannot be handled exclusively by the home care coordinator**
    F. Evidence of conflict between patient and the family to which he plans to return that may interfere with discharge planning or medical follow-up

---

*Submitted by John Suttinger, ACSW.
**Home care coordinators are part of the nursing staff and are primarily responsible for visiting nurse and public health referrals.

G. No family member available to assist patient in completing plans

H. Need for assisting family to make transportation arrangements to leave hospital and/or keep return clinic appointments

II. Protocol for social work intervention
 A. Assessment
  1. Process
   a) Review patient's chart
   b) Obtain information from physician and relevant staff
   c) Interview patient and family
  2. Information to be obtained about
   a) Level of self-care and nursing needs
   b) Problems precipitating referral
   c) Anticipated discharge date and confirmation that patient and/or family have been informed of discharge date and plans
   d) Patient's prior living arrangements and life-style
   e) Adequacy of family's ability to care for patient and commitment to caring for patient
   f) Financial resources
   g) Available community resources
   h) Patient and family's understanding of medical problems, nursing needs, and their ability to plan adequately
   i) Patient and family's existing posthospital plan and adequacy of that plan
 B. Goal setting
  1. Major problems needing resolution specifically identified and discussed with family, hospital, and involved agencies
  2. Discharge objectives identified and discussed with patient, family, agencies, and hospital staff
 C. Implementation of plan
  1. Assist patient/family in evaluating the feasibility of their posthospital plans
  2. Assist family in determining whether they can meet the patient's physical, emotional, and nursing needs. If not, discuss alternatives such as obtaining needed equipment

and making modifications in living arrangements or placement in a nursing care facility. (See Appendix D, Protocol
for Adult Nursing Home Placement.) If necessary, contact
physician for referral to home care coordinator for provision of home nursing services or referral to Vocational
Rehabilitation for modification of home situation

3. Instruct patient and family regarding application for financial benefits to which they may be entitled
4. Assist patient and family to plan and accommodate to
needed changes in their roles in the family and community
5. Determine with patient and family their transportation
plans for discharge and follow-up appointments. Make
tangible arrangements if family cannot

D. Recording
1. Summary of assessment and plan in medical chart
2. Progress toward goals or resolution of major problem(s)
noted in medical chart
3. Documentation in chart of recommendations made to patient or family regarding community resources (including
names of agencies, name of contact person, addresses,
phone numbers)

III. Unexpected complications
A. Family uncooperative in making plans or resistant to dis-
charge
B. Family difficult to contact for necessary interviews
C. Medical change in patient that alters previous plan
D. Patient/family refuses social work service

IV. Criteria for termination
A. Assessment of patient and family reveals that they are able
to plan adequately or have already planned for discharge
without assistance
B. Discharge plans successfully completed and/or patient discharged

APPENDIX D
Protocol for Adult Nursing Home Placement

I. Criterion for referral
A. Placement in an extended care facility identified as most appropriate discharge plan by staff, family, and/or patient. So-

cial work protocol for discharge planning to be used for initial assessment and determination of plan (Appendix C)

II. Protocol for social work intervention
   A. Assessment
      1. Process
         a) Review medical chart
         b) Contact referring physician to determine family and patient's knowledge and understanding of medical conditions necessitating transfer to a nursing care facility
         c) Interview patient and family
      2. Information to be obtained
         a) Medical chart, medical and nursing staff
            (1) Medical diagnosis and prognosis
            (2) Anticipated discharge date
            (3) Level of nursing care required (e.g., skilled or basic, ambulation status, mental status, hygiene requirements)
            (4) Medications
            (5) Mode of transportation
            (6) Extent of medical follow-up expected by this institution
         b) Family and patient
            (1) Understanding of medical condition, recommended care plan
            (2) Ability to plan adequately
            (3) Patient and family's attitude about and adjustment to diagnosis, prognosis, and need for extended care
            (4) Adequacy of financial resources and coverage for extended care
            (5) Any preference regarding particular facilities
            (6) County in which patient resides
   B. Goal setting
      1. Nursing home placement identified as mutually accepted goal by patient, family, social worker, and medical staff
      2. Tasks for completion of arrangements identified and discussed with patient, family, and medical staff
      3. Date of transfer set after consultation with physician, patient, family, and nursing care facility

4. Redefine goals or reset transfer date due to
   a) Change in medical status
   b) Lack of beds in chosen facility
   c) Lack of cooperation and participation by involved parties
C. Implementation
   1. Obtain authorization for release of information from patient and/or family
   2. Counsel patient and/or family regarding adjustment to illness, change in life-style, and long-term care
   3. Contact significant community agencies currently involved with patient and/or family for explanation of patient's needs, anticipated plans, and information sharing
   4. Place patient transfer form on chart for completion by medical staff
   5. Determine which available nursing care facilities in patient's county meet care requirements
   6. Provide explanation of extended care coverage to patient and family
      a) If insurance is inadequate, instruct family regarding application for medical assistance (Medicaid) at the Department of Social Services in county of nursing care facility
      b) Have public health form R-19 completed by physician or nurse and sent to state agency for determination of level of care when coverage is provided through Medicaid
   7. Assist family in determining selection criteria for choosing a facility
   8. Have family and patient, if possible, contact and visit facility for approval
   9. Contact nursing care facility chosen to provide relevant information
   10. Confirm with medical staff, family, nursing care facility, and ambulance service appropriate transportation arrangements
   11. Send with patient
      a) Transfer form

b) Recent chest X-ray report
c) Discharge summary (if required)
d) Other medical information requested by facility
12. Refer to appropriate community agency when counseling or ongoing contacts are needed
D. Recording
  1. Note in progress notes of patient's medical chart social work involvement within 24 hours of receipt of referral and/or request for assistance
  2. Record relevant assessment data and plans in medical chart, and progression of these plans with explanation of any unexpected complications that may delay disposition
  3. Final recording to include
    a) Name, address, and telephone number of nursing care facility
    b) Financial coverage
    c) Key resource person within client system
    d) Transfer date and transportation arrangements
    e) Medical information required from staff upon transfer
III. Unexpected complications
A. Change in medical condition
B. No beds available in nursing care facility (which may result in an unavoidable extension of patient's hospitalization)
C. No family member to assist with transfer or family refusal to participate in arrangements
D. Patient and/or family refusal of social work services
E. Lack of insurance coverage
IV. Criteria for termination
A. Successful transfer to nursing care facility
B. Successful completion of alternative discharge plans (see Appendix C, Protocol for Adult Discharge Planning)
C. Withdrawal of request for social work assistance
D. Death of patient

Clinical Social Work
with Young Adult Inpatients:
Perspectives of Patients,
Parents, and Clinicians

Mollie C. Grob, MSW, ACSW
Susan V. Eisen, PhD
Golda M. Edinburg, MSW, ACSW

SUMMARY. This article describes an empirical study designed to identify the unique role of the clinical social worker as a member of the hospital team in the treatment of young adult psychiatric inpatients. Fifty-five patients, their parents and social workers were interviewed at admission and 60 days later to ascertain: (1) initial attitudes and expectations regarding social work services, (2) specific services desired by clients, (3) actual services provided, and (4) helpfulness of the services. Results indicated that the services most frequently desired were those most often provided. These included providing information to families about patients' progress, helping families deal with hospital procedures and helping with aftercare planning. Most services provided were viewed as helpful. Social workers were seen as more helpful to families than to patients and more so by parents than by patients. Clients who felt the social worker understood their needs and was available when needed, felt he/she was more helpful to them. The implications of these findings for definition of the social worker's role are discussed.

At the time of writing Mrs. Grob was Director of the Evaluative Service Unit, McLean Hospital, 115 Mill Street, Belmont, MA 02178. Dr. Eisen was Coordinator of Patient Care Evaluation in the Evaluative Service Unit and Ms. Edinburg was Director of Social Work, McLean Hospital.

The authors wish to acknowledge the enthusiasm and support of Dr. Helen Reinherz, Chairperson, Research Department, Simmons College School of Social Work and the second-year graduate students who participated in the project.

Reprinted from *Social Work in Health Care*, Volume 8(2), Winter 1982.

606 SOCIAL WORK IN HEALTH CARE: A HANDBOOK FOR PRACTICE

An ongoing debate taking place among our colleagues today concerns the unique focus of clinical social work intervention. This dialogue is a healthy indication of the continuing effort within the social work profession to reaffirm basic values with respect to its historic role and evolution in response to social, economic and cultural needs (Goldstein, 1980; Meyer, 1979; Weick, 1981).

In the past role definition has been primarily conceptualized by the professional as part of his/her theoretical sophistication and practice. More recently its exploration has been pursued with the use of a more empirical approach. Beginning steps are being taken to include participants in the treatment process as collaborators in this endeavor; for example, the consumer who is central to the process and the ultimate determinant of outcome (Warfel, Maloney & Blase, 1981). That consumerism in social work practice can embrace families as well as the identified client or patient expands the potential value of an empirically based approach to role definition by utilizing multiple sources of information.

With this orientation McLean Hospital and the Simmons College School of Social Work undertook an investigation of the role of the social worker from the joint perspective of patients, families, and clinical social workers.[1]

Among the questions to be answered by our study were the following:

1. What concept of the social worker's role is implied in the services desired by patients and their families?
2. What are the actual services provided and views of the social worker's helpfulness?
3. What factors influence views of helpfulness, e.g., initial reactions to the social worker, earlier experiences, patient's outcome?
4. What are the implications of these findings for definition of the social worker's role?

---

1. Preliminary data have been included in Beck et al., *An Evaluation of the Delivery of Social Work Services to Young Adult Psychiatric Patients and Their Families: Part I*, 1978, and Ashley et al., *Part II*, 1979. Unpublished masters dissertations, Simmons College School of Social Work.

METHOD

Treatment Setting

At McLean Hospital, a private psychiatric hospital with 280 beds and 17 inpatient units, social work intervention for patients and families is recognized as a method for facilitating successful coping of families and enabling the identified patient to improve optimally. The critical assumption behind this viewpoint is that most families need help in dealing with the crisis of mental illness and the hospitalization experience.

At or about the time of admission, patients and their families are routinely provided with a social work evaluation and treatment plan by the social worker on the unit to which the patient is assigned. The extent to which the social worker is actively involved varies; families are usually seen by appointment on a regular basis, and patients also by formal agreement or informally on the hall. Within the hospital setting, the social worker is a member of the treatment team, and his/her functions vary according to differences in philosophy, treatment style, and patient population. These may include supportive case work, individual group, marital or family therapy.

Sample

The sample consisted of consecutive admissions to the adult service of unmarried adolescents and young adults ages 14 to 23 (N = 55). Young, single patients were chosen to provide a homogeneous sample of patients and family members receiving social work services.

Almost 70 were 19 years of age or under; more than two-thirds were male. All but five were living with their parents at the time of the admission; the rest were in school dormitories. Almost three-quarters were from two-parent families, the rest, single-parent families. The most common admitting diagnoses were schizophrenia (35%), personality disorder (27%), and transient situational disorder (20%). Approximately one-third had not experienced a previous psychiatric hospitalization; another one-third had three or more. The median duration of the current McLean hospitalization was 58 days.

Procedure

Data collection involved the use of structured interviews administered separately to patients, their mothers and fathers one to two weeks after admission and again at discharge, or two months after admission, whichever came first. Patient and family interviews were completed in person or by telephone by social work graduate students who had no clinical involvement with the informants. The McLean Hospital clinical social workers assigned to each case participated in the data collection by completing mailed questionnaires parallel in content to the interviews administered to the patients and their parents.

At the initial interview all informants were asked a number of specific questions to identify their views about the type and extent of social work involvement desired. In addition, patients and parents were asked to assess their understanding of the social work role in the hospital and their expectations as to whether or not social work services would be helpful to them. Also included were questions about prior experience and satisfaction with social work intervention and initial reactions to the current social worker. The later interview reviewed the extent of contact and type of services actually received. Patients and parents were also asked to assess the helpfulness of each specific service and the overall helpfulness of the intervention.

RESULTS

A total of 377 interviews were conducted, yielding an overall response rate of 86%, with all categories of informants well represented (six fathers and one mother were not available due to death/divorce/separation).

Seventy percent of the patients and parents had met their social worker at the time of the admission, the rest shortly thereafter. Included among those who did not see a social worker at admission were readmitted patients. Plans were made for regularly scheduled appointments with almost all of the parents (91%) and about one-half of the patients (46%), with the rest to be seen on an informal basis as needed. A majority of all the respondents reported that they found these arrangements satisfactory.

In the initial interview, a greater proportion of mothers than fathers or patients reported that they understood the role of the social worker, that a social worker might be helpful, and that the social worker understood their needs (see Table 1). Patients and fathers were more skeptical, particularly in response to the question, "Do you think the social worker understands your needs?" Less affirmative responses reflected uncertainty rather than negativity (only 11% of responses across all informants were unfavorable).

Fourteen areas of service to patients and families had been identified by the social work department prior to the investigation as relevant for social work intervention. In most of these areas the social worker functioned as a liaison between patients and their parents or between the hospital and the family. Nine services focused exclusively on work with family only; two involved patients and their families; three patients alone.

When asked to indicate which of these services they would like to receive, more than one-half of the informants wanted 12 of the 14 services (Table 2). Least desired services were help with resolution of parents' marital problems (36%) and with other family problems (50%). Thus, while services for the family were clearly indicated,

Table 1

Percentage of Informants with Favorable
Initial Views of the Social Worker

Area of Inquiry	Informant Category		
	Mother	Father	Patient
Do you understand the social worker's role?	94%	79%	75%
Do you think social worker might be helpful?	75%	63%	61%
Does social worker understand your needs?	65%	53%	40%

Table 2

Extent to Which Specific Social
Work Services Were Desired

		Informant Category			
Service	Total	Patient	Mother	Father	Social Worker
Provide information to family about patient's progress	91%*	83%	96%	95%	92%
Help family deal with hospital procedures	85%	74%	83%	88%	96%
Help with after-care planning	83%	73%	92%	88%	81%
Help family understand patient	79%	71%	81%	70%	87%
Help family become less worried	79%	77%	83%	81%	75%
Give family recommendations on how to relate to patient	77%	71%	85%	80%	73%
Help patient deal with hospital procedures	76%	71%	80%	85%	67%
Help family cope with stress	75%	67%	77%	76%	81%
Help patient understand family	73%	64%	79%	80%	69%
Help resolve patient's problems	70%	64%	74%	87%	54%
Provide family with information about mental illness	65%	61%	64%	72%	63%
Someone to talk to about one's own problems	63%	60%	70%	59%	--
Help resolve other family problems	50%	62%	50%	51%	39%
Help resolve parents' marital problems	35%	37%	33%	43%	29%
Average of all services	71%	67%	75%	76%	69%

*Percentages are proportion of each group desiring to receive (or provide) that service; services are arranged from most to least desired.

the areas of intervention focused on those relating to the patient's illness.

When we examined the informant's view at the later interview of actual services provided, those most frequently desired were also most frequently provided; similarly, those least frequently wanted were least frequently provided. The highest agreement between social workers and all informants about services provided was in the area of (1) informing family about patient's progress and (2) helping with aftercare planning. Very high agreement between social workers and other informants also occurred regarding help in resolving marital issues; they agreed that it was not provided. Least agreement was reported in the area of helping the patient deal with hospital procedures; ambiguity seems to be greater here.

Across respondents, most specific services received were judged to be "quite" helpful, although patients generally felt the services were less helpful than did either fathers or mothers. Social workers were seen as more helpful to families than to patients by all family members; parents were more favorable in their ratings of the social worker's general helpfulness (to both patients and families) than were patients (see Table 3).

The majority of patients and parents agreed that the social worker had been available to them when needed; similarly, they agreed that the social worker "understood their needs." Perceptions of the social worker's understanding of the clients' needs were usually related to personal qualities ("sensitive and likable" — "listens well and is available" — "insightful, understanding") or to skills and

Table 3

Mean Ratings of General Helpfulness
of Social Worker

Respondent	Helpfulness to Patient	Helpfulness to Family
Patient	3.25*	2.92
Mother	2.04	2.43
Father	2.60	2.42

*Scale: 1 = extremely, 2 = quite, 3 = moderately, 4 = somewhat, 5 = not at all

activities ("tried hard to find solutions" — "goes to morning report and talks with the doctors" — "helpful in trying to figure out our individual needs" — "listens to our complaints" — "thorough and knowledgeable"). A central theme that emerged in this view of the social worker was that of provider and coordinator of social services for the patient and the family. Frequently when family members reported dissatisfaction with the social worker, there were expressions of dissatisfaction with the hospital system in general.

Factors Influencing Satisfaction

A question often raised relates to the identification of factors that influence consumer satisfaction. With this objective, we examined the relationship between a number of variables and views of the social workers' helpfulness. In the initial interview, the social workers' understanding of the clients' needs was significantly related to later views of helpfulness ($p < .01$). Clients who felt the social worker understood their needs within two weeks of their first meeting, judged them as more helpful two months later. Ratings of helpfulness were significantly correlated with social worker's availability and understanding of needs at the later interview as well. Social workers who were available when needed and who understood their clients' needs during the course of hospitalization were seen as more helpful ($p < .01$). By contrast, the extent of intervention, hospital length of stay, and clinical outcome were not related to views regarding the social workers' helpfulness.

SUMMARY AND DISCUSSION

This report presents the results of an investigation exploring the role of the clinical social worker with young adult inpatients and their parents. With the increase in the number of young people seeking or requiring psychiatric hospitalization in the last two decades, services were created to meet their special needs. A number of investigators have reviewed the hospital experiences and follow-up outcome of this population with some attention to the characteristics and involvement of their families, yet relatively little has been reported on the process and effectiveness of the social work intervention carried out in their behalf (Garber, 1972; Gossett, Lewis, Lewis & Phillips, 1973; Grob & Singer, 1974; Hartmann, Glasser, Greenblatt, Solomon & Levinson, 1978). Our study provides an empirical view of the social worker's role from the perspective of patients, parents and the professionals.

The young adult sample was predominantly male with schizophrenia or personality disorder as the more common diagnosis. Among the priorities identified for social work activities were helping the family deal with issues around the hospitalization and the patient's illness, helping the family understand the patient, and relieving family stress. The major focus in expectations about service was on work with the family with the basic need relating to aspects of the patient's illness.

The burdens placed on families of the mentally ill and the need for further efforts on their behalf have been highlighted elsewhere as well (Hatfield, 1978; Kreisman & Joy, 1974). Hartman (1981), recognizing the potential of families, urges that the delivery of services be carried out to strengthen rather than to undermine the families. Reporting on family intervention with severely disturbed inpatients, Anderson (1977) emphasizes the importance of a patient-oriented family approach, the goal being to reduce family stress and enhance the patient's potential for achieving the treatment goals. One of the mothers interviewed in our study expressed this idea in personal terms, "The social worker was extremely helpful to me so that I in turn could be more helpful to my daughter."

Respondents also gave priority at the initial timepoint to aftercare planning as a major aspect of the social work role. This finding echoes Adelson and Leader's (1980) conclusion regarding its significance following a recent survey of 26 private psychiatric hospitals in which social work directors were asked to identify the relative importance of various professional duties. In their words, "Social work has always represented the link between the patient and the community in the broadest sense" (p. 780).

By an examination of the relationship among variables, some indicators were identified that might be influencing client satisfaction (here derived from the rating of helpfulness). The social worker seen as more accessible during the intervention was viewed as more helpful. In addition, how well the social worker understood the client's needs was predictive. This correlation between the perceptions of understanding of the client's needs and of the professional's helpfulness may derive from an underlying process centering on the quality of their relationship. Additional data from the study describing the social worker's attributes further serve to strengthen the idea that the ability to form an alliance is a key factor in the success of the social work intervention.

Increasing recognition is being given to the rights of the client to be involved in decision making and evaluation of treatment modes and outcome (Maluccio, 1979; Prager & Tanaka, 1980). The inclusion of patients and families enhances our ability to broaden the empirical base of our understanding of the intervention. With this in mind the goal of a true collaboration between the social worker and the client in the planning and delivery of service may yet become a reality.

REFERENCES

Adelson, G. & Leader, M. The social worker's role: A study of private and voluntary hospitals. *Hospital and Community Psychiatry*, 1980, *31*, 776-780.

Anderson, C. Family intervention with severely disturbed inpatients. *Archives of General Psychiatry*, 1977, *34*, 697-702.

Garber, B. *Follow-up study of hospitalized adolescents.* New York: Brunner/Mazel, 1972.

Goldstein, E.G. Knowledge base of clinical social work. *Social Work*, 1980, *25*, 73-178.

Gossett, J., Lewis, S., Lewis, J., & Phillips, V. Follow-up of adolescents treated in a psychiatric hospital: A review of studies. *American Journal of Orthopsychiatry*, 1973, *43*, 602-610.

Grob, M.C. & Singer, J. *Adolescent patients in transition: Impact and outcome of psychiatric hospitalization.* New York: Human Services Press, 1974.

Hartman, A. The family: A central focus for practice. *Social Work*, 1981, *26*, 7-13.

Hartmann, E., Glasser, B., Greenblatt, M., Solomon, M.H., & Levinson, D.J. *Adolescents in a mental hospital.* New York: Grune and Stratton, Inc., 1978, 197 pp.

Hatfield, A. Psychological costs of schizophrenia in the family. *Social Work*, 1978, *23*, 355-359.

Kreisman, D. & Joy, V. Family response to the mental illness of a relative: A review of the literature. *Schizophrenia Bulletin*, 1974, *10*, 34-57.

Maluccio, A. *Learning from clients: Interpersonal helping as viewed by clients and social workers.* New York: Free Press, 1979.

Meyer, C.H. What directions for social work practice? *Social Work*, 1979, *24*, 267-272.

Prager, E. & Tanaka, H. Self-assessment: The client's perspective. *Social Work*, 1980, *25*, 32-34.

Warfel, D.J., Maloney, D.M., & Blase, K. Consumer feedback in human service programs. *Social Work*, 1981, *26*, 151-156.

Weick, A. Reframing the person-in-environment perspective. *Social Work*, 1981, *26*, 140-143.

Predicting Patterns
of Social Work Staffing
in Hospital Settings

George I. Krell, MS, ACSW
Gary Rosenberg, PhD

SUMMARY. One long-standing problem of social work departments in acute care hospitals has been their diverse patterns of staffing. The lack of a standard or guide has tended to diminish the utilization of social work services in hospital settings. Over a period of six years, the Society for Hospital Social Work Directors of the American Hospital Association developed and revised a guide for inpatient staffing. The guide is designed to assist hospital and social work administrators establish an inpatient line staffing plan which is based on the number of hospital beds, the number of patients to be served and the number of functions carried. The logic of the inquiry and the findings can serve as a base for future research in inpatient, ambulatory care and other settings that serve special populations.

At the time of writing George I. Krell was Director, Department of Social Work, The Mount Sinai Medical Center of Greater Miami, Miami Beach, FL 33141. Gary Rosenberg was Director, Department of Social Work Services and Associate Professor of Community Medicine (Social Work), The Mount Sinai Medical Center, New York, NY 10029.

This work emanates from the interest of both authors as well as the work of the Society for Hospital Social Work Directors. Of particular importance to the development of some of the thinking are the contributions of a number of individuals who participated in the process: Barbara Berkman, Claudia Coulton, Abraham Lurie, Helen Rehr, Robert Spano, Salie Rossen, Robert Stepanek.

Reprinted from *Social Work in Health Care*, Volume 9(2), Winter 1983.

INTRODUCTION

The purpose of this article is to provide a framework for studying and predicting patterns of social work staffing in hospital settings. It can be useful to social work managers in assessing their current and projected staffing patterns. Hospital managers, concerned with the provision of social work services and the overall allocation of scarce resources, can use it to obtain a rationale on how many social workers are necessary to meet the missions and goals of the setting.

History

Although there were many state standards for social work, it had not achieved a major official place in national health care until the conditions of participation of Medicare established a standard. These acknowledged the need for social health services and identified social work as one of the main providers of these services. Except in the major academic teaching centers characterized by their low income, multi-problem population, hospital managers have been reluctant to commit extensive resources to social work services. This diffidence is linked with less than clearly defined hospital missions; with the question of how much the provision of social health services belongs in the community-based practice as opposed to hospital-based practice; and with the fact that social workers have not had the tools to demonstrate their services in out-come/output, cost-efficiency/cost-effectiveness or cost-benefit terms. The literature which suggests that social work can provide useful systems of support for the patient, family and team members is not well known to hospital administrators.

Thus, the picture at the present time is one of great unevenness. Between 3,000 and 4,000 hospitals have organized social work departments. Most of them are staffed by one to two persons. The major Medicare conditions of participation, which at least refers to social work, is now under a review which may result in the removal of social work as well as other professions from the standards. In studies of health care providers, social work productivity is not even mentioned.

It is in a complex scene of conflicting values, policies and programs that a step towards rational approaches to staffing patterns is required. The development of staffing patterns in health care has not been a particular strength in the professions which are the major providers in health care. Thus, social work need not be defensive with regard to the development of its standards so far. There are a number of national studies which represent serious efforts of the social work profession to deal with this issue.

Relevant Literature

The pertinent literature consists of accumulated studies all of which are *descriptive* rather than *analytic* or *experimental*. They suggest some guidelines for in-patient staffing. For example, it is projected that 55-60% of patients in hospitals need psychosocial intervention. Assuming that a social worker gives 60-70% direct service time to patients,

- for a 60-bed acute medical/surgical unit, two MSWs and one BSW are needed;
- for high risk groups, one MSW for each 25 beds;
- for psychiatry, two MSWs for 20 beds where the MSW is involved in the primary delivery psychotherapy;
- for psychiatry, two MSWs for 24 beds when this is a shared responsibility. (Lurie, 1976)

The literature on out-patient staffing is less clear. However, for outpatients the following staffing patterns are suggested:

- of each 10,000 patients that generate approximately 35,000 visits, it has been determined that 85% need psychosocial services; therefore, 3 MSWs and 3 BSWs for each 10,000 patients is a suggested staffing ratio;
- for emergency room visits, 30,000 patients require 3 MSWs on staggered shifts. (Lurie, 1976)

Other professions have attempted to deal with staffing patterns. Physicians per person in a population is one standard sometimes used to project numbers of physicians needed in underserved populations. The need for psychiatrists is viewed in terms of incidence and prevalence by regions so that distribution patterns can be seen. Frequently, however, the statistics utilized have to do with national distribution patterns and not with distribution patterns within a particular health care facility. Nursing has come the closest to having a reasonably well-developed staffing patterns formula developed in conjunction with the federal government and Medicus. Its key notion is the level of patient "acuity," that is, the complexity of care the patient requires. Social work has used this idea, too, although in a parallel way, with mutual benefit of interaction between the two professions absent. Social work's patient "acuity" factor is that of high social risk which identifies individuals at risk and aggregates populations at risk (Productivity and Health, 1980).

Factors Which Influence Staffing Patterns

There are factors which are key in influencing staffing patterns. Some are more significant than others, but all help explain the variations in different settings and need to be applied to current work and future research.

1. Institutional Factors

The size of the health care setting is a major factor relevant in social work staffing. Included in size are number of beds, average daily census, average length of stay, number of ambulatory care visits, number of registered ambulatory care patients and number of clinics.

The purpose of the hospital is another crucial variable. Is it a chronic or acute care setting? Do its missions and functions include teaching and research in addition to service?

2. Patient Factors

This is a second major area. What is the nature of the population served: ethnicity, socio-economic background, race, culture? The mix of patient illnesses, sophistication of patients and families about social work, their requests for social work services, the number and severity of their social problems related to illness, their premorbid psychosocial problems all influence staffing.

3. Physician Factors

Physicians' attitudes and beliefs about social work are crucial factors. Do they recognize the psychosocial component as important in care? Do they control the entry or exclusion of social work services for patients? Can social work itself identify the population it will serve?

4. Department Factors

Departmental factors such as the mission of the department, the functions it carries, the current or proposed level of staffing, the size of the support staff, the organization of the department, the ordering of priorities, the sanctions regarding case entry and pickup and the extent of its primary treatment functions are all crucial to staffing.

Predictors to Staffing Patterns

This paper identifies a set of factors and variables, and their use in establishing staffing patterns. It summarizes three studies conducted to test their usefulness as good predictors of staff needed. Their rationale is based on deductive logic and the logic of stepwise multiple regression analyses. Although the formula approaches are not problem free, they are usable, objective ways to arrive at staffing needs. They are described in detail because they establish the foundation of thinking and study on which further efforts to refine and perfect them can be built.

DEVELOPING A STAFFING GUIDE

The long overdue need for some standard of uniformity was no more aptly illustrated than by a 1975 survey of 79 acute hospitals (Salary Survey, 1975). Thirteen hospitals with 125 beds or less had staffing patterns ranging from a low of one to a high of 6 professionals; 27 hospitals with 126-249 beds had professional staff ranging from one to 21 plus; 27 hospitals with 250-499 beds had staffs ranging from one to 21 plus; and 12 hospitals with 500+ beds ranged from a low of 7 to more than 21 plus. The latter group included hospitals with staffing patterns of 40 to 50 plus. In 1975 the Society for Hospital Social Work Directors, American Hospital Association began to develop a plan for determining social work staffing for acute care hospitals.

The Board charged an ad hoc committee to develop such a guide by 1976. However, a usable plan was not finalized and agreed to until 1981, some six years later. The involvement of 252 hospitals and 2 studies were needed to complete the project. The long delay, despite the sustained effort maintained over the years, speaks to the complexity of the problems inherent in developing any plan that purports to be a national guide for the hospital field. The process also speaks to the difficulties in quantifying the delivery of human services, difficulties which become even more monumental when the services are provided in settings where social work often is viewed as a guest.

The project moved in three phases. Phase One saw the development of basic concepts and the testing of these concepts in 10-12 leadership hospitals in 1975-1976. Phase Two used a national research forum to conduct a scientific testing of the original concepts; and saw the evolution of a new approach developed from 1976-1979 from the test results of 67 hospitals. Phase Three saw the substantiation of the original concepts and the simplification of the formula as the result of data obtained through a national study and agreement of the final formula in 1979-1981.

Phase I: The Deductive Formula

The committee approached the task with this objective: to develop a gross formula which could be refined in the years ahead but which could be immediately applied to any general hospital. Key goals were set. The formula should reflect the staffing patterns of the leadership hospitals; but at the same time consider the realities in the entire hospital field. The formula should be usable by the administrator of the hospital which did not have an existing structured department as well as by the administrator of the hospital which did have a department, and who, in concert with the social work director, needed assistance in planning and revising a staffing pattern. Formulae were needed which could establish a minimum service level and yet allow for consideration of a maximum of service to meet the special needs of an individual institution. These concepts were enunciated as critical to the development of an effective staffing plan.

1. The scope of functions which constitute a social work program must be identified and agreed to for staffing purposes. While all hospitals do not have to provide the full range of functions, each hospital should specifically identify each service it planned to provide from a list of social work functions.
2. The number of functions provided by a social work department relates directly to the size of the staff required. Functions relate to program services and the more functions the department carries, the greater the time demands upon staff, and the greater the number of staff required.
3. For inpatients, the total number of patients to be served at any given point in time is limited by the number of hospital beds. It is necessary to approximate the number of patients requiring social work from the total inpatients being served by the facility.
4. It is possible to extract a service population by identifying and agreeing to a certain number of high risk factors that tend to characterize those in need. High risk factors would include patients 65 years of age or older, low income patients, especially those on public programs, and certain categories of high medical and/or psychosocial need, i.e., illnesses such as cancer, stroke, heart disease. An agreed upon set of percentages for patients at risk would be applied to the total patient population to extract a social service "at need" population. The formula to be devised would predict for the general hospital only the line staff needed, regardless of educational level, and would make no attempt to identify supervisorial and administrative staffing levels. Utilizing these concepts, the first inpatient formula developed is shown in Figure 1.

The significant features of this first generation formula were:

Figure 1

First In-patient Formula

STEP I	Total of all hospital patients by month	÷	Number of hospital beds	=	Monthly turn-over ratio
	1,013 patients	÷	377 beds		2.7

STEP II	Establish percent of patients to be served	×	Total of all hospital pa-tients by month	=	Patients re-quiring social work (active case ratio)
	25% base plus 15% high risk = 40%	×	1,013	=	405

STEP III	Patients requiring social work (active case ratio)	÷	Monthly turn-over ratio	=	Active cases per period
	405 patients	÷	2.7	=	150

STEP IV	Active cases per period	÷	Staff caseload (based on num-ber of func-tions)	=	Number of line staff required
	150	÷	25 (or 15 or 35)	=	6

1. The *active case ratio* (ACR) was an approach to determine the percent of patients who required social service. The formula used a base percent developed for the major medical service areas of the hospital, i.e., surgical services beds, out of the experience of the ad hoc committee members. The hospital was then allowed to increase the percentages of patients to be served beyond the base percentage by taking into account high risk factors. It was possible under this system to project up to 100% of the patient population as a service group and to plan the size of staff accordingly.

2. The *staff/caseload ratio* was an approach to determine the number of functions the hospital wanted to carry out; it provided a weight value of these functions in line with the significance of the functions. These were 11 basic functions such as

psychosocial counselling and 11 optimal functions such as patient health consultation, spread over four categories.

The hospital social work department checked the functions it desired to provide; this achieved a point value. The higher the point value, the greater the number of staff required. This was achieved in the formulae by allowing a staff ratio of one worker to 15 cases (1-15) for maximum functions; a staff ratio of one worker to 25 cases (1-25) for medium number of functions; and a staffing ratio of one worker to 35 cases (1-35) for minimum functions. The actual numbers used were based on the following considerations.

1. The use of the one worker to 15 cases ratio derived from social work experience in psychiatric settings, often regarded as providing the most intensive level of professional services. In those settings the worker to case ratio is low in order to allow more time per case and staffing ranges from one worker to 10-15 active cases.
2. The use of the one worker to 35 case ratio was based on federal reimbursement standards to state/county welfare departments for family and children programs. This ratio was regarded as the maximum number of cases a worker could carry at a given point in time and maintain an acceptable level of professional practice.
3. The ratio of the one worker to 25 cases was based on aware- ness that in most social agencies actual practice falls somewhere in between the high and low caseload ratios and level of contact intensity.

Positives and Problems — Phase I Formula

During 1975-1976, the initial formula was revised three times to reflect the knowledge gained by the input of data from the hospitals where the committee members worked; and by the testing of data from 12 hospitals in three categories of bed size (small, medium, large) which were seen as "leadership" institutions because of "manpower" ratios and program reputation (AHA, 1977). A large number of respondees found the application of the formula relatively accurate as it called for a size of staff that reflected the respondees' personal observations of their institutional needs. Major problems which reduced the effectiveness of the formula arose from the tendency of many directors to be unrealistic in the number of functions they indicated their departments provided and in their projections of high risk cases beyond the base number.

Some small one member departments indicated that they carried many functions more congruent with that of a large well staffed hospital. The results of formula application thus overstated the number of staff required. When the formula was recomputed with data which accurately reflected functions carried, the staffing results came closer to expectations. It became obvious that the formula concepts needed to be clarified and simplified. The formula allowed too much flexibility and could propose overstaffing. Another major concern related to the use of the formula in out-patient settings where it resulted in projecting staffing out of line with reality. The effectiveness of the formulae in this area was seriously questioned. Because it mathematically utilized volume as a factor, the formula was not reflecting the reality of most settings which provided only nominal social work services to its ambulatory patient population.

Phase II: The Analytic Formula

The second major phase of the formulae development was initiated in 1977 when the Society entered into an agreement with the Program Evaluation Resource Center, (PERC), an independent research team in Minneapolis, Minnesota, for the development and evaluation of staffing pattern formulae for hospital social work departments.

The beginning point for the study was to be the January, 1977 report.

> The primary objective of the research is to determine the degree to which the initial version of the staffing formula compares with established practice in social work. A secondary objective is to examine possible modifications in the formula to enhance its predictive accuracy. (Sherman, 1978)

The method used by PERC involved the development of a questionnaire germane to the determination of social work staffing needs. This was sent to a random sample of 100 general medical/surgical hospitals of moderate size (100-999 beds) drawn from the membership list of the Society for Hospital Social Work Directors. The questionnaire was completed and mailed October, 1977. Sixty-seven (67) questionnaires were returned with sufficient information to allow application of the proposed staffing formula. The final report from PERC was completed November, 1978.

The study revealed that the initial formula (the Deductive Formula) provided estimates that considerably exceeded current staffing practice. A revised or second generation version was proposed which involved a simplification of the initial formula; that is, algebraically it was possible to reduce the formula to only three variables: the active case ratio, the staff case ratio and the number of beds. The Active Case Ratio fixed at 0.40 to provide staffing estimates which would compare more realistically to actual practice. The revised formula reads as follows:

$$\text{Staff Required} = \frac{0.40 \ (\text{Active Case Ratio}) \times \# \text{ of Beds}}{\text{Staff Case Ratio}}$$

PERC's formula was based on a model suggested by statistical analysis called the Analytic Formula. The two instruments were remarkably close in estimating staffing need, but the analytic formula had features "that seem to favor it over the deductive formula for further development and refinement" (Sherman, 1978).

The basic assumptions and concepts of this alternate formula is that other things being equal, the social work staff requirements will be proportional to the following: the *size* of the hospital's patient population; the *need* in the patient population and the *extent* of services offered. Actual social work staff size will tend to stand in some fixed ratio to the social work staff need.

The assumptions resulted in the development of a multiplication model built around the following variables: social work size, annual number of hospital admissions, average length of stay, number of services provided, level of patient population, and adequacy of existing service population. After an assessment of each variable "using standard least squares analysis" it was determined that "annual hospital admissions (AHA), average length of stay (ALS) and number of services provided (NSP) related significantly to the size of the actual social work staff required." The analytic formula is as follows:

$$\text{Staff Required} = \frac{\underset{\text{Admissions}}{\overset{\text{Annual Hospital}}{\text{AHA}}} \times \underset{\text{NSP}}{\overset{\text{Functions}}{}} \times \underset{\sqrt{\text{ALS}}}{\overset{\substack{\text{Square Root of} \\ \text{the Average} \\ \text{Length of Stay}}}{}}}{100,000}$$

By early 1979 the study committee faced a dilemma. Neither of the two major formulae met all the criteria that had been initially set. The initial deductive formula, based on data of leadership hospitals participating in the test, did not conform to actual hospital social work practice and produced staffing estimates somewhat in excess of the actual practice. The formula was congruent with hospital staffing patterns of the "leadership" hospitals. The value of the formula lay in its ability to determine what a quality staffing pattern should be based on: its adaptability to differential manpower needs within an institution; its fit to leadership hospitals; and as a guideline to other hospitals trying to reach a standard. Although its concepts and approach had produced a positive membership response, its greatest weakness lay in the still unproven percentages used in the formula to determine the patient population requiring social work and the worker caseload.

The analytic formula which had not been tested by the membership but which was developed around a "best fit" regression line for the hospitals in the PERC survey, mirrored staffing practice as it actually existed in the field. It introduced and gave mathematical considerations in the formula to such factors as total in-patient volume and average length of stay.

Phase III: Revised Deductive Formula

At this point in time an independent activity provided the "rescue" of the staffing formula. In response to federal legislation calling for a "uniform reporting" system in hospitals, the Society for Hospital Social Work Directors and the National Association of Social Workers joined forces to carry out a comprehensive survey of hospital social work practice. By the summer of 1979 complete data was collected for 173 hospitals, representing all regions of the country and sizes of hospitals. Survey instruments on 4,381 patients were completed (Coulton, 1979).

The significant aspect of this study was that it provided a wealth of data that related to and could be utilized by the deductive formula to enhance its predictive reliability, to simplify its application and reduce the margin for error in its use. It provided the deductive approach with proven data that could be inserted into the formula: this negated one of the remaining criticisms of the formula. What was even more remarkable was the ease with which the data fit the deductive formula and the similarity of the studies. The following data obtained by the nationwide survey of hospital social work practice was considered pertinent for the revitalization of the deductive concept.

— The median staff size for a small hospital (1 to 200 beds) was 1 to 2 social workers; the mean number of functions was 12.77; and the mean of in-patient admissions served by the social work department was 15%.
— The median staff size for medium hospital (201 to 500 beds) was 3 to 9 social workers; the mean number of functions was 14.47; and, the mean of in-patient admissions served by the social work department was 26%.
— The median staff size for a large hospital (501 to 1,000 beds) was 10 to 19 social workers; the mean number of functions was 14.66; and, the mean of in-patient admissions seen by the social work department was 23%.
— The median staff size for very large hospitals (1,000 plus beds) was 20 plus social workers; the mean number of func-

tions was 17.62; and, the mean of in-patient admissions served by the social work department was 46%.

FURTHER REVISION

The deductive formula was further revised for predicting the number of in-patient admissions to be served by a social work department. Following the PERC concept that in estimating patients to be served (ACR), an agreed upon and set percentage (PERC suggested 0.40 as valid related to their testing findings) should be used rather than the original approach of estimating at-risk percentages; it was decided that the National Survey data allowed for a refinement that would enable three (3) percentage factors to be utilized, based on the size of a hospital:

1. For a small hospital 28% was selected as characteristic of the patients requiring social work services; 28% was the average of the base percentages for leadership general hospitals without a high risk consideration in the Phase I Deductive Formula. In the National Survey Data 27.5% was the mean between the in-patient admissions served by the smallest hospital and those by the largest hospital. In addition, the workers in the combined small through medium hospital categories served a high of 26% of hospital admissions.
2. For a medium sized hospital, 34% was selected as characteristic of the patients requiring social work service. This figure was derived from data in the National Survey Data: it combined the 26% mean of the admissions seen by the medium size hospitals with the 46% mean of admissions seen by the large size hospitals to achieve an average of 36% patients requiring social work services. In the PERC Study the highest mean of patients to be served was 40%; when this was averaged with the 26% mean for National Survey Data medium size hospitals a 33% average was derived.
3. For a large size hospital, 40% was selected as characteristic of the patients requiring social work services; this specific percent built around the PERC suggested maximum. The Na-

tional Survey Data for admissions seen by large hospitals and very large social work departments was 46%.

The Deductive Formula concept was validated; increased functions mean increased services and require a greater number of line staff to provide these services. The number of functions a department serves is significantly related to the department size; the difference is most striking between the very small and the very large hospitals (Coulton, 1979, p. 23). In order to reflect these new data, the Deductive Formula included the 19 functions characteristic of a social work department. These are described in Appendix I.

The revised deductive formula is applied by deciding how many of the 19 functions will be carried. Once the number of functions is determined, the formula factors in a social worker to caseload ratio that takes into account the number of functions chosen. The National Survey provides comprehensive data by hospital bed size and makes it possible for an institution to develop its functions using the experience of hospitals as a group (Coulton, 1979), as below.

Functions and Hospital Bed Size

1. From one to 13 of these 19 functions are carried by social work departments of small (1-200 beds) hospitals, according to the National Survey Data, with a mean of 12.77 (scale of 19 functions); or 67.2% of the total functions. The Phase I Deductive Formula used an approximate range based on points of 1 to 11.1 functions (scale of 22 functions) or 50.4% of the total functions.

2. From 14 to 17 functions are carried by social work departments of medium size hospitals; the National Survey Data indicated a mean of 14.47 functions or 76% of the total functions. The Phase I Deductive Formula used 11.3 to 18 functions as the range for medium hospitals and 15.09 or 69% was seen as the mean of the total functions.

3. Eighteen plus functions are characteristic of a large hospital; Coulton indicated 14.66 functions for large and 17.62 functions for very large hospital social work departments; 16.14 or 84.9% of the total functions (Coulton, 1979). Phase I Deduc-

tive Formula indicated that 19.1 or 86.8% of the total functions were characteristically carried by departments in large hospitals.

While the actual numbers finalized in the adjustments were decided upon arbitrarily, the numbers both in the Active Case Ratio and functions carried fall within the range of the data developed in three separate surveys: the "leadership" hospital data reflected in January, 1977 report; the PERC data as reflected in Phase I report; and the data as reflected in the 1979 report of the National Survey.

The staff caseload ratio, which in the original plan was applied to the number of functions based on points, is now applied to the number of functions based on hospital size. A small hospital with 1 to 13 functions now picks up to 1 to 35 caseload ratio to determine staff, a medium hospital with 14 to 18 functions a 1 to 25 caseload ratio and a hospital with 18 plus functions a 1 to 15 caseload ratio.

The Revised Deductive Formula

The foregoing factors revise the deductive formula to that depicted in Figure 2.

Figure 2

Revised In-patient Formula

$$\frac{\overset{A}{\text{(Number of Beds)}} \times \overset{B}{\text{(Percentage of Patients to be Served:}} \ [\text{Active Case Ratio}])^*}{\underset{\text{(Staff Caseload Ratio [SCR]}^{**} \text{ by Functions Carried)}}{C}} = \text{\# of Staff Needed}$$

*ACR   **SCR

28% (1 to 200 beds)   1 to 13 functions = 1 staff to 35 cases
34% (201 to 500 beds)   14 to 18 functions = 1 staff to 25 cases
40% (501 plus beds)   18 plus functions = 1 staff to 15 cases

A - The number of beds is multiplied by:
B - The percentage of patients to be served. This figure is divided by:
C - The staff caseload ratio applicable to the functions carried, to give the figure of:
D - The staffing required.

USING THE FORMULA

As illustration, the formula is applied here to a 400 bed hospital:

Step 1. Establish the number of beds to be served
(a) Total beds = 400
   or
(b) Total beds adjusted for one year utilization experience-80%
   = 320 beds
   or
(c) Total beds by major service areas
   or
(d) Beds by Service Areas Adjusted one year utilization

	(c) Total Beds	(b) Bed Occupancy	(d) Bed Occupancy Percent
Medical	180	142	78%
Surgical	150	125	83%
Pediatric	20	18	90%
OB/GYN	30	15	50%
Specialty Psychiatric	20	20	100%
TOTAL	(a) 400	(b) 320	(b) 80.2%

Step 2. Establish the in-patient population to be served
Multiply the number of beds by one of the following averages of active case ratio:

— In 1 to 200 bed hospitals 28% of the in-patient population is characteristically served.
— In 201 to 500 bed hospitals 34% of the in-patient population is characteristically served.
— In 501 plus bed hospitals 40% of their in-patient population is characteristically served.

In the case of this 400 bed hospital, 34% would be applied as the active case ratio.

Step 3. Determine the worker to caseload ratio by functions carried

Divide the results of multiplying Steps 1 and 2 with one of the following:

— 1 to 200 bed hospitals tend to carry out 1 to 13 social work functions which the formula applies as one worker to 35 cases.
— 201 to 500 bed hospitals tend to carry out 14 to 17 social work functions which the formula applies as one worker to 25 cases.
— 501 plus bed hospitals tend to carry out 18 plus social work functions which the formula applies as one worker to 15 cases.

In the case of this 400 bed hospital, the one worker to 25 cases would apply.

Step 4. Establish the staffing pattern
(a) Total Beds 400 = 5.4 staffing need
    or
(b) Beds adjusted 320 = 4.3 staffing need for one year utilization experience
    or

	(c) Total Beds by Major Service	Staff by Service	(d)Beds Adjusted One Year Utilization	Staff Needed by Service
Medical	180	2.4	142	1.9
Surgical	150	2.0	125	1.7
Pediatric	20	0.3	18	0.2
OB/GYN	30	0.4	15	0.2
Specialty* Psychiatry	20	0.8	20	0.8
TOTAL	400	5.9	320	4.8

*100% of patients require service

FORMULA VARIATIONS AND REFINEMENTS

The formula allows for variations and refinements in its use to accommodate institutional differences:

1. The formula is more discriminately utilized when the total number of patients to be served is computed on a service/ward basis; large hospitals are encouraged to utilize the patient population to be served on a unit by unit basis.
2. In the event that every patient on a given service area is to receive social work services because of the nature of his/her medical problems, i.e., psychiatry, oncology, etc., then the base percent of patients to be served can be adjusted up to 100% for those particular beds. However, it should be regarded as unlikely that an acute general hospital as a whole should be adjusted higher than 40% for small hospitals, 46% for a medium size hospital and 52% for a large hospital.
3. Hospitals with a bed size close to the dividing point between the hospital categories may find their risk/service population percent more characteristic of another category; if so, the other category, either higher or lower, should be used.
4. Hospitals with special functions, i.e., trauma center, public hospital role, high risk populations, etc., may find their risk/service population more characteristic of the *next highest* category; if so, the next highest category should be used.
5. Hospitals which tend to carry the number of social work functions characteristic of another bed category should also try the formula weight of that category; these functions should be those carried on an ongoing regular basis.

SUMMARY

Until now the social work profession has not had a staffing standard or guide for its work in acute hospitals. Institutions similar in program and size have operated with staffing levels that are so dissimilar as to make social work practice and the meaningful meeting of the hospital patient and family psychosocial needs an uneven enterprise. This has been true for many years and the increases in the health care needs of individuals as reflected by an aging population, chronicity, and the high costs of in-patient hospital care intensify the need for an organized, uniform system of social work services delivery. The literature to date reports no approaches which have been tested or have universal applicability.

The work begun in 1975 under the auspices of the Society for Hospital Social Work Directors, American Hospital Association, has resulted in the development of a usable guide for staffing in-patient service areas of acute hospitals. The formula developed considered bed size, special in-patient services, the number of social work functions to be provided, and the number of patients to be served as the basis for projecting a social work staffing pattern for an institution. The formula offers a staff norm that has universal application but allows flexibility for individual institutional situations. The formula promotes more accurate hospital and departmental planning which relates the size of social work staff to a variety of professional and administrative factors. The deductive formula approach provides a significant step forward for the establishment of social work standards in hospitals and sets the foundation for further work, refinements and the development of new approaches.

REFERENCES

An Approach for Determining Uniform Social Work Staffing in Acute General Hospitals, January, 1977. Draft. George I. Krell with the Ad Hoc Committee of the Board on Staffing Patterns, Society for Hospital Social Work Directors, American Hospital Association.

An Approach for Determining Uniform Social Work Staffing in Acute General Hospitals, July, 1981. Society for Hospital Social Work Directors, American Hospital Association.

Coulton, Claudia J., et al. *Nationwide Survey of Hospital Social Work Practice*, Human Services Design Laboratory, Case Western Reserve University, Cleveland, Ohio, 1979. Unpublished.

Lurie, Abraham "Staffing Patterns: Issues and Program Implications for Health Care Agencies," *Social Work in Health Care*, 2(1), Fall, 1976, pp. 85-94.

Sherman, Robert E., Lund, Sander H. and Kiersuk, T. *Survey on Staffing Patterns for Hospital Social Service Departments*, Program Evaluation Resource Center, Minneapolis, Minnesota, November, 1978. Unpublished.

OTHER SUGGESTED READINGS

Barker, Robert L. and Briggs, Thomas L., *Differential Use of Social Work Manpower*, National Association of Social Workers, New York, 1968.

Berkman, B., Rehr, H. and Rosenberg, G. "A Social Work Department Develops and Tests a Screening Mechanism to Identify High Social Risk Situations," *Social Work in Health Care*, 5(4), Summer, 1980, pp. 373-385.

Clark, Eleanor *High Social Risk-Audiotape*, Society for Hospital Social Work Directors, 1980.

Kim, Paul H. K., Hasan, S. Zafar, Egli, Dan *Mental Health Professionals Perceive Knowledge and Skills Need*, College of Social Work at the University of Kentucky: Kentucky, 1981.

Productivity and Health—A Review and Evaluation of Health Personnel Productivity, Medicus Systems Corp., Washington, D.C., August, 1980.

Rehr, H., Berkman, B. and Rosenberg, G. "Screening for High Social Risk: Principles and Problems," *Social Work*, 25(5), September, 1980, pp. 403-406.

Salary Survey, October 29, 1975, Massachusetts Chapter of the Society for Hospital Social Work Directors. Unpublished.

APPENDIX I**

A) *NINETEEN SOCIAL WORK FUNCTIONS*

* 1. *INFORMATION AND REFERRAL*

Information provided to the patient and family about the types of community resources available; connection made with resource so identified.

* 2. *FACILITATING COMMUNITY AGENCY REFERRAL*

Assistance beyond information is provided to ensure patient access to appropriate resources; i.e., applications are completed in behalf of patients and processed; conferences and visits are carried out to agencies in behalf of or with patients; representation of patient and patient interest is directly made

---

*The 5 functions most common to social work departments.

**(An Approach to Determining Uniform Social Work Staffing in Acute General Hospitals.) Society for Hospital Social Work Directors, American Hospital Association, 1981.

to community social agencies; escort transportation and child care are provided.

* 3. *PRE-ADMISSION PLANNING*

Counseling on patient and family problems directly related to planning and arranging for hospital admission.

* 4. *CASE FINDING OR SOCIAL RISK SCREENING*

A structured ongoing outreach program geared to identifying those patients potentially in need of social work services and arrangements for the provision of those services.

* 5. *DISCHARGE PLANNING*

Counseling on patient problems directly related to planning and arranging for post hospital care in order to consolidate gains made during hospitalization.

6. *FACILITATING USE OF HOSPITAL SERVICES*

Advocacy role is assumed within hospital in behalf of patient and family with all departments and hospital personnel.

7. *COUNSELING OF PATIENTS AND FAMILIES*

Counseling directed toward helping patients and their families deal with their situations more effectively as these situations relate to health and medical care.

8. *PSYCHOSOCIAL EVALUATIONS*

The gathering of information about the patient's social, psychological, cultural, environmental and financial situation and utilizing this information for a psychosocial assessment and treatment plan or formal report.

9. *HEALTH EDUCATION*

The enhancement of patient knowledge through a structured program geared to provide factual knowledge to patients and/or families; i.e., family planning, birth control, sickle cell anemia, alcoholism, etc.

10. *FINANCIAL ASSISTANCE*

Financial or other concrete aid is *provided directly* by the hospital social work department; transportation assistance, medications, prosthetic devices, etc.

11. *UTILIZATION REVIEW*

Participation in the formal concurrent review process of the hospital related to the P.S.R.O. requirements.

12. *CASE CONSULTATION TO HOSPITAL STAFF*

A structured meeting which provides specialized knowledge to other health care personnel regarding patient psychosocial problems, procedures or services. It can be of an individual and/or team nature.

13. *CASE CONSULTATION TO COMMUNITY AGENCIES*

A structured meeting which provides specialized knowledge to health care personnel of an outside agency regarding the psychosocial problems of a patient active with the outside agency.

14. *PROGRAM CONSULTATION TO HOSPITAL STAFF*

Assesses patient population to determine unmet needs, investigates and channels information about patient care problems to appropriate departments, identifies and makes recommendations for changes in hospital policy and procedure as related to patient/family rights.

15. *PROGRAM CONSULTATION TO COMMUNITY AGENCIES*

A structured meeting which provides specialized knowledge to institutions.

16. *HOSPITAL PLANNING ACTIVITIES*

Involvement in the structured activities and mechanisms of the institution which relate to short term and long term planning and program development that relates to outreach and community services.

17. *COMMUNITY HEALTH PLANNING ACTIVITIES*

Working with the community and its agencies to develop necessary programs and uncovering community resources to meet patient needs.

18. *COMMUNITY SERVICE ACTIVITIES*

Responsibility to represent the hospital to the community on matters pertaining to social work; participation with community groups in carrying out appropriate programs.

19. *RESEARCH*

A structured system of study of the psychosocial factors of patient care and needs. A structured system of review of the quality of social work services provided as part of both the hospital's and the department of social work's patient care evaluation and peer review program.

A Survey of Patient
and Family Satisfaction
with Social Work Services

Leslie Garber, ACSW
Susan Brenner, ACSW
Diane Litwin, ACSW

SUMMARY. Client satisfaction can be an important indicator of the quality of social work services. This article reports the results of a survey conducted by a social work department of a large urban teaching hospital to elicit patient and family reaction to its services. A random, proportionate sample of in- and out-patient cases in medical and psychiatric programs was used. In general, staff was seen as helpful, although with interesting variations depending on the social work function performed. The findings have implications for education, supervision, quality assurance, levels of staffing and staff's perception of their usefulness.

What do our clients think of us? The answer to this question must be included in any thorough assessment of the value of social work services and in planning for future service delivery. Client satisfaction, if it can be demonstrated, can speak for us to the money managers in our agencies. In 1982, these considerations led a department of social work in a large urban voluntary medical center to conduct a consumer survey. The project was an aspect of a Quality

---

At the time of writing Leslie Garber, ACSW, was Supervisor; Susan Brenner, ACSW, Assistant Director; and Diane Litwin, ACSW, Social Worker, Department of Social Work, St. Vincent's Hospital and Medical Center of New York, New York, NY 10011. An earlier version of this article was presented at the 19th Annual Meeting of the Society for Hospital Social Work Directors, New York, NY, March 26, 1984.

Reprinted from *Social Work in Health Care*, Volume 11(3), Spring 1986.

Assurance Program and a part of the department's effort to meet the hospital and professional objective of maintaining quality care.

GOALS AND ASSUMPTIONS

The goals of the project were to maintain a high quality of social work services and to convey to clients, both patients and families, our interest in and respect for their opinions. We began with the following assumptions: (1) there is a relationship between clients' perceptions of staff attitudes and their perceptions of staff effectiveness; (2) clients see the provision of tangible services as a more significant social work function than counseling; (3) clients prefer to see social work staff at point of entry into the hospital system, rather than when a crisis develops, and more frequently than they had been seen; (4) the level of satisfaction varies with the service provided, and is lowest in those areas where resources are limited; (5) the level of satisfaction is lower among in-patient clients, who are in an acute care setting with bed-utilization restrictions, than among out-patient clients, who have a more extended period to decide on their options; and (6) clients referred by non-social work staff have not received a specific explanation of the nature of social work services, may have been led to have unrealistically high expectations and are, therefore, less satisfied.

LITERATURE REVIEW

Both social work and mental health practitioners have published client survey results comparing client satisfaction to outcome (Edwards, 1978); to staff perceptions of the impact of their services (Maluccio, 1979); and to demographic data.

The literature highlights several issues that were of particular relevance to our survey: (1) the difficulty obtaining a representative sample from an inner-city population (Ogren, 1975); (2) the prevalence of over-positive responses (Edwards, 1978); (3) clients' perceptions of improvement of specific target symptoms (Fineberg, 1982); and (4) the correlation between clients' reactions and their perceptions of practitioners' affective behaviors, for instance, "devotion," "time," and "interest" (Ben-Sera, 1976).

METHODOLOGY

Tools

Our tool was a telephone questionnaire. A letter was sent to potential respondents to prepare them for the questionnaire and reassure them about confidentiality. Mail questionnaires were sent only when we were unable to reach clients by phone, and a stamped, self-addressed envelope was included.

Case Selection

We selected a proportionate random sample of the 533 cases closed in the Department of Social Work in May, 1982. Within four groupings (In-Patient and Out-Patient, General Hospital and Psychiatry), every third case was selected for a total of 168 cases (31% of closed cases). This was done to assure a statistically significant response rate of at least 15% of closed cases. In drawing the sample, we excluded 22 cases and selected the next case on the list. The cases excluded were: (1) eleven in which the clients' whereabouts were unknown—i.e., A.M.A. discharges, street people who refused to accept planning or give information; (2) five in which contact might have been harmful or especially painful to the client—i.e., some victims of sexual abuse, including children; (3) four in which the patient had died or had significant organic impairment, and there had been no available family; and (4) two in which the patient had a pending legal suit against the hospital.

The 168 cases fell into three groups: (1) one hundred one (60%) in which only the patients could be surveyed, because there had been no family available for social work intervention; (2) twenty-eight (17%) in which both the patient and family were surveyed; and (3) thirty-nine (23%) in which only the family was surveyed, because of the patient's extreme youth or age, major organic impairment, or death. The sample of 168 cases produced 196 potential respondents—129 patients and 67 family members.

Process

This 813 bed metropolitan area hospital serves a heterogeneous patient population, including some hard-to-locate clients. To keep our sample representative of this population, we retained among our potential respondents 23 who went to shelters or single-room occupancy hotels, 3 who went to other treatment facilities, and 18 who had no phone.

Since response rates are higher for phone surveys than for mail surveys, we attempted to phone as many clients as possible. However, 64 mail questionnaires were sent to clients who could not be reached by phone. Telephone surveys were initiated three months after cases were closed, and two weeks after pre-survey letters were mailed. Phone interviewers were available, when needed, in Spanish, Italian, and Chinese.

Phone interviews were conducted by seven social work staff members other than those who had provided the service. We attempted to insure uniformity by instructing them to conduct the survey by reading the questions precisely as they were written, while still allowing for free expression by respondents.

RESPONSE RATE

We received responses in 87 of 168 cases (52%), and from 96 of 196 potential respondents (49%). The response rate was higher for family members (67%) than for patients (40%), and substantially higher on phone surveys (68%) than on mail surveys (7%).

SURVEY RESPONSES

Responses were reviewed in four categories: (1) perception of staff attitudes; (2) perceptions of staff effectiveness in specific areas; (3) perceptions of service delivery system; and (4) overall perceptions of the helpfulness of social work services. The question about their expectations of social work services prior to contact did not elicit responses that could be analyzed, and will not be reported.

Within each category, we also compared patient/family responses and in-patient/out-patient responses.

Clients' Perceptions of Staff Attitudes

Two questions were used: (1) "Did the social worker seem to understand what you wanted?" and (2) "Did the social worker seem to care about what happened to you?" Overall response rates were 78% positive, 7% negative, and 16% unsure (Table 1).

There were only slight variations between patient and family responses and between in-patient and out-patient responses.

Clients' Perceptions of Staff Effectiveness in Specific Areas

Clients were asked to rate staff effectiveness in any or all of 13 service categories (Table 2). Clients viewed staff as most effective in providing those services not dependent on the availability of community resources: counseling, providing information about hospital services, group work, and providing information and education about the illness. Staff was also viewed as effective in arranging follow-up care.

Clients viewed staff as somewhat less effective in providing services for which hospital social work staff most often have to turn to community agencies, i.e., medical insurance problems, arranging

TABLE 1

CLIENTS' PERCEPTIONS OF STAFF ATTITUDES

QUESTION #2 Did the social worker seem to understand what you wanted?	YES	NO	UNSURE
	75 (78%)	6 (6%)	15 (16%)
QUESTION #6 Did the social worker seem to care about what happened to you?	74 (77%)	8 (8%)	14 (15%)

TABLE 2

CLIENTS' PERCEPTION OF STAFF EFFECTIVENESS

	Counseling	Plan for Care of People at Home	Information or Services In Hospital	Information or Education Re: Illness	Medical Insurance Problems	Arranging Home Help	Housing Problems	Applying for Financial Assistance	Arranging Follow-Up Services	Arranging Transportation	Referral to Residential Facility	Something Not Mentioned	Don't Remember
QUESTION #3 — What did you and the social worker work on?	50	21	41	35	27	20	4	18	22	16	21	14	5
QUESTION #4 — Was the social worker able to help?	YES 46 (92%)	YES 15 (71%)	YES 36 (88%)	YES 28 (80%)	YES 21 (78%)	YES 14 (70%)	YES 0 (0%)	YES 9 (50%)	YES 20 (91%)	YES 12 (75%)	YES 12 (57%)	YES 11 (79%)	
	NO 2 (4%)	NO 3 (14.5%)	NO 2 (5%)	NO 2 (6%)	NO 4 (15%)	NO 3 (15%)	NO 2 (50%)	NO 6 (33%)	NO 1 (4.5%)	NO 3 (19%)	NO 4 (19%)	NO 2 (14%)	
	Par-tially 2 (4%)	Par-tially 3 (14.5%)	Par-tially 3 (7%)	Par-tially 5 (14%)	Par-tially 2 (7%)	Par-tially 3 (15%)	Par-tially 2 (50%)	Par-tially 3 (17%)	Par-tially 1 (4.5%)	Par-tially 1 (6%)	Par-tially 5 (24%)	Par-tially 1 (7%)	
QUESTION #12 (If you or your family attended a group led by a social worker), was it helpful?			YES 17 (81%)							NO 4 (19%)			

646

transportation, planning for care of people at home, and arranging home help.

Social work staff were viewed as least effective in referral to residential facilities, applying for financial assistance, and housing problems. We speculate that both lack of availability of resources and attitudes at some community agencies influence these responses.

Patients were more satisfied than families with effectiveness of service in the areas of care of people at home, arranging transportation, and referral to residential facilities. They were less satisfied than families in the areas of applying for financial assistance and arranging follow-up services. We noted that 90% of family members were satisfied with group work services, as compared with 73% of patients.

In-patient clients and their families consistently found social work service more effective than did out-patient clients — most notably in the areas of planning for care of people at home, providing information about hospital services, medical insurance problems, arranging home help, and referral to residential facilities. This may be because discharge planning often requires more intense and/or frequent client contact. Further, out-patients may be less satisfied because they are not in a protected environment while waiting for important community services — i.e., food stamps, home help.

Clients' Perceptions of Service Delivery System

Clients were asked to respond to questions on the source of their referral to social work, and on the timeliness and frequency of social work contact (Table 3). The majority of referrals, 65%, came from physicians, social workers, or clients themselves.

Slightly more than half of our clients (53%) were satisfied with the timeliness of the initial social work intervention. A somewhat higher number (76%) was satisfied with the frequency of social work contact. Patients were less satisfied than family members with both the timeliness and frequency of social work intervention. Out-patients were less satisfied than in-patients in both areas.

TABLE 3

CLIENTS' PERCEPTIONS OF SERVICE DELIVERY SYSTEM

QUESTION #1
Who told you about or referred you to the social worker?

NURSE	DOCTOR	SOCIAL WORKER	YOU, FAMILY OR FRIEND	OTHER HOSPITAL STAFF	OTHER	DON'T KNOW
9 (9%)	23 (24%)	20 (21%)	19 (20%)	3 (3%)	4 (4%)	18 (19%)

QUESTION #7
Do you think it would have been helpful to see the social worker sooner?

YES	NO	UNSURE
20 (21%)	51 (53%)	25 (26%)

QUESTION #8
Why?

NO RESPONSE	WOULDN'T HAVE PREFERRED TO SEE SOCIAL WORKER SOONER	WOULD HAVE PREFERRED TO SEE SOCIAL WORKER SOONER	WOULD MIGHT HAVE PREFERRED TO SEE SOCIAL WORKER SOONER
57 (59%)	14 (15%)		25 (26%)

QUESTION #9
If yes, when would you have preferred seeing the social worker?*

BEFORE STARTING CONTACT WITH HOSPITAL	DURING FIRST DAYS OF CONTACT WITH HOSPITAL	OTHER
5 (25%)	9 (45%)	6 (30%)

QUESTION #10
Would you have liked to see the social worker? (92 of 96 clients responded):

MORE OFTEN	LESS OFTEN	THE SAME
24 (26%)	6 (7%)	62 (67%)

QUESTION #11
Did you or your family attend a discussion group led by a social worker?

YES	NO
21	74

*Question 9 was not completed by everyone who responded "Yes" to Question 7; was completed by others - thus the slight discrepancy in numbers.

Clients' Overall Perceptions of the Helpfulness of Social Work Services

Clients were asked to comment on the helpfulness of seeing a social worker, and if they would refer themselves or others to a social worker in the future (Table 4). There were positive response rates to both questions (81% and 80%, respectively). Clients were also asked if there was any way the social workers at this hospital could improve their services. Of the 80 clients who answered this question, 63% said "No," and 37% said "Yes." In the latter group of 31 respondents, 7 (23%) noted problems in the area of staff attitudes, 5 (16%) in staff effectiveness, 7 in timeliness and frequency of social work intervention. Twelve (39%) gave answers that were non-specific or inconclusive.

Patients and families showed similar positive response rates (80% and 82%, respectively) to the question about the overall helpfulness of social work services. Family members showed a slightly higher positive response rate (84%) than patients (76%) on the question of future referrals to a social worker. There was virtually no difference in positive response rates on both questions between in-patient and out-patient clients.

FINDINGS AND CONCLUSIONS

1. This similarity of positive response rates to questions on staff attitudes and overall helpfulness of social work services reinforces the importance of an empathetic attitude and of conveying one's understanding of what the patient wants, thus validating our initial assumption.

2. Clients perceived social work staff as more effective in counseling, groups, and information/education services than in community resource services. Moreover, clients who received services without counseling were twice as likely to be dissatisfied as clients who received these services along with counseling. This finding did not validate our initial assumption.

3. Forty-seven percent of clients were not fully satisfied with the timeliness of the initial social work intervention and would have preferred earlier intervention; thirty-three percent would have pre-

TABLE 4

CLIENTS' REACTIONS TO SOCIAL WORK INTERVENTIONS

QUESTION #13	YES	NO
Overall, was it helpful for you to see a social worker?	75 (81%)	18 (19%)

(93 respondants of a potential 96)

QUESTION #14	YES	NO	UNSURE
If you, a friend, or relative had a problem would you advise seeing a social worker?	76 (80%)	10 (11%)	9 (9%)

(95 respondants of a potential 96)

QUESTION #15	POSITIVE RESPONSE	NEGATIVE RESPONSE	QUALIFIED RESPONSE
Why?	62	5	12

(79 respondants from potential 96)

QUESTION #16	YES	NO
Is there any way you feel the social workers at St. Vincent's Hospital could improve their services?	30	50

(TOTAL RESPONSES: 80 of 96 POTENTIAL)

ferred to see the social worker more frequently. These figures, which validate our initial assumption, imply a need for adequate staff to provide timely services.

4. Perceptions of staff effectiveness varied with the specific service provided. Staff was seen as least effective when the service requested was for a limited community resource, such as housing or financial assistance. This validates our initial assumption.

5. In- and out-patient clients reported similar levels of satisfaction in all categories surveyed, a finding which does not validate our initial assumption.

6. Seventeen of the 18 clients who did not find social work services helpful were self-referred or referred by other hospital staff. This supports our initial assumption that clients referred by non-social work personnel have a less realistic understanding about what social workers can provide and as a result may be less satisfied with services.

IMPLICATIONS AND USES

Consumer surveys have implications for hospital social work departments in the areas of staff education and training, management of staffing resources, and demonstration of the value of social work services to hospital administration.

Survey results were presented at a departmental meeting, with follow-up discussion in individual and group supervision. Based on the findings noted above, three issues were highlighted. First, clients who perceive staff as empathetic and understanding may be generally satisfied even when particular services cannot be provided. Second, clients *do* value and appreciate the counseling aspect of the social work role. Both findings provided a boost for staff morale and emphasized the importance of a caring attitude. Third, the lower level of satisfaction among clients referred by non-social work staff indicates the need for social workers themselves to define for clients the nature of the social work role.

Survey findings about the timeliness of social work intervention support the need for social work departments to take the initiative in case-finding through pre-admission screening, patient-care rounds, and high-risk screening mechanisms. The Department was already participating in patient-care rounds, and had developed high-risk screening tools which continue to be used effectively. Pre-admission screening is being explored. In addition, the positive perceptions of the effectiveness of social work groups (albeit in our small sample) supports the Department of Social Work emphasis on groups. Several new groups have been initiated since the survey was reported to staff.

Finally, the survey was distributed to hospital administration, and the findings reviewed with the administrator to whom our Department is responsible in order to demonstrate the effectiveness and value of social work services, and to point out that the positive image of social work staff has an important public relations value to the hospital. The survey finds were among the factors contributing to more rapid approval of open social work positions.

REFERENCES

Ben-Sera, Zeer. The function of the professional's affective behavior in client satisfaction. *Journal of Health and Social Behavior*, March, 1976, *17*.

Edwards, D.W., Yarvis, R.M., Mueller, D.P., & Langsley, D.G. Does patient satisfaction correlate with success? *Hospital and Community Psychiatry*, March, 1978, *29* (3), 188-190.

Fineberg, Beth L., Kettlewell, Paul W., & Sowards, Stephen, K. An evaluation of adolescent in-patient services. *American Journal of Orthopsychiatry*, April, 1982, *52* (2), 337-345.

Maluccio, Anthony N. Perspectives of social workers and clients on treatment outcome. *Social Casework*, July, 1979, 394-401.

Ogren, Evelyn H. Sample bias in patient evaluation of hospital social services. *Social Work in Health Care*, Fall, 1975, *1* (1) 55-63.

Commentary

Social workers have struggled to overcome the roles defined for them by others and to replace them with professional contributions that they themselves define as needed components in patient care. As they do in all organizations, professional social workers in hospital settings encounter tensions between the sometimes conflicting needs of the institution, its other constituencies, and those of the consumers it services. The resultant strain may engender the role ambiguity that Butrym has noted as "a continuous feature of the history of the profession" (1967, p. 22).

Cannon acknowledged that in the early years the special function of social service was not clearly defined in the minds of the social workers (1952). As professional social work in health care settings expanded and evolved there was diminished satisfaction with early roles of augmenting the doctor's care of patients in a "facilitating service role" (Teague, 1971). Social workers began to define and extend their roles to include those of preventing and reducing psychosocial factors that exacerbate illness or impede appropriate use of resources for care or cure. These often include organizational and system barriers to access and use; as well as attitudinal barriers about social work held by physicians, nurses, and hospital administrators who may define the social work role narrowly. Influencing these impediments calls for skills and time as the processes are interpersonal, developmental, and political. As Freidson notes, the collaboration and positive interest of physicians are vital ingredients in the development of greater autonomy for health care workers as are acceptance of their services by patients (1970).

In a setting where health care administrators or professional colleagues of other disciplines often have defined and limited the services that social workers provide, one consequence has been that professional authority and autonomy have been limited as well, so that some sociologists have termed social work a "semi-profession" (Toren, 1972; Etzioni, 1969; and Carr-Saunders, 1955).

A more autonomous professional role, with the authority to define functions and services that will be provided, requires a distinct knowledge base and strong systems of accountability and internal controls (Goode, 1969) as well as a primary commitment to clients. As Epstein notes about professionals in social work agencies in general, "although practitioners and agencies agree in principle that service to clients is paramount, their interests do not necessarily coincide" (1973).

In the wake of stringent cost-containment policies of the past decade, external requirements for accountability have provided a stimulus to social workers to identify what is unique in their contribution to total patient care. Autonomous practice is predicated on assuming professional responsibility for accountability, documented via mechanisms established for quality assurance (Germain, 1980).

A strong professional identity is essential to deal with the impact of institutional and regulatory constraints that derive from cost-containment measures such as DRGs and the competition for functions traditionally assigned to the social worker. Changes in legislation have led to opportunities for power inherent in the institutional role of discharge planning coordinator, which was mandated by cost-containing legislation in the '70s. The process of helping patients plan for care after their hospitalization is clearly an appropriate professional function (Caputi and Heiss, 1984) and social workers have developed new approaches to demonstrate their effectiveness in fulfilling this role in the best interest of the patient and at the same time promoting the hospital's interests. The task of balancing these interests can be accomplished when social workers are in charge of defining the nature of their services and of the procedural systems basic to efficient implementation.

MANAGEMENT AND ACCOUNTABILITY

The stresses experienced by social work departments in health care during times of tightened budgets and calls for increased accountability have reinforced social work's search for increased autonomy and self-definition and have led to reexamination of priorities, choices of targets, and methods for intervention and relationships to other health care professionals. This search has stimulated the development of new case-finding mechanisms, systems for early intervention, attempts to develop uniform standards of practice, redeployment of staff, and modifications in staff training and development (Carrigan, 1978).

The need to be accountable to many constituencies, to clients, employers, governmental and regulatory agencies, colleagues in other disciplines, and the social work profession itself has stimulated study and research in management systems. The process of reexamining what social workers in hospitals do, how effectively they meet their goals, how well they communicate what they are doing to colleagues, and how well they prepare staff for changing responsibilities has confirmed many established practices. It has also promoted new ventures in areas such as systems for resource location, quality assurance, educational and supervisory programs, and documentation systems, including medical chart recording (Kagle, 1982; Rosenberg, 1980; Biagi, 1977; Spano, Kiresuk, and Lund, 1977; Spano and Lund, 1976; Kane, 1974; Volland, 1976).

Seeking to improve the quality of their programs, to increase their visibility, and to demonstrate their value to the health care system and its clients, social work departments have developed accountability systems that demonstrate effective professional practice grounded in knowledge and ethical principles (Rosenberg and Weissman, 1981). The achievement of these important goals has required the active participation of social workers at all levels (Chernesky, 1981). Sophisticated business management and accountability systems also provide a secure fiscal base for social workers in these settings. Their acceptance and use depend on molding these structures to fit the shape of social work's practice and principles.

Administrators of social work departments in health care settings provide direction, resources, education, and other supports to the social work staff practicing in a challenging and complex health care system. Management programs are designed to help staff develop competence for effective practice, even in a context of declining resources and diminished support for social work programs, and to insure availability and retention of adequately trained, skilled, and committed staff who can work with the independence necessary for current professional responsibilities.

REFERENCES

Biagi, Ettore. "The Social Work Stake in Problem-Oriented Recording," *Social Work in Health Care, 3*:2, Winter 1977, pp. 211–222.

Bracht, Neil. *Social Work in Health Care: A Guide to Professional Practice*. New York: The Haworth Press, 1978.

Butrym, Zofia. *Social Work in Medical Care*. London: Routledge and Kegan Paul, 1967.

Cannon, Ida. *On the Social Frontier of Medicine*. Cambridge: Harvard University Press, 1952.

Caputi, Marie A., and Heiss, William A. "The DRG Revolution," *Health and Social Work 9*(1). Winter 1984, pp. 5–12.

Carrigan, Zoe H. "Social Workers in Medical Settings: Who Defines Us?" *Social Work in Health Care 4*(2), Winter 1978, pp. 149–163.

Carr-Saunders, Alexander M. "Metropolitan Conditions and Traditional Professional Relationships" in Robert M. Fisher (Ed.), *The Metropolis in Modern Life*. New York: Doubleday, 1955, pp. 279–288.

Chernesky, Roslyn H. "Attitudes of Social Workers Toward Peer Review," *Health and Social Work 6*(2), May 1981, pp. 67–73.

Epstein, Laura. "Is Autonomous Practice Possible?" *Social Work 18*(2), March 1973, pp. 5–12.

Etzioni, Amitai (Ed.). *The Semi-Professions and Their Organizations*. New York: The Free Press, 1969.

Ferguson, Kristi; Bowden, Leora; Halman, Marc; Huff, Arlene; Langlie, Joann, and Morgan, Gladys. "Social Work Quality Assurance Based on Medical Diagnosis and Task: A Second-Stage Report," *Social Work in Health Care 6*(1), Fall 1980, pp. 63–71.

Freidson, Eliot. *Professional Dominance: The Social Structure of Medical Care*. Chicago: Aldine, 1970.

Germain, Carel B. "Social Work Identity, Competence and Autonomy: The Ecological Perspective," *Social Work in Health Care 6*(1), Fall 1980, pp. 1–10.

Goode, W. J. "The Theoretical Limits of Professionalization," in Amitai Etzioni (Ed.), *The Semi-Professions and Their Organizations*. New York: The Free Press, 1969, pp. 266–313.

Kagle, Jill Doner. "Social Work Records in Health and Mental Health Organizations: A Status Report," *Social Work in Health Care 8*(1), Fall 1982, pp. 37–46.

Kane, Rosalie A. "Look to the Record," *Social Work 19*:4, July 1974, pp. 412–419.

Lurie, Abraham, and Rosenberg, Gary (Eds.), *Social Work Administration in Health Care*. New York: The Haworth Press, 1984.

Rosenberg, Gary. "Concepts in the Financial Management of Hospital Social Work Departments," *Social Work in Health Care* 5(3), Spring 1980, pp. 287–297.

Rosenberg, Gary, and Weissman, Andrew. "Marketing Social Services in Health Care Facilities," *Health and Social Work* 6(3), August 1981, pp. 13–19.

Spano, Robert M., and Lund, Sander H. "Management by Objectives in a Hospital Social Service Unit," *Social Work in Health Care* 1(3), Spring 1976, pp. 267–276.

Spano, Robert M.; Kiresuk, Thomas J., and Lund, Sander H. "An Operational Model to Achieve Accountability for Social Work in Health Care," *Social Work in Health Care* 3(2), Winter 1977, pp. 123–141.

Teague, Doran. "Social Service Enterprises: A New Health Care Model," *Social Work* 16(3), July 1971, pp. 66–74.

Toren, Nina. *Social Work: The Case of a Semi-Profession*. California and London: Sage Publications, 1972.

Volland, Patricia. "Social Work Information and Accountability Systems in a Hospital Setting," *Social Work in Health Care* 1(3), Spring 1976, pp. 277–285.

Additional Readings

Bennett, Claire, and Beckerman, Nancy. "The Drama of Discharge:
Worker/Supervisor Perspectives," *Social Work in Health Care*
11(3), Spring 1986, pp. 1–12.

Berkman, Barbara, and Rehr, Helen. "Seven Steps to Audit," *Social Work in Health Care 2*(3), Spring 1977, pp. 295–303.

––––––. "Social Work Undertakes Its Own Audit," *Social Work in
Health Care 3*(3), Spring 1978, pp. 273–286.

Blackey, Eileen. "Social Work in the Hospital: A Sociological Approach," *Social Work 1*(2), April 1956, pp. 43–49.

Brody, Stanley J. "Common Ground: Social Work and Health
Care," *Health and Social Work 1*:1, February 1976, pp. 16–31.

Chernesky, Roslyn, and Lurie, Abraham. "The Functional Analysis Study: A First Step in Quality Assurance," *Social Work in
Health Care 1*(2), Winter 1975-6, pp. 213–223.

Christ, Winifred R. "A Method for Setting Social Work Staffing
Standards Within a Psychiatric Setting," *Social Work in Health
Care 8*(2), Winter 1982, pp. 87–103.

Coulton, Claudia J. *Social Work Quality Assurance Programs.* Sil-
ver Spring, Md.: National Association of Social Workers, 1983.

––––––. "Confronting Prospective Payment: Requirements for an
Information System," *Health and Social Work 9*(1), Winter
1984, pp. 13–24.

Coulton, Claudia J., and Butler, Nathaniel. "Measuring Social Work
Productivity in Health Care," *Health and Social Work 6*(3), August 1981, pp. 4–12.

Davidson, Kay W. "Evolving Social Work Roles in Health Care:
The Case of Discharge Planning," *Social Work in Health Care
4*(1), Fall 1978, pp. 43–54. (See Part II of this volume.)

Haber-Scharf, Michele. "Costing Social Work Services in a Hospital Setting," *Social Work in Health Care 11*(1), Fall 1985, pp.
113–129.

Harris, Dorothy V., and Allison, Elizabeth Keith. "Performance Management and Professional Development as Separate Functions of Supervision," *Health and Social Work* 7(4), November 1982, pp. 283–291.

Hirsch, Sidney, and Schulman, Lawrence C. "Participatory Governance: A Model for Shared Decision Making," *Social Work in Health Care* 1(4), Summer 1976, pp. 433–446.

Jansson, Bruce S., and Simmons, June. The Ecology of Social Work Departments: Empirical Findings and Strategy Implications," *Social Work in Health Care* 11(2), Winter 1985-6, pp. 1–16. (See Part 9 of this volume.)

_____. "The Survival of Social Work Units in Host Organizations," *Social Work* 31(5), September-October 1986, pp. 339–343.

Kulys, Regina, and Davis, Sister M. Adrian. "Nurses and Social Workers: Rivals in the Provision of Social Services?" *Health and Social Work* 12(2), Spring 1987, pp. 101–112.

Lister, Larry. "Role Expectations of Social Workers and Other Health Professionals," *Health and Social Work* 5(2), May 1980, pp. 41–49.

Lurie, Abraham. "Staffing Patterns: Issues and Program Implications for Health Care Agencies," *Social Work in Health Care* 2(1), Fall 1976, pp. 85–94.

Nacman, Martin. "Reflections of a Social Work Administrator on the Opportunities of Crisis," *Social Work in Health Care* 6(1), Fall 1980, pp. 11–21.

Olsen, Katherine M., and Olsen, Marvin E. "Role Expectations and Perceptions for Social Workers in Medical Settings," *Social Work* 12(3), July 1967, pp. 70–78.

Reamer, Frederic G. "Facing up to the Challenge of DRGs," *Health and Social Work* 10(2), Spring 1985, pp. 85–94.

Rehr, Helen. *Professional Accountability for Social Work Practice: A Search for Concepts and Guidelines*. New York: Prodist, 1979.

Reinherz, Helen; Berkman, Barbara; Ewalt, Patricia L., and Grob, Mollie C. "Training in Accountability: A Social Work Mandate," *Health and Social Work* 2(2), May 1977, pp. 42–56.

Segal, Brian. "Planning and Power in Hospital Social Service," *Social Casework 51*(7), July 1970, pp. 399–405.

Spano, Robert M., and Lund, Sander H. "Productivity and Performance: Keys to Survival for a Hospital-Based Social Work Department," *Social Work in Health Care 11*(3), Spring 1986, pp. 25–39.

Ullmann, Alice, and Kassebaum, Gene. "Referral and Services in a Medical Social Work Department," *Social Service Review 35*(3), September 1961, pp. 263–264.

Wax, John. "Developing Social Work Power in a Medical Organization," *Social Work 13*(4), October 1968, pp. 62–71.

_____. "Power Theory and Institutional Change," *Social Service Review 45*(3), September 1971, pp. 274–288.

_____. "Clinical Contributions to Administrative Practice," *Social Work in Health Care 8*(3), Spring 1983, pp. 129–142.

PART 7
SPECIAL POPULATIONS
AND CONTEXTS

Introduction

With the explosion of biomedical knowledge and the revolutionary advances in diagnostic and treatment methods, specialty practice, a continuous trend in medical care since World War II, has proliferated, divided, and subdivided into ever more discrete units of expertise.

As social workers respond to the multiple and changing needs of clients of all ages, and ethnic, cultural, and socioeconomic status when medical and psychiatric problems affect their lives, core planning and practice principles are applicable universally when adopted for the particular characteristics of programs as diverse and specialized as home care, emergency trauma, in vitro fertilization, coronary bypass, organ transplant, pediatric oncology, renal dialysis, and care for chronically ill psychiatric patients, to name only a few.

Program models developed for one specialized area of practice or one set of special needs have obvious relevance for work with similar populations and settings.

Caregivers of patients with chronic illness and disability, whether they are young or old, have spina bifida or Parkinson's disease, need a similar range of support, respite, and counseling services available over extended periods of time to help them in their accommodation to long-term social dislocations. Thus social workers in many settings can review the reported experiences of their colleagues who serve special populations for program ideas with potential for adaptation and replication.

As health care technology expands, new populations and new contexts for social work practice emerge. Out of new technologies that provide life-saving treatments for the acutely ill, such as trauma victims, premature infants, and even the unborn in embryo states, new populations develop whose special needs challenge social workers to design new approaches and adapt traditional ones. For older chronically ill patients, current policies, implemented through the PPS program, shift the focus of care outside the hospital to home and ambulatory care systems. Different models of continuing care such as home care, foster care, and institutions for long-term care need to be revamped to fit better with basic quality-of-life issues. A range of potential models is needed to assist clients with their management of social needs over a continuum of time, as needs change.

In addition to those populations whose special needs derive from their prolonged survival in the face of chronic illness and disabilities that require complex, exhaustive, and exhausting medical care, other groups have psychosocial needs that derive from ethnic and cultural characteristics. Sensitive social work practice can enable these clients to make better use of health care services that in all probability were not designed with concern for adapting their systems to patients of differing cultural roots.

Chronically ill patients who are treated in settings that utilize high levels of technological intervention present particular challenges and pressures for staff. Rarely having the satisfaction of seeing a cure, they witness on a daily basis their patients' deterioration and the erosion of families' endurance. Staff are in the position of initiating and administering rigorous medical requirements and may have little time, emotional energy, or ability to provide comfort and relief.

Seven articles were selected to illustrate these issues. Berman and Rappaport's report on patients with Alzheimer's disease details the phases of this progressive, devastating illness and its powerful impact on patient and caregiver alike. It spells out the range of services needed and interventive methods that social workers can use to help patients and families adapt to the chronic and exhausting effects of this deteriorating disease. Applicability to other progressive conditions is identified.

In their review of the nature of AIDS and its effects on its victims, Furstenberg and Olson highlight the generic and specific elements of social work practice needed by this growing population of patients and their friends, families, and staff caring for them. They map out an expanded role for social workers in the development of needed social policies for this population.

The critical topic of cross-cultural and ethnically sensitive practice is addressed by Guendelman. Her analysis of social work activities responsive to the special needs of Hispanic families in a hospital setting illustrates the expanded professional knowledge and skills entailed in work with various ethnic and cultural groups.

The special context of a reverse isolation unit treating children with life-threatening illness and immune deficiency problems is the subject of Kutsanellou, Meyer, and Christ's analysis of the role of social work practice in a particularly complex and technologically sophisticated setting. Although this article does not focus on practice methodology, it does define the need for a systems approach to practice, with differential interventions to help patients, families, and staff cope with the extreme stress of the medical situation. Since this paper appears to have broken new ground in reporting on social work in an evolving medical specialty, the authors turned to literature from fields other than social work in developing their analysis of a new and highly specialized area of practice.

Moonilal's article on trauma centers analyzes the multiple social work roles called for in situations of complex traumatic injury and high-tech lifesaving treatment. The article applies concepts of crisis theory useful in assisting patients and families deal with actual or threatened loss of life, limb, or function.

Williams and Rice illustrate other aspects of social work practice with the critically ill, in this case with families of patients on intensive care units. The special nature of care on such units, their unique impact on families, and their needs for service are the basis for the comprehensive proposed plan of care, which includes crisis intervention and mobilization of multiple supports within the setting.

Brochstein, Adams, Tristan, and Cheney's article demonstrates an expanded role for social work developed within the context of primary care setting. The authors build on earlier work, such as that of Nason and Delbanco (1977), to develop new definitions of social work services as an integral component of primary health. A strong role for social work is further developed in the Clarke, Neuwirth, and Bernstein article included in Part 9.

Social Work and Alzheimer's Disease: Psychosocial Management in the Absence of Medical Cure

Stephen Berman, ACSW
Meryl B. Rappaport, LCSW

SUMMARY. Because the illness erodes and destroys an individual's humanness and personality, patients and families affected by Alzheimer's Disease have particularly critical needs for help with its psychosocial sequelae. This article develops a model of psychosocial management and details specific interventions to help patients and caregivers develop and maintain adaptations during the long course of the disease.

INTRODUCTION

Alzheimer's disease, fifth leading killer in this country, destroys the human personality and creates social problems of magnitude. Sometimes referred to as the silent epidemic, it is the most frequent cause of irreversible dementia in an estimated 1.2 to 4 million Americans age 40 and older, including about half of the population in nursing homes. The statistical spread reflects different epidemiological studies (Thomas, 1983). At present there is no cure or medical treatment for Alzheimer's Disease (U.S. Department of Health & Human Service, 1983). Recent investigations suggest biochemical changes, viral agents, aluminum intoxication, genetic defects,

At the time of writing Stephen Berman, ACSW, was Assistant Chief, Social Work Services and Coordinator, Extended Care Services; Meryl B. Rappaport, LCSW, was Coordinator, Hospital Based Home Care Program, Veterans Administration Medical Center, Palo Alto, Menlo Park Division, 3801 Miranda Avenue, Palo Alto, CA 94304.

Reprinted from *Social Work in Health Care*, Volume 10(2), Winter 1984.

and changes in the immune system as possible causative factors (Schneck, Reisber and Ferris, 1982) but a specific cause is not known. The consequences of the illness are well known: gradual and unrelenting deterioration of memory, intellect, and self-care ability. "By altering, and, in some cases, destroying the personality, dementia strikes the patient at the core of his humanness, his ability to relate to the world around him" (Cath, 1978).

With its history of helping the chronically ill mobilize inner and outer resources to cope with problems of living, social work is uniquely suited to the "case management" of Alzheimer's disease. This paper defines social work practice with Alzheimer's disease as psychosocial management in the absence of medical cure. The model described outlines social work practice within each of three phases. The phases, forgetfulness, confusional, and dementia, are not distinct with finite and predictable beginnings and endings, but reflect irregular and progressive deterioration of functioning over a period of time.

The model gives the social worker two primary roles. In one role the social worker coordinates the interdisciplinary treatment of the patient, ideally as a case manager. Because the resources needed for optimal management of Alzheimer's patients and family are frequently not in place, this ideal will be difficult to achieve in most health care delivery systems without significant changes in national policy for reimbursement for psychosocial support and programming for those with dementing and other chronic illnesses. Therefore, for the present, it is likely that the social worker, or several social workers over the course of time, will become involved with the family intermittently. The model presented here can help social workers at different entry points understand the psychosocial upheavals and issues taking place at that time.

In the second role, the social worker is the direct practice generalist who gives a broad spectrum of psychosocial services to patients and families. Many of the principles and functions described in the model are applicable to other progressive dementing illnesses such as multiinfarct dementia, Pick's disease, and Huntington's chorea.

Throughout the three phases of the illness, the social worker is instrumental in two areas: values clarification and working with the emotional impact of the disease. Value questions arise around specific issues which are noted in the paper. Where societal values are unclear, social workers need to assist families in clarifying their own values and making decisions consonant with them. The progressive downhill course of the illness necessitates a keen sensitivity to issues of loss, grief and bereavement. The social worker plays a vital role in supporting the patient and family in working through anger, frustration, guilt and mourning they may experience. Counseling and grief work are key interventions to be implemented intermittently through the duration of the illness.

THE FORGETFULNESS PHASE

During the forgetfulness phase (Schneck, Reisber and Ferris, 1982) which can last from one to ten years, the patient experiences subjective cognitive deficits. The major area of impairment is recent memory: there is a tendency to forget where things are placed, difficulty remembering names; the person starts to write things down in order to remember them. Family and social disruptions, increased marital conflict, employment problems, and patient abuse of alcohol and medications may occur. During this period of uncertainty, the major social work functions are to provide support and counseling to the patient and family, to facilitate an interdisciplinary work-up and to develop a psychosocial assessment.

Diagnosis

Until the assessment and work-up are completed, there is no diagnosis of Alzheimer's disease. All the symptoms and problems described mimic many other disorders which have to be ruled out in this "prediagnosis phase" before Alzheimer's disease can be diagnosed (Easterly, 1981). The only time that a diagnosis of Alzheimer's disease can be made with absolute certainty is upon autopsy (U.S. Department of Health and Human Services, 1980). Because this diagnosis carries with it such a dismal prognosis, the primary care physician needs to take great care in evaluating the work-up before deciding that the patient has Alzheimer's. The patient and family need to know that Alzheimer's diagnostic work is a process in which the health care team backs into a differential diagnosis by systematically discounting all the other conditions and illnesses that might cause "senile" symptoms. In line with this, the initial social work task is to help the patient locate a primary care physician who is accessible, knowledgeable about dementing illness, and willing to spend the necessary time with the patient, family, the other members of the treatment team. The next step is to help them move through the tedious, frustrating, and embarrassing evaluation process which typically includes evaluation by an internist, a neurologist, a psychiatrist, a psychologist, and a social worker. The patient and caregiver need to receive help from the social worker in developing the emotional and practical resources to travel to many examinations and be asked a multitude of questions, some of which can feel humiliating. Because this is an exhausting experience, scheduling the evaluation over eight to twelve weeks can make it less hectic and fatiguing.

Psychosocial Assessment

The psychosocial assessment, which takes place concurrently with the evaluation, is a critical part of the work-up since the decline of memory and intellectual functions characteristic of the irreversible dementias are also characteristic of certain reversible conditions that can be identified by the social worker. The following is an example:

> An 80 year old man living alone in a rooming house was referred for placement in a nursing home by his landlord, who thought he was senile and could no longer understand what people were saying to him. The social worker thought she detected a hearing impairment, later confirmed by an audiologist. His "senility" vanished when he was fitted with a hearing aid.

This emphasizes the importance of reviewing sensory, psychological, emotional, and functional dimensions in the psychosocial assessment. Older persons with hearing impairments are frequently misunderstood as having poor understanding and poor memory. A person who cannot hear what other people are saying cannot possibly remember, understand, or respond to what is said. Too, malnutrition caused by a variety of psychological, economic and social factors sometimes causes symptoms which mimic dementia.

The most common cause of forgetfulness, confusion, and disorientation in the aged is drug intoxication which can be reversed if recognized and treated (U.S. Department of Health and Human Services, 1980). An inventory of the prescribed and over-the-counter medication the patient is taking can be relevant. Frequently older persons accumulate medications from several different physicians and begin to use them in combination with each other without medical supervision. Although the "retired" comprise 11% of the population, they receive 25% of dispensed prescriptions. A recent study showed that about 70% of an elderly population used nonprescription drugs without knowledge of the primary care physician (Graedon, 1980). Sleeping pills, sedatives, tranquilizers, antianxiety agents, and a host of other nervous system depressants are among the medications that have been most frequently associated with confusion in the elderly. The social worker is in a good position to alert the patient and family to the importance of bringing this information to the primary care physician.

The most frequent psychological cause of cognitive impairment is depression, and depression masked as dementia (pseudodementia) is a frequent finding among elderly patients (Wells, 1979). Along with symptoms that mimic senility, these patients manifest clear depressive symptoms, usually have a history of affective illness, and exhibit relatively rapid onset and progression of cognitive disability.

An excellent tool for differentiating pseudodementia from irreversible dementia is the Wells Comparative Table (Table 1). In depression the onset of symptoms is more precisely dated, the symptoms progress more rapidly after onset, and there usually is a history of previous dysfunction. The depressed patient's complaints about cognitive losses are more detailed and specific than those the demented patient can describe. The depressed patient has a pervasive affective change and communicates a strong sense of distress, whereas the demented patient has a shallower affect and seems less concerned about his cognitive condition. The social worker trained in this task may complete such an evaluation or the patient can be

TABLE I

THE MAJOR CLINICAL FEATURES DIFFERENTIATING PSEUDODEMENTIA FROM DEMENTIA

(Wells, C. Am. J. Psychiatry 136:7, July 1979)

Pseudodementia	Dementia
Clinical course & History	
Family always aware of dysfunction and its severity	Family often unaware of dysfunction & its severity
Onset can be dated with some precision	Onset can be dated only within broad limits
Symptoms of short duration before medical help is sought	Symptoms usually of long duration before medical help is sought
Rapid progression of symptoms after onset	Slow progression of symptoms throughout course
History of previous psychiatric dysfunction common	History of previous psychiatric dysfunction unusual
Complaints and clinical behavior	
Patients usually complain much of cognitive loss	Patients usually complain little of cognitive loss
Patients complaints of cognitive dysfunction usually detailed	Patients complaints of cognitive dysfunction usually vague
Patients emphasize disability	Patients conceal disability
Patients highlight failures	Patients delight in accomplishments, however trivial
Patients make little effort to perform even simple tasks	Patients struggle to perform tasks
Patients do not try to keep up	Patients rely on notes, calendars, etc., to keep up
Patients usually communicate strong sense of distress	Patients often appear unconcerned
Affective change often pervasive	Affect labile and shallow
Loss of social skills often early and prominent	Social skills often retained
Behavior often incongruent with severity of cognitive dysfunction	Behavior usually compatible with severity of cognitive dysfunction
Nocturnal accentuation of dysfunction uncommon	Nocturnal accentuation of dysfunction common
Clinical features related to memory, cognitive, and intellectual functioning	
Attention and concentration often well preserved	Attention and concentration usually faulty
"Don't know" answers typical	Near miss answers frequent
On tests of orientation, patients often give "don't know" answers	On tests of orientation, patients often mistake unusual for usual
Memory loss for recent and remote events usually equally severe	Memory loss for recent events usually more severe than for remote events
Memory gaps for specific periods or events common	Memory gaps for specific periods unusual
Marked variability in performance on tasks of similar difficulty	Consistently poor performance on tasks of similar difficulty

referred to a psychologist or psychiatrist. Because behaviors considered eccentric or unconventional but normal in younger people are often considered abnormal and evidence of dementia in older people, the psychosocial assessment should link current behavior with past life patterns, behavior, quality of relationships and family interaction.

Counseling

When the diagnosis of Alzheimer's disease is made, the focus shifts to helping patients and families absorb and deal with what has happened. Families need information from the primary care physician about the disease and its probable course as well as help in coping with the psychosocial problems the diagnosis brings. Easterly has described graphically the shock, the confusion, and the fear of a newly diagnosed patient, "There are so many unanswered questions I have to face. What will happen to my health, my spouse, my relatives, my savings, my world, my everything? What will happen to me?" (Easterly, 1981). The patient's family faces a heavy burden once this diagnosis has been made. "It may mean a lot of physical work, financial sacrifice, and changes in roles and relationships while you are learning to accept the reality that someone you love will never be the same" (Mace and Rabins, 1981). During this time the social worker plans with patients and families for the individual or family therapy they will need, probably on an intermittent basis, either at the institutional site or by referral to a counseling agency.

This is the time when the social worker begins to work with the patient and family as they look at their lives and plan for what lies ahead. Planning for the future proceeds at a pace in sync with patient and family readiness to face the implications of altered life. An early value issue families need to consider is whether care provision and decision making should remain the domain of the family, or be shared with formal sources of support. The social worker can offer some counter-balance to the sense of hopelessness and futility the diagnosis generates by helping patients and family understand that even after a diagnosis has been made, the rate of degeneration is variable and is partly dependent on the patient's support system.

Because the progression of the disease is highly idiosyncratic, there is no way to predict what an individual patient may still be able to do many years after the diagnosis has been made (U.S. Department of Health and Human Services, 1980). A recent review reports that the progression of patients from Phase I (forgetfulness) to Phase III (dementia) varies as much as ten years (Schneck, Reisber and Ferris, 1982). Consequently, in this first phase, the focus is on enabling patients to develop the social, environmental, and emotional supports which can keep the individual employed, mobile, and in a position to interact with others as long as possible. If engaged, families, friends, and employers can use social work support to help the patient perform to his fullest potential and maintain intact cognitive functions.

Mr. C was a married man, top executive of a computer company, and supervisor of 35 employees. After two years of increasing memory problems and mild confusion, Mr. C was diagnosed as having Alzheimer's disease. Mr. C's work performance gradually deteriorated because of his forgetfulness. Although still oriented and sociable, Mr. C had to rely on constant note taking in order to remember conversations, details of recent transactions, and names of close associates. After many months of this, Mr. C's employer suggested he retire. This angered Mr. C who initially denied any problems and said he was too young to retire.

In several sessions with him, the social worker helped Mr. C acknowledge his sense of loss and disappointment. He was then able to compare the financial and emotional pros and cons of retiring as opposed to seeking a less demanding job in the company. He decided to continue working and apply for a non-supervisory position.

With help, he discussed his problems with his boss and the company agreed to reassign Mr. C to another job. This patient was helped to manage his problem so that catastrophic losses in personal worth, financial security, and social stimulation were avoided. Job reassignment represented a loss of status and was not easy but Mr. C was able to maintain a work role, financial support of his family, and relate to a variety of persons outside the home. He worked successfully at this job for eight years before he retired.

During the forgetfulness phase, families should make business decisions, wills and conclude other legal business which must involve the patient before his judgement becomes too impaired.

THE CONFUSIONAL PHASE

Although the length of time it takes varies, patients with Alzheimer's disease will gradually develop increased impairment of cognitive functioning until the confusional phase (Schneck, Reisber and Ferris, 1982) which may last from one to ten years, is reached. Initially, the patient's cognitive deficit is particularly severe for memory of recent events and orientation and concentration are significantly impaired. Vocabulary is spared, although the patient will have some difficulty recalling appropriate words. The patient gradually gets worse in all of these areas and will have increased difficulty with both recent and remote memory and recognizing names and faces. Intellectual functioning, particularly abstract thinking, gradually declines. The patient becomes less able to discern common themes, essential differences or use good judgement. He cannot apply experiences to new situations or separate the significant from the trivial; ideas become meager and he is unable to grasp new ones (Roth, 1980). Self-care abilities will progressively deteriorate and the patient will find it more difficult to eat with the appropriate utensils, select appropriate clothing, and use the bathroom.

The two major objectives of psychosocial management of Alzheimer's disease in the confusional phase are developing care plans for the functionally impaired patient and preserving the caregivers and family. Even in the early stages of confusion, losses in memory, orientation, and social skills impair the patient's ability to communicate and to function without supervision. Yet with guidance from others, he can still function in some areas.

Persons living alone can no longer continue to do so. Then the social worker needs to help the patient come to terms with the need to live in a supervised setting. This may mean moving in with such family or friends available and willing to care for the patient, or placement in a boarding home, an adult foster home, or a nursing home, depending on the patient's abilities and limitations. This decision raises a new value concern: should the physical security of the patient take precedence over his psychosocial needs? Each family has its own way of handling stressful situations and making difficult decisions. The social worker can help them to clarify value considerations and promote decision-making which is comfortable because it is consistent with the family's values.

Elderly individuals who have always lived alone may vehemently resist giving up their independence. When the patient's cognitive functioning permits this, the social worker can help the patient make the transition from independent living to a supervised setting gradually, in stages, through the use of homemakers, meals-on-wheels, day care programs, and volunteer visitors in his own home.

Role of Caregiver

The well being of the Alzheimer's patient depends directly on the well being of the person who is providing his or her care (Mace and Rabins, 1981). Thus, the functionally impaired patient who lives with caregivers and families will need social work assistance in preserving this support system. As the patient has more difficulty in understanding others and in making himself understood, incidents such as home accidents, abuse of medications, altered sleep patterns, and wandering, increase. This puts a tremendous strain on the patient, the caregiver, the family and their interactions with each other. Members of families develop reciprocal relationships in which they share responsibilities and roles which ensure that the work of the family gets done and its stability is maintained (Kapust, 1982). Within this delicately balanced system, a stress in one family member affects everyone. Shifts in the traditional ways family members share work and relate to each other must occur because Alzheimer's so profoundly alters the patient's physical, mental, and emotional characteristics. The employed spouse of an Alzheimer's patient may have to do the cooking and laundry as well as go to work every day. A wife may now have to take on the role of nurse and parent to her demented husband. Years of interactive patterns and precedents are undone. Psychosocial management requires that the caregivers and the patient are treated as one system. Ways of helping the patient are also geared to helping the caregiver and vice versa.

Optimal Living Arrangement

The environmental design of the patient's living quarters requires evaluation. The goals are to make the home safer and at the same time conserve caregiver emotional energy. Very few homes, apartments, condominiums, or group living facilities are designed for mentally or physically impaired persons. Living quarters need to be made safe to eliminate accident hazards in the location of heating and cooking appliances, stairs, excessive furniture, hot water taps, and steep embankments. If these adaptations are not feasible, a move should be considered while the confused person is still able to adjust. As the disease progresses and the patient has fewer cognitive skills, any environmental change, even minor rearrangement of furniture, can be upsetting, disorienting and disruptive to his functioning. The social worker alerts the family to potential safety hazards and suggests way of coping with these problems. It may be unsafe for the confused person to smoke when alone. Developing a relatively nonflammable smoking area and installing a smoke alarm helps reduce the danger and the supervision needed without restricting the patient's activity completely.

When the family has a patient who wanders, good management includes setting up a system such as placing bells on the doors or locks in unnoticeable places to reduce the risk of wandering or helping the patient obtain an identification bracelet inscribed with name, home address, phone number, and memory impairment. This increases patient safety and decreases family's need for worry, vigilance, or search for a lost patient.

Social Activities

The social worker can help the Alzheimer's patient and family develop new ways to spend time together. The goal is to promote continued functioning as a couple for as long as possible. Previous pastimes need to be restructured to accommodate the patient's cognitive changes and new activities may also be needed. Listening to music, reading aloud, dancing, walking, attending church, going on drives, or visiting a shopping center may still be possible in this phase. To provide stimulation without frustration, these activities should take into account the confused person's stamina, tolerance for unfamiliar surroundings, and comfort with groups of people.

> Mr. and Mrs. J always enjoyed watching situation comedies on television. Even though Mrs. J no longer understood the story, she still enjoyed laughing with her husband and the laugh track. She still seemed to look forward to watching the shows with her husband.

The ability to communicate with others about Alzheimer's is a critical skill in the caregiver's network building repertoire. Caregivers may feel embarrassed, resentful, or puzzled by some of the things the confused person may do in public and avoid such activities. The social worker provides emotional support to the caregiver's feelings of alarm and anxiety that the patient does not always know what is expected, and is unable to control all of his actions. The caregiver may need help in developing and practicing explanations of the patient's condition to others, and in achieving comfort in this necessary and painful task. Role playing may help the caregiver become more comfortable in explaining this disease to family and friends. Caregivers may be taught cognitive therapy techniques to remind themselves that the patient does not understand what he is doing.

Sexual Functioning

The maintenance of sexual intimacy for as long as possible is important for an Alzheimer's couple. It is one area that may still define the relationship as a marriage in which mutual satisfaction is possible (Mace and Rabins, 1981). Alzheimer's disease varies in how it affects the sexuality of patients: some become sexually demanding, others lose interest in sex. The Alzheimer's patient may have the desire and ability to make love, but may forget sex happened after it is over, leaving the spouse distressed. In some cases, neuroleptic drugs are used to reduce behaviors such as paranoia, combativeness, sleep disturbances, and hallucinations which make intimacy or sexual contact impossible.

Promoting Residual Functioning

How can the confused person's connection with the world around him be maintained? Some can benefit from structured cuing which stimulates long-term memory and evokes habitual patterns of functioning. Simple steps such as informing the impaired person where she is going and cuing her in on names and contexts ("Jane, you remember Mr. Smith from church"), may help the confused person feel more comfortable.

Structured cuing, labeling, and signals can curb negative behaviors and help the confused person adopt new behavior patterns.

> Mrs. H would become agitated when her daughter left her alone to run errands. She would tell her next door neighbor that her daughter was missing and insist she call the police. Sometimes she would wander down the street looking for her.
>
> The social worker suggested her daughter place a note on the door stating where she had gone and the time she would be back. Mrs. H was told that the note on the door signified that her daughter was gone on an errand and not missing. Presence of the note was a cue to catch her mother's attention and served to keep her indoors and reassured when her daughter left the house.
>
> Mr. S would constantly ask his wife when he could have another cigarette. She solved the problem by setting a timer and teaching him that he could only have a cigarette on cue when the timer rang once an hour.

The social worker may role model several techniques for the caregiver to use in communicating with the patient. Although impairment increasingly prevents patients from understanding all that is going on around them, many of them remain sensitive to the emotional affect of others and retain some ability to express their own emotions of joy, fear, anger, etc. While they may not understand the complete content of a conversation they do comprehend the tone and understand parts of what is being said. The use of non-verbal gestures to augment words can be particularly helpful in conversations with the patient: a smile, eye contact, holding a hand out, and use of body position are methods to relate to persons who have problems with words (Bartol). In many cases a combination of these non-verbal techniques with continual stimulation, cuing, simplified sentences, and reminders make it possible for the confused person to relate to what is going on.

As the patient gets more confused, caregivers will need assistance in making difficult judgments about the impaired person's functioning. The family must decide when the confused person is no longer capable of driving safely, cooking independently, or being alone. Decisions which restrict the patient's span of control and personal freedom can be difficult for the caregiver because they may not be easily accepted by the patient. Families may be reluctant to restrict the impaired person's activities, and may feel guilty or upset when they do so. The social worker facilitates the family's problem solving processes of making sound though difficult decisions and dealing with the resulting problems. When patients forget to open mail, pay bills and lose bankbooks, caregivers have to organize searches for bank statements, insurance policies, income tax records, and legal correspondence. When the patient can no longer manage property or financial affairs the social worker can support the family work in the psychologically painful process of establishing a conservatorship or guardianship of both property and person so that the conservator can take responsibility for medical treatment or placement.

Families need help to balance roles and responsibilities, to make decisions about how to distribute their time and energy and to arrange for regular respite periods. As the confusional phase progresses, the focus of work is on preserving the caregiving family unit. Families care for the majority of the Alzheimer's patients in this country (Rabins, Mace and Lucas, 1982) and for most demented patients the family can be a comprehensive and successful multiservice agency. Thus, it follows that the social worker focuses on their needs and on helping family members maintain their physical health, emotional strength and financial solvency, and on strengthening the network of family, friends, and others who can provide strong social bonds and practical resources. Persons caring for demented patients are more likely to maintain their mental health if they have an emotionally intimate relationship with at least one other person. The social worker can serve in this role. Other significant sources of psychological sustenance are self-help groups of other Alzheimer's families. Some support groups are sponsored by the Alzheimer's Disease and Related Disorders Association, and others by hospitals, community mental health centers, brain injury rehabilitation programs, and family service agencies. Regularly scheduled times away from the care of the confused person enables the caregiver to replenish diminished physical and emotional resources; they have been identified as a key factor in facilitating home care of persons with debilitating illness (Baulch, 1980).

Sources of caregiver respite must be organized to maintain service to the patient in the absence of the primary caregiver. A resource inventory can be developed in which the caregiver lists all the tasks that might be appropriate for respite care and then matches these tasks with persons or agencies that might provide respite care resources. One neighbor might help with shopping while another might agree to look in on the confused person when the caregiver goes to a movie. The social worker supports the caregiver's right to ask others for help and offers assistance to organize this supportive social network. The caregiver can convene periodic "caregiving discussions" with family, friends, and others in which caregiving responsibilities are divided up among the participants. This can create a team approach as well as a shared appreciation for the demanding role of caring for a confused person.

Caregivers who have not had respite or time out for many years may need help in identifying an inventory of activities that will provide diversion and enjoyment. They may also need "permission" to take some time out to have fun. Recent research indicates that depression can be reduced if the caregiver can have four daily events they define as pleasant (Lewinsohn and Amenson, 1978). Help with scheduling these can be particularly useful with those caregivers who overidentify with the patient to the extent that they consider their well being and that of the Alzheimer's victim as one and the same. Agencies that offer assistance with nursing care in the home, chore assistance, occupational and physical therapy, and income maintenance can supplement the help of family and friends in making respite periods possible.

Helping to preserve family financial solvency is a critical goal.

Familiarity with each family's financial situation helps the social worker make appropriate use of SSD, SSI, Medicare, food stamps, and tax assistance, tax shelters and disability insurance. Families often need social work advocacy to receive these benefits.

Geriatric day care programs are a good resource for Alzheimer's families. If the patient can adjust to day care, this gives the caregiver an opportunity to work, earn money and develop social contacts outside the home. Some mildly confused Alzheimer's patients have reported positives about geriatric day care since it puts the patients in the company of others who have similar problems (Geiger and Berman, Jan., 1983).

Throughout this confusional phase the social worker helps the family make continuing and appropriate use of the primary care physician as even a minor illness can exacerbate the impaired person's behavior and create more confusion. Urinary tract infections deserve special mention since they can be responsible for incontinence that is reversible. Continuing medical care should include careful evaluation of new symptoms to determine whether a superimposed treatable illness is the cause. Since the confused person may be increasingly unable to communicate what is wrong, the caregiver needs to learn the signs and symptoms to watch for: for example, rubbing dentures and pressure points can develop into complicated problems; drug intake needs careful monitoring since delirium is a common side effect of over-medication.

As the confusional phase progresses, caregivers need continuing psychological support in dealing with the painful losses they experience as the afflicted person's functioning declines. Caregivers may feel angry or trapped in the situation, and then feel guilty about these feelings. They may become depressed over the loss of friends, favored pastimes, and the isolation which results from the increasing demands of the caregiving role.

THE DEMENTIA PHASE

Alzheimer's patients will ultimately deteriorate, sometimes over a period of many years, and move into the final dementia phase of the disease in a constant state of severe and significant decline. (S)he is severely disoriented, often to the point of mistaking a spouse for a parent and being unable to identify other family and friends. Behavioral problems such as paranoid ideation, agitation, combativeness, and psychotic-like symptoms may develop. Neurological disabilities, abnormal reflexes, incontinence, and wandering become more pronounced. The person eventually becomes non-ambulatory and bedridden as the brain no longer is able to direct many aspects of functioning. This phase has been called the "funeral that never ends" (Kapust, 1982). By this time Alzheimer's patients have usually lost the unique personality traits which defined them as individuals, though many live on for years.

As the patient requires help with all activities of daily living, activities to preserve the caregiver accelerate. The social focus is on helping spouses who are usually the main caregiver cope and adjust to the final change in the marital relationship. Since the patient can no longer recognize people, the other partner is faced with the dilemma of being alone but not single. The caregiving spouse needs help in redefining the marriage as a new relationship, with different rules and with a different person. Rabins, Mace and Lucas (1982) illustrate the moral, ethical, and spiritual issues this raises.

> One husband said "I will always take care of her but I've started dating again. She is no longer the person I married." Another husband said "For me caring for her, keeping my promise, is most important. It is true that she is not the same but this too is a part of our marriage. I try to see it as a challenge."

Families must make difficult, painful decisions during this final stage of dementia as they try to achieve a balance between the responsibility to care for the patient and the need to maintain the strength of the family.

Families who decide to try to manage demented patients at home may need assistance in developing daily structures and supports needed to care for persons so severely disabled. Nursing care is a critical service for the patient at this stage of the illness. This care should be supervised by a professional nurse through a home health agency. The nurse can train the caregiver or assistant in the functions of needed care. For example, a regular toileting schedule may be established to help with incontinence; when this no longer controls the problem, disposable diapers may be used. Also, if possible, a regular schedule of in-home help through regular homemaker visits can support home management.

Managing a demented person at home means that caregivers have to cope with the unexpected, jump from one job to another, and accept interruptions as a way of life. Rather than rely on memory, a patient care chart which tracks medications and nursing needs aids the family to stay in control of the situation (Baulch, 1980). It is also a tangible record of the care provided. A major issue is that the decision to care for the patient at home is reversible. Throughout this phase the social worker helps the family reevaluate whether the plan remains tenable and feasible. When the home care plan is no longer viable, the social worker should be active in helping the family change it. The social worker repeatedly serves as a consultant, providing crisis intervention and triage. When home management is not workable, the family must consider placement of the patient in a nursing home. Usually a complex interplay of physical, psychological, and practical pressures lead to the caregiver fatigue that necessitates placement.

Mrs. Y had cared for her husband for seven years, the last three years of which Mr. Y had been incontinent and needed help with bathing and feeding. A home health aide who gave sixteen hours a week left because of agency budget cuts. No one else was available to help Mrs. Y who quit her part-time job. The income from this job supplemented the family's limited pension income and provided an important source of social stimulation for Mrs. Y.

Mr. Y began waking up more frequently at night and wandering. Mrs. Y complained of severe anxiety, exhaustion, and dizziness. Her blood pressure elevated and she was no longer able to manage Mr. Y's incontinence. She was very dejected because Mr. Y no longer seemed to know who she was.

Mrs. Y wanted to place him in a nursing home but a daughter from Mr. Y's first marriage, who lived 500 miles away, berated Mrs. Y for neglecting her duty.

The social worker called the daughter, helping her realize the importance of visiting and seeing the situation first hand. The daughter did visit, saw her father and participated in family conferences with the social worker and Mr. Y. After this both Mrs. Y and her step-daughter could agree that nursing home placement was the only care alternative for Mr. Y.

Caregivers served by one hospital identified these major reasons for placement of demented patients: (1) physically assaultive behavior; (2) increasing needs for physical care or medical care; (3) incontinence; (4) physical and emotional illness of the caregiver; and (5) lack of financial resources to purchase supportive services to maintain the person at home (Geiger and Berman, May, 1983).

In addressing the psychosocial problems in the decision to place the demented person in a nursing home, the social worker integrates understanding of family dynamics and the needs of the patient with a knowledge of community resources. Sustained, supportive and problem-solving counseling is a pivotal need of families at this time. For the older couple, institutionalization may be the first separation in years of marriage, and is likely to be a final one. Caregivers need help in coping with anger about experiencing this loss. Some need psychological support in working through the guilt of "abandoning" a spouse in a nursing home. Nursing home costs may drain a couple financially and mean a changed lifestyle for the healthy spouse. A caregiver who gives up a large home or apartment when the demented person is institutionalized faces relocation at a time when financial, physical, and emotional resources may be depleted. Loss of the caregiving role can leave a huge void in the caregiver's life.

The caregiver needs the opportunity to mourn once again the loss of the demented relative. This is essential since, long before dementia proves fatal, a psychological death occurs with the deterioration of the personality of the patient. Toynbee (1968) has said that the premature death of a human spirit in advance of the death of the body is more appalling than any premature death in which spirit and body die simultaneously. Social workers play an essential role in facilitating resolutions of this complicated and protracted mourning process. Grief work, supportive therapy and self-help groups are useful in facilitating the healing process (Kapust, 1982).

The caregiving spouse often needs help in letting go of the caregiver role, in learning to limit visits to the nursing home and in becoming reinvolved in former activities and hobbies. The social work role here is to help the spouse develop a renewed sense of engagement in life. A new fit between person and environment needs to be developed, organized around wellness instead of illness. New patterns of living are needed to alleviate the dysphoria that has probably occurred from years of caregiving for a demented spouse (Yalom, 1980).

COMMUNITY ACTION ROLE FOR SOCIAL WORKERS

Social workers can fulfill a vital community role as advocates and developers of services for the demented and their families. Organized respite services, geriatric day respite, day health programs, chore and companion services for this population are scarce, and there is decreasing coverage by private insurance and Medicare. As the social brokers of resources, social workers can identify gaps in services and work to develop alliances and political support for the creation of the needed programs. The Family Survival Project for Brain Damaged Adults in San Francisco and the Palo Alto Veterans Administration Medical Center offer programmatic examples of the directions such efforts may take.

The Family Service Project for Brain Damaged Adults (FSP) is a nonprofit organization which helps those who care for adult victims of chronic and degenerative brain disorders. Its purpose is to build services where none exist, to assist families directly, and to be a public voice for those facing related emotional and financial problems. FSP offers services such as a clearinghouse of statewide and national information and advice for families and professionals, family support groups, family consultations to help plan and coordinate resources and services, respite care and legal and financial advice. Professional training, publications, conferences, speakers and technical assistance to organizations are also offered.

The Veterans Administration Medical Center, Palo Alto offers a continuum of care for Alzheimer's patients and support for their families. Interdisciplinary teams in the geriatric outpatient clinic, inpatient consultation service and Hospital Based Home Care offer full scale assessments to establish the diagnosis. The outpatient clinic offers continuing medical care and case management once the diagnosis has been established. The Elder Veterans Day Center transports Alzheimer's patients to a program regularly offering day respite, socialization and recreational activities, health maintenance and service referrals; psychosocial support, family counseling and caregiver network building opportunities are also provided. Hospital Based Home Care uses an interdisciplinary team to provide coordinated, comprehensive short-term medical and psychosocial management services to Alzheimer's patients at home. The patient and caregiver are viewed as the unit of care and receive assistance in problem solving and decision making around patient management issues, long term care planning, counseling and referral linkages. Separate support groups for Alzheimer's patients and families are offered at this facility, as well as opportunities to participate in research on Alzheimer's disease. An inpatient respite program provides time out to caregivers and 24 hour care to Alzheimer's patients one week out of every eight. Finally, several long term care wards specifically care for Alzheimer's and demented patients; support groups for relatives of nursing home patients assist in working through issues of role transition and loss. Further program development efforts are under way to meet other patient care needs.

CONCLUSION

The social treatment of demented people and their families presents diverse and demanding challenges to our profession. It requires a full range of social work skills, including counseling and support; resource referral; case management; grief work; family therapy and group work; patient, professional and community education; political action and advocacy; program development; and research. These tasks require strength, stamina, flexibility, and creativity as we apply our helping skills to both patients and their caregivers who carry such depleting and draining social responsibilities.

REFERENCES

Bartol, Mari Ann, RN, *Nursing Care of the Patient with Alzheimer's Disease*. Unpublished guideline, Veterans Administration Medical Center, Tacoma, Washington.
Baulch, Evelyn M., *Home Care—A Practical Alternative to Extended Hospitalization*. Millbrae, California: Celestial Arts, 1980, 106.
Cath, S. H., The Geriatric Patient and His Family: The Institutionalization of a

Parent: A Nadir of Life. *Journal of Geriatric Psychiatry*, 1978, *1*, 25-46, 125-146.

Easterly, Warren, *The Alzheimer Caregiver's Disease*. Unpublished guide, June, 1981.

Geiger, Deborah and Stephen Berman, *Respite Care*, videotape produced by the Veterans Administration Medical Center, Palo Alto, California, January, 1983.

Geiger, Deborah and Stephen Berman. Personal interviews with spouses of Alzheimer's disease patients at the Veterans Administration Medical Center, Palo Alto, California, May, 1983.

Graedon, Joe, *The People's Pharmacy—2*. New York: Avon Books, 1980, 354.

Kapust, Lissa Robins, MSW, Living With Dementia: The Ongoing Funeral. *Social Work in Health Care*, Summer, 1982, 7(4), 82.

Lewinsohn, P. M. and C. S. Amenson. Some Relations Between Pleasant and Unpleasant Mood-Related Events and Depression. *Journal of Abnormal Psychology*, 1978, 87, No. 6, 644-654.

Mace, Nancy L. and Peter V. Rabins, MD. *The 36-Hour Day*. Baltimore and London: The Johns Hopkins University Press, 1981, 139.

Rabins, Peter V., MD, Nancy L. Mace, MA, and Mary Jane Lucas, RN. The Impact of Dementia on the Family. *Journal of the American Medical Association*, July 16, 1982, Vol. 248, N. 3,333.

Roth, Sir Martin, Senile Dementia and its Borderlands. *Psychopathology in the Aged*. Jonathan Cole and James Barrett, eds., New York: Raven Press, 1980, 211.

Schneck, Michael K., MD, Barry Reisber, MD, and Steven H. Ferris, PhD. An Overview of Current Concepts of Alzheimer's Disease. *American Journal of Psychiatry*, February, 1982, *139*:2, 170-171.

Thomas, Lewis, MD, Chancellor, Memorial Sloan-Kettering Cancer Center. Testimony presented at a Joint Hearing of the House Energy and Commerce Subcommittee and the House Aging Committee, August 3, 1983.

U.S. Department of Health and Human Services, *Alzheimer's Disease: A Scientific Guide for Health Practitioners* (Public Health Service National Institutes of Health Publication No. 81-2251). November, 1980, 2.

Wells, Charles E., MD, Pseudodementia. *American Journal of Psychiatry*, July, 1979, *136*:7,896.

Yalom, Irvin D., *Existential Psychotherapy*. New York: Basic Books, Inc., 1980, 482.

Social Work and AIDS

Anne-Linda Furstenberg, PhD
Miriam Meltzer Olson, DSW

SUMMARY. AIDS (Acquired Immune Deficiency Syndrome) is a new contagious disease for which no cause or cure is known at present. The majority of people who have contracted AIDS are gay men. This paper examines individual and societal responses to this illness and to homosexuality that create issues for social work practice. These are unique to AIDS and at the same time exemplary of issues in all of health care. General principles of practice are applied to the specifics of dealing with AIDS and social work tasks with patients, families and significant others, health care staff, the community and policy makers are identified.

This paper is concerned with social work practice dealing with the health problem AIDS. It operates from the premise that general principles of social work in health care are applicable to the specifics of social work practice with people with AIDS and that there are lessons to be drawn from the AIDS situation that have bearing on social work practice throughout the health field.

Because the incidence of AIDS has been highest in gay men, and

At the time of writing Anne-Linda Furstenberg was Assistant Professor, University of Pennsylvania, School of Social Work, 3701 Locust Walk C3, Philadelphia, PA 19104. Miriam Meltzer Olson was Associate Professor, Temple University, School of Social Administration, Ritter Hall Annex, Philadelphia, PA 19122.

This paper is based on papers the authors presented at a conference on AIDS and Social Work: Issues, Information, Intervention, held September 22, 1983 at Graduate Hospital, Philadelphia, PA.

The authors acknowledge the generous assistance of Robert Schoenberg, MSW, Roger Stephens, MSW and Joseph Tramo, MSW in the preparation of this paper.

Reprinted from *Social Work in Health Care*, Volume 9(4), Summer 1984.

because the lessons to be drawn come from the association of AIDS with this population, the focus of this paper is primarily on AIDS and gay men. Most of the ideas discussed, however, can be applied as well to the other groups contracting AIDS.

AIDS THE DISEASE

AIDS, Acquired Immune Deficiency Syndrome, is a condition in which there is a breakdown of the body's immune defenses. As a result, individuals become prone to developing one or more serious diseases. The most common are Kaposi's Sarcoma, a rare skin cancer previously seen only in older people; and a variety of severe infections, called opportunistic infections because they would not be serious in people with normally functioning immune systems. The most common of these is pneumocystis carinii pneumonia (PCP), but severe infections by viruses, fungi and parasites also occur (Philadelphia AIDS Task Force, 1982; Conte et al., 1983).

AIDS was first identified and named in the United States in 1981, but the first cases had been seen in 1978 (Bazell, 1983). The cause of AIDS is presently not known, but current data point to a virus that plays some role in the development of the syndrome. It is thought to be a new disease, "to which human beings had never previously been exposed" (Bazell, 1983), but several already known viruses are also suspected. Ninety-five percent of AIDS cases in the U.S. fall into one of four groups:

1. Sexually active homosexual and bisexual men with multiple sex partners, who make up about 71% of all reported cases
2. Abusers of intravenous drugs, 17% of reported cases
3. Persons with hemophilia, 8% of reported cases
4. Haitians, 5% of reported cases (U.S.P.H.S., 1983) (There is doubt that being Haitian in itself is a risk factor: rather, poor methods of interviewing are thought to have resulted in Haitians' denial of the other risk factors (Bazell, 1983; Altman, 1983; Sullivan, 1983)

Based on available data, scientists have concluded that AIDS is not spread by casual contact, but is transmitted only through sexual contact with a person with AIDS, and through contact with tissues, blood or other body fluids of a person with AIDS. The incubation period appears to range from a few months to approximately two years. While there are treatments of varying efficacy for the cancers and infections, there is no cure for the underlying condition. Weakened by repeated overwhelming infections, most people with AIDS eventually succumb to one of them. Early observations indicated that a year and a half following diagnosis, 75% of the victims were dead (Bazell, 1983). As of February, 1984, 3500 cases of AIDS had been identified, of whom 1,400 had died (USPHS, 1984).

This new, contagious, presently incurable disease has drawn a great deal of public attention and evoked a broad range of lay and professional responses. Widespread concern about the disorder has firmly established it as a public health problem. However, as with most diseases, the concerns which shape the specific responses to the problem come from many sources. As with cancer, T.B., epilepsy, heart disease and others, responses to AIDS are affected not only by scientific information and rational appraisal, but by myth, superstition, stigma and their attendant attitudes and feelings. Because gay men are the primary group at risk of contracting AIDS, attitudes, beliefs and feelings about homosexuality have played a significant part in the responses to AIDS. Reactions have ranged from overt hostility to intense commitment to treatment and cure. Hostile responses have included outright expressions of hope that AIDS will wipe out the homosexual population, and belief that the disease is deserved punishment for the sin of sexual perversion, brought upon themselves by those who, choosing to engage in illicit sex, forfeit any claim to society's concern (Morgenthau et al., 1983; Beauchamp, 1983).

Other rejecting responses have been made under the guise of concern for the public health. The proposal made by Rev. Jerry Falwell, spokesperson for the "moral majority," that all homosexual blood donors be registered (Murphy, 1983), the medically contraindicated transfer of an AIDS patient from a Florida hospital to San Francisco (*Philadelphia Inquirer*, 10/9/83) and the refusal of some hospital, home health, social agency and other personnel to provide services to people with AIDS are examples.

At the other end of the spectrum from the hostile reactions to

AIDS are responses which have come from among the gay population itself. The recognition that the largest group with AIDS has been gay men and that the stigma attached to homosexuality negatively affected the quality of care of patients with AIDS generated considerable social activism within the gay community. In many cities, AIDS "task forces," organized by gays and other concerned people, have formed patient care networks and support groups, raised funds, publicized health information and referral sources, and lobbied for proper care, research on AIDS and increased protection of the civil rights of gays and lesbians (Collins, 1983; McKeown, 1983; Byron, 1983).

With the help of gay activists, concerned professionals and others, there have also been informed and informative responses in the media and the health field that have advanced efforts to understand and deal with the disorder and its effects. Television, newspaper and magazine reports as well as professional articles, workshops and symposia have focused attention on the multiple impact of AIDS. This attention has encompassed the progressively debilitating physical course of the illness, its emotional trauma, disruption of family and social relationships, employment and housing dislocations and financial hardships, as well as the stress which treating people with AIDS places on health care providers and the epidemic scale fear of AIDS both within the gay and the larger community.

AIDS AS A MULTIDIMENSIONAL PHENOMENON

The critical circumstances of AIDS and the attention given to it vividly demonstrate a proposition that underlies all of social work in the health field, that health and health care are not just matters of biology and physiology, or of medicine and medical technology. The situation surrounding AIDS serves to bring into sharp relief that fact that every health condition, good health, illness and disability, is at once a physical, psychological, social, economic and political phenomenon.

The politics of health involves more than governmental policies and regulations. Politics involves power relationships. Disparities in power among individuals and groups affect who gets how much of what resources and under what conditions to meet their health needs. Everything from the control that physicians may exercise over the information patients get about their own medical conditions, to poverty and racism which result in, among other things, higher infant mortality rates and lower life expectancies for the poor and minorities, speaks to the role of politics in the health arena. The deleterious effects of power inequities, when combined with the vulnerability to feelings of powerlessness which illness often evokes, makes politics a particularly significant dimension of health and health care.

In addition to dramatizing that health is a multidimensional phenomenon, AIDS has also illuminated another principle basic to social work in the health field: that understanding of culture is essential in health care. Discussions of AIDS have emphasized the association between the disorder and the "gay life-style." The term "life-style" itself lacks precise meaning, but serves generally as a popular substitute for aspects of culture. Our society is comprised of numerous subgroups with different subcultures. Each has its own set of norms, values, beliefs, customs and environments, some of which are necessarily developed in response to pressures from the dominant culture, that bear on the health of group members. Such cultural patterns shape people's definition of and susceptibility to health problems, their use of lay and professional health care resources, their access to services, their responses to treatment and more.

The term "life-style," when applied to gay men, refers variously to their sexual orientation, sexual practices and/or the social milieu. Gay men, estimated to be about 10% of the male population, are highly diverse in personality, age, race, ethnicity and socio-economic status. Some are married and have children (Bell and Weinberg, 1978). Yet, as members of a minority population unacceptable to the majority, they have had certain common experiences and a number of shared ways of dealing with them. One commonality has been a need for secrecy in work and/or family life to protect against discrimination and rejection. One response to this which bears on the situation with AIDS is that it has been through leisure activities primarily that many gay men have sought acceptance, companionship and sexual partners (Warren, 1974). Particularly in large cities, to which they have gravitated because of the greater possibility of keeping the different segments of their lives separate, bars (and baths to some extent) have served as social centers (Bell and Weinberg, 1978). In many communities, home ownership has been highly valued by gays for the privacy and protection it affords. Here, home gatherings have been important in providing opportunities for gays to meet one another (Warren, 1974). Associated with this pattern of socializing is also acceptance among many gays of casual sexual encounters and sexual activity with numerous partners. Even gays in stable couple relationships tend to regard sex with others as less of a threat to their stability than do heterosexual couples (Bell and Weinberg, 1978).

These aspects of gay "life-style" are implicated in the transmission of AIDS, because the number of people interacting sexually contribute to the spread of any communicable disease (Bazell, 1983). Indeed, there is some speculation that the frequent bouts with a variety of sexually transmitted infections may reduce the resistance of an individual when the AIDS-producing agent attacks (*Sexual Medicine Today*, 1983). Engaging in anal intercourse, with consequent opening of small lesions, is also thought to be an important factor in transmitting AIDS (Bazell, 1983; Seligmann and Gosnell, 1983).

Other shared experiences also shape the response of the individual to his disease. Being gay affects the relationships and resources available for his physical and emotional sustenance, and the reactions by "straight" health care and other workers to him. The concern with the relationship between AIDS and the gay "life-style" can serve as a paradigm, then, for the concern of social workers with the role culture generally plays in health.

Given the fact that AIDS, like all health conditions, is a multidimensional phenomenon, it follows that health care for people with AIDS requires, as does all health care, intervention into the complete system of interacting physical, psychological, social, economic and political forces. Social workers obviously cannot perform all of the necessary health care tasks, and cannot perform many of them alone. We will discuss some tasks that social workers are uniquely equipped to perform and others in which they play a vital part. Common social work tasks involve activities with patients, their significant others, health care providers, the community and policy makers.

WORK WITH PATIENTS

Emotional Reactions of Patients

Social workers in health settings, particularly hospitals and home health agencies, normally see people who have already come into the system for treatment of an illness or injury. They help patients deal with the physical impact of their disorder, with difficulties in gaining access to and making use of medical treatment, with the emotional reactions to their condition and with changes required by it in role performance and relationships with others. AIDS patients may share all these needs.

The diagnosis of AIDS and its subsequent course place severe demands on the coping capacities of the patient. Suspected AIDS patients often endure a long period of uncertainty before the diagnosis can be made. People diagnosed with AIDS then face a usually terminal illness, with limited possibilities for treatment, which will probably proceed through repeated but unpredictable acute episodes over a course of several years. They will probably suffer considerable pain, debilitation, bodily change and possibly physical disfigurement, and eventual death.

The youth of AIDS patients makes coping with this diagnosis particularly difficult and painful. The median age of people with AIDS is 35 (NASW News, 1983). For many, this is the first experience with serious, much less life-threatening, illness, shattering the illusion of immortality they may have held until this time. As a result, many respond with massive denial of the diagnosis or its implications (NASW News, 1983). Anger and depression are also common feeling reactions.

Many sick people struggle with the question, "Why me?" People with AIDS confront the association of this disease with an alternative sexual orientation, usually accompanied by contact with many different sexual partners, both patterns severely censured by much of this society. Because social attitudes so often are internalized, many people with AIDS also experience guilt and self-blame.

Those who have not yet fully accepted their homosexuality may experience even greater self-rejection. One social worker "says his patients have told him, 'I've heard my whole life that I'm going to be punished for being gay. And now it has happened'" (*NASW News*, 1983). With the feelings about their sexual orientation unresolved, dealing with an illness that lends itself so easily to definition as a punishment presents a painful challenge to people with AIDS. These features complicate the normal lowering of self-esteem resulting from the stigma attached to all illness and from the sick person's inability to perform usual valued roles.

Related to the issue of comfort with his homosexuality, the person with AIDS may not have been "out," i.e., public about his sexual orientation, in one or more of the arenas of his life. As his illness becomes known to others, he is forced "out," and must face all the negative reactions to homosexuality which induced him to remain "in the closet."

To add to these stresses, the AIDS patient often encounters isolating behavior from those around him. Illness, particularly severe illness, usually creates a sense of distance, difference or isolation. The seriousness of AIDS, coupled with its association with socially disapproved sexual behavior, and capped by uncertain risks of contagion often produces extreme isolation and ostracism. The person with AIDS may find himself avoided by associates in the workplace, friends and family members. Even intimate friends and lovers may distance themselves, and relationships may flounder under the challenges posed by this disease. Forced to face the resulting feelings of abandonment, to deal alone with the changes in his life and to make critical decisions without support, the usual coping mechanisms of the person with AIDS may be easily overwhelmed (Hausmann, 1983).

Powerlessness

Under these circumstances, social workers may find the person with AIDS experiencing a profound feeling of immobilization and loss of control, loss of control of his body, his relationships, and his future. Other external factors in the course of his treatment do much to aggravate this sense of powerlessness. In the initial stages of the disease, patients can most easily be rendered powerless by a lack of information. During the diagnostic period, there is considerable ambiguity. Some physicians, in their effort not to label the illness as AIDS prematurely, avoid providing much information at all until the case is full-blown and the diagnosis unambiguous. The patients' stress may increase even more as physicians order tests or treatments with little or no explanation of their purpose. Many of these tests are painful and frightening, and patients should be prepared for them. A San Francisco source reported: "Many patients have felt violated by having violent reactions to tests and treatments that they were not psychologically prepared for" (Shanti Project, undated). While some physicians are careful about giving all possible information and some are also scrupulous about encouraging the patient to exercise choice about undergoing tests and treatments, many are not. Often there are alternative treatments or diagnostic tests, which are never offered to the patient. Instead, procedures are decided on by the physician(s) without any explanation to the patient. There have even been instances when treatments, such as placing the patient on a respirator, were carried out even though the patient had specifically requested this not be done.

Terminally ill patients often feel quite dependent on their physicians, who seem their last hope for any amelioration whatsoever. Under these conditions, patients may have trouble resisting or making demands, for fear that their physicians will abandon them. While all of these conditions are commonplace in the treatment of serious and terminal diseases, the lack of much previous knowledge of or familiarity with AIDS increases its mysterious character. For most people, information contributes to the emotional mastery of uncontrollable situations. Even the doctor's acknowledging to the patient the degree of uncertainty can have an orienting effect.

Other aspects of his treatment can further increase the patient's sense of powerlessness. When hospitalized, the person with AIDS may find that services or treatments are delayed or omitted because nursing staff refuse to come into his room or make physical contact with him (Daley, 1983). The usually complex responses patients have to dependence on hospital staff can therefore be further complicated by the increased confrontation with helplessness that occurs when needed help is not provided.

Interventions

These various issues faced by people with AIDS and their responses to them differ, of course, in their particulars from patient to patient; thus social work interventions need to be tailored to each unique situation. But interventions invariably will call for affording the patient opportunities to exercise some autonomy and experience some mastery over his circumstances.

Ventilation or discharge of the strong feelings of patients faced with a terminal illness may be the first and most pressing need the social worker has to help with. Continued attention to the patient's affective responses can then provide assistance in the working through of denial, in the management of anger and in the cognitive processing of the events of his life.

The social worker may also need to assist the patient with reality testing in relation to self-blame based on his homosexuality as well as with possible unresolved issues in accepting his homosexuality or being forced to make it public in areas of his life he had previously chosen not to.

By assisting with devising solutions to the many problems created by the illness, the social worker can help the person with AIDS regain some sense of control over his life. The social worker may need to help him to partialize, i.e., to break a large, complex and overwhelming situation into small, manageable tasks. She might work with him on adhering to regimens or diets, or support his work on a series of small decisions and plans. S/he may help him in gaining access to and paying for treatment or in dealing with health professionals.

The social worker may also have to act to help the patient exercise as much control over his diagnostic workup and treatment as he wants. Direct and straightforward communication with the patient to encourage and support his efforts to communicate with physicians and other health care staff may be required. Rehearsal for such exchanges or the offer to be present during discussions between patient and physician to ask questions or help the patient ask questions and review afterwards may also be indicated. The social worker also has to advocate for the right of the patient to participate to the maximum degree in the decisions affecting him, and to have his wishes regarding treatment adhered to.

Planning

Periodically or permanently, the person with AIDS may become unable to work, straining his financial situation. He may lack the resources to pay for long and costly care. He may become weak and unable to care for himself and his living situation may dissolve around him because of the stigma the disease carries. "Many AIDS patients who don't require constant care have 'no place to go,'" and discharge following hospitalization is often problematic (Management Rounds, 1983). In New York City, which has had about one half of all of the cases of AIDS, it was not until December, 1983 that a nursing home agreed to accept a patient with AIDS (*New York Times*, 12/6/83).

The social worker also assists the patient to prepare for the difficulties that lie in the future: continuing illness, impaired functioning and death. To facilitate this, the social worker can help the person with AIDS find and use needed resources, both within the health care setting and in the community. Planning for care following discharge may require referrals for financial and legal help as well. The disposition of property and the provision for loved ones may be sources of concern. As will be discussed later, there are possible conflicts that occur between the patient's family and his lover, if he has one, and the social worker may help him to anticipate them. The patient might, for example, find it useful to draw up a will.

In the larger cities, the social worker should be able to draw on the resources of the gay community and of local AIDS task forces. These groups, which include both health professionals and lay people, have raised money (the New York group raised several hundred thousand dollars). They have organized and trained groups of volunteers and "buddies" to reduce the isolation of people with AIDS (Collins, 1983). They provide assistance to the individual with AIDS as he becomes weak and debilitated, and needs help with the basic activities of daily living. In Philadelphia, the AIDS Task Force designates service managers who coordinate and advocate for services for individuals with AIDS. These volunteers remain close to the person with AIDS to monitor new needs as they develop (McKeown, 1983). Social workers within health care facilities work out clear allocation and coordination of tasks with such service managers.

In the cities where the larger number of cases of AIDS has occurred, patient groups provide another vital resource for reducing isolation and the sense of powerlessness. Where such groups are linked to AIDS task forces, patients may not only work on the issues discussed but may also be able to join in the social activities of the organizations and to further their experience of empowerment.

WORK WITH FAMILIES AND SIGNIFICANT OTHERS

Social workers often work directly with the patient's family members, as well as with the patient. Family situations can pose many kinds of difficulties, but that of the AIDS patient may be particularly complex. As noted, many gay people keep their homosexuality from their family. Because family members share societal standards, gays may anticipate rejection or castigation by family members, or may know that their family would be pained by knowledge of their sexual orientation. Coppola and Zabarsky (1983) report that four out of five urban gay males interviewed for a 1982 marketing survey had not revealed their homosexuality to their families. Consequently, family members may face a dual crisis, having to deal with the disclosure not only of a diagnosis of terminal illness, but of the patient's homosexuality as well. Under these circumstances, some families have been known to abandon their ties and withhold support from their family members with AIDS (Hausmann, 1983), while others remain involved.

Whether separated from family by his difference, or simply having established adult independence, the gay person may have a stable relationship with a lover, and/or a well-developed intimate network of gay friends that serve as kin. A disease like AIDS presents a severe crisis for whichever "family" system the person with AIDS interacts with. Any catastrophic illness threatens the existing ways of meeting the emotional, financial or other needs of family members. The needs of the patient place new and often unfamiliar demands on those involved in his life. "Significant others" are called on to change important roles to deal with the changed situation, and often, to develop new coping skills.

In this situation, as with patients, social workers need to encourage and support the ventilation by family members of their own strong feelings of pain, anger, grief and fear. As they do with patients, they need to help family members to mobilize their strengths and capacities to deal with the situation. With intervention, some of the retreating network members may be helped to remain engaged with the person with AIDS. The social worker may have to assist the patient and his significant others to open or reopen lines of communication so that mutual problem-solving can take place. With the social worker's support, friends and family members may develop new personal and interpersonal resources, find and use social and community services, plan for new tasks and work on old business. These are common social work tasks with family members, but the situation of the gay person with AIDS adds yet other complications.

In addition to the normal fears felt by the family of a terminally ill patient, those close to the person with AIDS confront a number of other fears. Parents uncomfortable with their son's homosexuality may fear the revelation to others that comes with knowledge of the patient's disease. The wives of those gay men who are or have been married face particularly difficult issues.

All of the people close to the individual with AIDS are likely to experience strong fears of contagion, sometimes to the level of panic. Such fear aggravates whatever impulses the family, friends or lover may have to withdraw from the sick person. The social worker can play a critical role in helping the fearful person to become aware of his/her fears. Sometimes the fear of contagion covers other anxieties and it is important for the person to understand correctly the basis of his/her reaction. It is important that the social worker help family and other involved people to gain and use essential information about avoiding or minimizing the risk of contagion.

Fears of contagion are not the only difficulty for the significant others of the person with AIDS. When he is hospitalized, his lover or his primary circle of friends may be excluded from visiting him by hospital rules limiting visiting, especially in intensive care units, to relatives by blood or marriage. They may also be harassed by hostile hospital staff. Unsuspecting or unsophisticated care providers may simply overlook the visitors' feelings, or their importance to the patient. In this situation, the social workers' role is to advocate for the access to the patient of *all* concerned with his care, "convinc(ing) hospitals to expand the definition of family to include the partners of gay AIDS victims" (*NASW News*, 1983). It is also their task to interpret to other professionals the important role of these people in the patient's life.

In working with adult patients who are married, social workers sometimes encounter situations in which spouses and in-laws conflict over issues in a patient's care. More commonly the two systems are articulated well enough to cooperate. Gay men, in contrast, may have kept their two "family" systems strictly compartmentalized, or there may be distance or resentment between them. Each circle may claim priority in visiting, in making decisions with or for the patient, or in communicating with the health professionals providing care.

Social workers need to be available to help *all* who care about the patient to deal with their reactions, whether to a newly disclosed identity or to the diagnosis. Social workers may need to help mediate between the patient and the two kin networks, and between the family of origin and the family of lover or intimate friends. Most importantly, the social worker needs to be concerned with helping those who care but are in conflict to move beyond their differences to attend to the needs of the patient and to identify tasks they can each carry out, resources they can offer and ways they can work together. The help family members give patients, "(the) strong commitment to their care and nutrition," seems to be a crucial factor in the length of survival of the person with AIDS (Hausman, 1983). To this end, techniques such as bringing together the whole network of friends and family can be most productive. As with patients, groups for family members are a resource for support and mutual problem-solving. Again, where AIDS task forces are organized and family groups linked to them, relatives have also been able to join in social action.

WORK WITH HEALTH CARE STAFF

Health professionals and health personnel, like other people, have strong feelings, attitudes and beliefs about health and illness.

Some react emotionally or negatively to specific diseases or specific groups of patients. Social workers commonly work at solving problems in the relationship between patients and the health care staff treating and caring for them.

Dealing with patients with AIDs can arouse two particular sets of problematic feelings: fear of contagion and rejection of the person not only for his disease, but also for his homosexuality. As noted earlier, medical personnel have been reported to refuse to treat or even enter the rooms of AIDS patients; caretakers leave meal trays at the door of the hospital room; service people refuse to accept anything handled by someone with AIDS (Hausman, 1983; Japenga, 1983; Starr and Gonzalez, 1983). One doctor interviewed said he had been washing some of his AIDS patients, since the hospital aides assigned refused to do the bathing (Collins, 1983). These problems have occurred even though there are clear, well-defined guidelines for health care personnel for protection from infection (Conte et al., 1983), which are the responsibility of the hospital administration and medical staff to implement. Some health care staff condemnatory of homosexuality communicate to the patient their blame of him for his illness and their view of the disease as a just punishment for his variant sexual behavior. There are three needs in this situation: for clear and specific information about the disease and about homosexuality, for a chance to work through feelings, and for continued support when working with patients in a threatening as well as painful and stressful situation.

Part of the social worker's mandate, therefore, is to initiate or help design in-service programs to inform health facility staff about all known facts about AIDS. These efforts have to include transport, maintenance and other non-professional staff. These personnel carry responsibility for day-to-day patient contact, but are often omitted from special training efforts. Social workers recognize that preparation for staff is not solely a question of *facts*, but of helping people to raise to consciousness, express, and begin to work through their feelings and fears. Moreover, people have to deal not only with their fear of the disease, but with their attitudes about gay people, feelings they may not have had to face previously.

Physicians with negative emotions and stereotyped attitudes may pose a particular threat to humane medical treatment and service delivery. Doctors control decisions about patient care and are the acknowledged authority and assigned leader for other health care personnel. We have already discussed the issue of communication with patients in an earlier section; there are other issues as well. Like other staff, physicians may fear contamination by the person with AIDS. They may also experience a threat to their sense of competence and mission betokened by the very poor prognosis for AIDS. Such experiences can sometimes result in unrecognized anger toward patients, withdrawal from them and their families, low morale, or disregard for ethical standards such as confidentiality or the patient's right to information. This behavior exacerbates the feeling of powerlessness of patients already debilitated and stigmatized.

In collaborating with physicians and other staff, social workers generally are required to educate them about the characteristics and needs of patients. When dealing with health care staff, just as when dealing with patients or others, the social worker needs not only to identify problems but also to mobilize people's strengths. By creating opportunities for ventilation of feelings, support from team members and the development of coping capacities, they make it possible for staff to treat patients competently and with compassion and commitment. Their relationships with others are important tools for these tasks.

One further issue, that of confidentiality and privacy, may require the attention of the social worker. How the hospital handles information can greatly increase or decrease the control the patient has over who knows either his diagnosis or his sexual orientation. Social workers may need to advocate within the hospital to guarantee that communications, both formal and informal, within the hospital or health care facility are avoided which "broadcast . . . the patient's diagnosis, medical condition, sexual orientation or personal habits" (Philadelphia Aids Task Force, undated). Existing hospital guidelines for protecting the confidentiality of patients with infectious diseases should be followed for notices posted on doors, the marking of specimens for lab work, etc. Where such guidelines are lacking or inadequate, this may become an area for advocacy. In this as in other issues, by finding and joining with other knowledgeable and concerned staff, the social worker can broaden his/her base of influence.

WORK WITH THE COMMUNITY

People in the community at large as well as the staff of social welfare agencies are also apt to experience the fear of illness and of ill people, hostility towards those with AIDS and ignorance of facts that health care personnel are susceptible to. The community's negative responses to people with AIDS make patients vulnerable to the arguments over jurisdiction and "buck-passing" which commonly occur between health, welfare and housing agencies when dealing with "problem" populations such as mentally impaired aged, the homeless, etc. Since it is the social worker who is the person in the health setting with responsibility for dealing with social agencies, it is necessary that s/he advocate with the web of community services on behalf of clients, find and mobilize the needed resources, develop and use relationships with staff in other agencies, identify barriers to care, identify and document gaps in service and stimulate the development of new services.

In addition to case-by-case problem-solving with community agencies, health care social workers may also have to take the lead in developing needed educational and support workshops for community health and social service workers who will be dealing with people with AIDS. In the cities with AIDS Task Forces, members of the gay and professional communities, including many social workers, have been carrying out some of these tasks. Health care social workers will therefore find already developed advocacy and community education efforts with which to collaborate.

A larger task confronts social workers in challenging community attitudes. The media attest to the frightened and destructive reactions to AIDS. Coworkers have demanded that an AIDS sufferer be isolated or fired. Funeral directors have refused to embalm the bodies of those who died from AIDS (Collins, 1983; Starr and Gonzalez, 1983). There have been bills to incarcerate gays "until and unless they can be cleansed of their medical problems" (Beauchamp, 1983); in more than one state there have been proposals to "recriminalize" homosexual behavior (Morgenthau et al., 1983). The number of calls to health departments and to a federal AIDS hotline, still 5,000 a day (Seligmann and Gosnell, 1983; *New York Times*, 8/22/83), indicate the level of public anxiety. Indeed, the panic of contagion is not limited to AIDs patients, but is transferred by many to include all gay men. People call hotlines to ask if "they can catch AIDS from a bus seat, from food served by a gay waiter . . . (or) . . . from documents handled by a gay co-worker" (Seligmann and Gosnell, 1983). *Newsweek* reports:

> In cities like San Francisco and New York . . . there have been reports of gays being told to leave restaurants, being refused ambulance service and being evicted from their apartments, all because they have – or might have – AIDS. (Morgenthau et al., 1983)

Social workers cannot be unconcerned with the impact that this heightened stigmatization carries for the entire gay population.

Social workers have to take an active part in educating the larger community through public forums and community groups. Special efforts might be taken to reach groups who have expressed specific concern about contagion, such as undertakers or the police and firefighters, who are called on in emergencies to give mouth-to-mouth resuscitation. Educational workshops can inform these groups about AIDS, dispel myths about people with AIDS and interpret the needs of patients and families. They can also educate about and advocate for the rights of all gays. Again, where AIDS Task Forces are engaged in community activity, health care social workers can contribute to or call upon their educational resources.

WORK IN THE POLICY ARENA

The final task for health care social workers is to wield influence in the policy arena. Legislators and policy makers, like their constituents, may be ignorant of health care needs and share some of the community's attitudes which have negative consequences for health care. Special efforts are needed to represent the health needs of poor or disenfranchised groups. Social work intervention in the policy arena requires advocacy, collaboration with other concerned health care providers and consumers and the development of coalitions for political influence. The effectiveness of such efforts to create political influence depends upon the visible presence of a constituency that is not only concerned but informed. Direct service health care social workers occupy a particularly advantageous position to gather data, case by case, on the impact of legislation and regulations on health and health care. Specific tasks social workers may perform such as writing letters or testifying at hearings also depend upon solid documentation.

In dealing with AIDS, social workers need to keep close records of their observations in order to be able to document obstacles to treatment and gaps in service. They may need to develop guidelines for recording that assure the systematic gathering and compiling of information about poorly met or unmet needs.

Social workers also need to keep informed and inform patients, families and other health providers of legislative and regulatory processes, of actions in progress and of organized efforts to advocate for the interests of those affected by AIDS. They need to join and assist others in joining lobbying efforts. The designation of $20 million by the Department of Health and Human Services (*Philadelphia Inquirer*, 8/18/83) and $5.3 million by the State of New York (Chira, 1983) for AIDS research are responses to political pressure. Continued pressure is needed so that funds are also allocated for health and social services. Based on the service needs they identify and their knowledge of health and social welfare systems, social workers may also be able to offer specific proposals for the allocation of funds or for changes in existing institutional programs and policies, thereby lending their special expertise to the effort to bring help to the AIDS situation.

SOCIAL WORK AND AIDS: CONCLUSIONS

All of these social work tasks have in common the goals of minimizing the negative impact of AIDS and of mobilizing the resources of individuals and institutions to deal with AIDS. The foregoing discussion has pointed up problems resulting from negative attitudes, beliefs and feelings. The presentation of the social workers' tasks is not meant to imply that social workers are less susceptible than others to the reactions described — that they do not fear exposure to a contagious disease, experience difficulty working with terminal patients or lack complete comfort and knowledge in dealing with homosexuality. Social workers differ, however, from the majority of others dealing with health in taking responsibility for developing and acting with self-awareness. In order to perform the tasks identified here, social workers must examine and bring into consciousness their own attitudes, beliefs and feelings, and the ways these affect their responses. Recognizing their own responses is necessary to assure that their interventions are guided by the clients' needs rather than their own. Understanding their own negative reactions also allows social workers to be more attuned to the fears and defenses of others.

Achieving and maintaining this self-awareness can be very demanding. Considering the complexities of AIDS, social workers should not expect to be able to meet this challenge alone. To assure self-aware practice, they ought to draw on individual and peer supervision, consultation, workshops, seminars and similar resources to examine feelings, increase knowledge, check out perceptions, work through concerns and garner support.

The responsibility for self-awareness, as well as the other tasks described, involves the application of general principles of social work practice to the specifics of the AIDS situation. The experience with AIDS has also provided some lessons applicable to all health issues.

Dealing with isolation and powerlessness is one example. Identifying and challenging discriminatory practices, exploiting the power of groups and linking patients and those close to them to organizations mobilized for social action are measures social workers can employ in a variety of circumstances. These reduce isolation and help people gain control over the conditions which affect their health and health care.

Collaboration is another example. The AIDS task forces have brought together patients and health care providers, professionals and lay people. By reducing barriers between groups and joining common interests, they have created a greatly expanded network of resources for all sorts of tasks, from direct patient care to lobbying. They also helped to reduce some of the power disparities that exist in relationships among health professionals and between health care providers and consumers. These task forces can serve as a model for dealing with other concerns, or at least as a reminder that there are common interests that can be served through such alliances.

Regard for the culture or "life-style" of patients is a third example. Attention to the vulnerability of the gay population to AIDS and to negative reactions to their differences is only one aspect of this situation applicable to work with other cultural sub-groups; recognizing and drawing on the strengths that exist within each group is another. Involving whatever people are close to patients and drawings on the assets of the subcultural community to which the patient belongs add to the total network of available resources. They also offset the alienation of disadvantaged patients from the "dominant-culture" health care system.

The focus on multiple targets to meet health care needs is a final example of the experience with AIDS useful to social workers dealing with other health care problems. Recognition of the social context of AIDS and the simultaneous intervention with both individuals and institutions within that context is a striking feature of the response to AIDS. This approach is needed in all health care, but particularly in that for stigmatized groups such as the poor, minorities and the aged.

As funding issues increasingly reverse the progress toward health care as a right, it becomes imperative that, as with AIDS, social workers practice in an advocacy mode. It is also necessary to move beyond a case-by-case approach to confront the politics of health care at every level.

REFERENCES

Altman, L. Debate grows on U.S. listing of Haitians in AIDS category. *New York Times*, 7/31/83.

Bazell, R. The strange history of a new epidemic. *The New Republic*, August 1, 1983.

Bell, A. P. & Weinberg, M. S. *Homosexualities: A Study of Diversity Among Men and Women*. New York: Simon and Schuster, 1978.

Beauchamp, W. A second AIDS epidemic. *New York Times*, 8/7/83.

Byron, P. AIDS and the gay men's health crisis of New York. *Gay Community News*, 8/6/83.

Chira, S. Cuomo says state will step up AIDS research and assist victims. *New York Times*, 6/23/83.

Collins, G. A moral epidemic. *Vanity Fair*, September, 1983.

Conte, J. E., Hadley, W. K., Sande, M., and the University of California & the San Francisco Task Force on the Acquired Immunodeficiency Syndrome. Special report: infection-control guidelines for patients with the acquired immunodeficiency syndrome, AIDS. *The New England Journal of Medicine*, 1983, *309*, 740-744.

Coppola, V. & Zabarsky, M. Coming out of the closet. *Newsweek*, 8/8/83.

Daley, M. AIDS anxiety. *New York*, 6/20/83.

Hausmann, K. Treating victims of AIDS poses challenge to psychiatrists. *Psychiatric News*, August, 1983.

Japenga, A. Life and death in the country's first AIDS ward. *Philadelphia Enquirer*, 8/7/83.

Krauthammer, C. The political uses of a deadly disease. *The New Republic*, 8/1/83.

Management Rounds, AIDS cited as major administrative concern. *Hospitals*, 8/1/83.

McKeown, P. No AIDS cure so buddies offer comfort. *Philadelphia Daily News*, 8/10/83.

McKeown, P. AIDS hot line: beacon in the darkness of panic. *Philadelphia Daily News*, 8/10/83.

Morgenthau, T., Coppola, V., Carey, J., Cooper, N., Raine, G., McCormick, J. & Friendly, D. T. Gay America in transition. *Newsweek*, 8/8/83.

Murphy, M. Newsmakers, *Newsweek*, 7/18/83.

NASW News, Workers help AIDS victims handle stress, guilt. May, 1983.

New York Times, 5,000 a day reach a federal telephone hot line, 3,000 more get busy signal, 8/22/83.

New York Times, First AIDS nursing home admission, 12/6/83.

Philadelphia AIDS Task Force. AIDS questions and answers, 11/10/82.

Philadelphia AIDS Task Force, Infection control guidelines for health care and related workers, 1982.

Philadelphia Inquirer, U.S. to add $20 million in AIDS war, 8/18/83.

Philadelphia Inquirer, Mayor angry at transfer of Florida AIDS case, 10/9/83.

Seligmann, J. & Gosnell, M. AIDS: fears and facts. *Newsweek*, 8/8/83.

Sexual Medicine Today, Facing AIDS, September 14, 1983.

Shanti Project, Psychosocial needs of AIDS patients, undated.

Starr, M. & Gonzalez, D. L. The panic over AIDS. *Newsweek*, 7/14/83.

Sullivan, R. City takes Haitians off list of high-risk AIDS groups. *New York Times*, 7/29/83.

United States Public Health Service. Facts about AIDS, August, 1983.

United States Public Health Service, toll-free AIDS hotline, 800-342-AIDS, 2/27/84.

Warren, C. A. B. *Identity and Community in the Gay World*. New York: John Wiley, 1974.

ADDITIONAL RESOURCE MATERIALS

Bergstrom, W. & Cruz, L. *Counseling Lesbian and Gay Male Youth*, National Network of Runaway and Youth Services, 1983. (Includes recommended readings and national resources.)

Fairchild, B. & Hayward, N. *Now That You Know: What Every Parent Should Know about Homosexuality*. New York: Harcourt, Brace, Jovanovich, 1979.
National Gay Health Directory. National Gay Health Education Foundation, P.O. Box 834, Linden Hill, N.J. 11354.
Siegal, F. & Siegal, M. *AIDS: The Medical Mystery*. New York: Grove Press, 1983. (Scientific. Written by M.D. and M.A.)
West, D.J. *Homosexuality Reexamined*. Minneapolis: University of Minnesota Press, 1977. (Good basic overview of fact and fiction.)
Woodman, N. J. & Lenna, H. R. *Counseling with Gay Men and Women*. San Francisco: Jossey-Bass, 1980). (Both authors are social workers. Includes annotated bibliography.)

Developing Responsiveness to the Health Needs of Hispanic Children and Families

Sylvia Guendelman, LCSW, DSW

SUMMARY. Admission to a tertiary care pediatric hospital is a stressful experience for the Hispanic child and family. The stress partially stems from the institutional barriers that conflict with the psychosocial needs of Hispanic families.

This article identifies six psychosocial needs of Hispanics and examines related risks for coping disturbances encountered during the hospitalization process. These risks can be reduced by increasing health providers' understanding of the psychosocial needs of Hispanics and by specifying culturally appropriate interventions. The development of cross-cultural committees, protocols, and hospital based Hispanic self-help networks represent distinct modalities for improving responsiveness to the health needs of Hispanic families in a hospital setting.

Admission to a pediatric hospital delivering acute and specialized care is a very stressful experience for the Hispanic child and his family. The source of stress lies not only in the child's diagnosis and response to treatment. It is also linked to institutional barriers which conflict with the psychosocial needs of Hispanic families.

The purpose of this article is to identify psychosocial needs and problems commonly encountered by Hispanic families when their

At the time of writing Dr. Guendelman was an Adjunct Assistant Professor in the Maternal and Child Health Program, 306 Earl Warren Hall, School of Public Health at the University of California, Berkeley, CA 94720. The material for this article is drawn from the author's experience as Clinical Social Worker, Social Service Department, Children's Hospital Medical Center, Oakland, California.
Reprinted from *Social Work in Health Care*, Volume 8(4), Summer 1983.

children are hospitalized. The author's experience and observations suggest that Hispanic families are at particular risk for developing disturbances in family functioning and coping behaviors that hamper delivery of medical care. These risks can be reduced by increasing health providers' awareness of the psychosocial needs of Hispanics and by specifying culturally appropriate interventions.

BACKGROUND

It is amply recognized in the health field that poverty and ethnicity are significant determinants of health status. Since Blacks are four times as likely and Hispanics are three times as likely to be below the poverty level as whites (U.S. HEW, 1977), it is not surprising that non-whites suffer more medical problems. Poor children are at a particular disadvantage. A child's health is vulnerable to overcrowded and inadequate housing, violence, poor nutrition and other health standards of his community. It is also affected by the behaviors of his caregivers, their responsiveness to his health needs and the resources available to them for care. A failure or delay in detecting, reporting or following up on a health problem by a parent may result in errors of prevention or treatment. Similarly, barriers that prevent a family from obtaining adequate care can result in poorer diagnosis or more severe prognosis. In fact, according to Budetti (Budetti, Butler & McMannus, 1982) poor children's greater medical needs can be partly explained because they receive less preventive care and enter the acute care system later than the non-poor. Late entry to specialized care systems leads to a more episodic, high-cost, high technology care.

High technology pediatric hospitals serve a high proportion of indigent non-white children. For example, compared to other hospitals in California, the seven children's hospitals throughout the state provide more specialized intensive care and a higher amount of care to indigent children. A higher proportion of youngsters are in the lower age groups, requiring more medical and patient care assistance. They require more exacting rates and precise doses of medication due to lower tolerances of intravenous administration. Young children also need more psychological and social services to help them as well as their families cope with a stressful environment away from home and with the disruptions in normal growth and development.

Although awareness of the psychosocial needs of children in hospitals is widespread, there is a tendency to overlook the multi-cultural needs of patients. Patients and families who have belief systems, language and cultural responses that differ from the mainstream are particularly vulnerable to encounter adjustment problems. Hence they require special attention from the health care providers. As part of an interdisciplinary team, social workers can make a significant contribution as change agents, helping health systems become more responsive to the needs of ethnic patients.

The material for this article is drawn from the author's experience as a Clinical Social Worker at Children's Hospital Medical Center (CHMC) in Oakland, California. CHMC is a teaching hospital that provides a range of primary, acute and specialty care services to approximately 6,800 in-patients and 89,000 out-patient children a year. Between 55 and 60% of the patients receive Medicare (Medicaid). Approximately 20% of the patients are Hispanic, primarily of Mexican descent. They are predominantly from poor, working class families who have migrated to the U.S. in the last decade or two. Many are undocumented immigrants and face legal, economic and educational barriers to proper utilization of the health system.

PSYCHOSOCIAL NEEDS OF HISPANIC FAMILIES IN A PEDIATRIC HOSPITAL

The Hispanic child admitted to the hospital is usually accompanied by his family throughout the experience. It can be a source of strain particularly if certain needs are not acknowledged by the providers of health care. What are some of these needs?

1. The Need for Maintaining the Family Together

When children don't feel well, they usually turn to their mothers for comfort. If in addition to feeling ill they are fearful of the unfamiliar surroundings and treatment, children normally turn to their parents for protection. Such behaviors are expected of hospitalized children. It is also expected that as they recover and become familiarized with the setting, attachment behaviors will subside. According to developmental theory, the older the child the easier the adjustment. However, frequently, this is not the case with Hispanic children. Not only do they seem to experience more separation anxiety, but they also demand continuous physical presence of the parent. Should the parent leave the bedside, Hispanic children get very upset. Very often, no other caregiver will be able to calm them down and they will not feel secure until the parent is back in sight.

These reactions can be understood within the context of culture and specifically of first generation Mexican American families. Mexican American children tend to be very dependent on their parents, particularly on their mothers who are the primary caregivers (Falicov & Karrer, 1980). Children are less pressured to achieve, develop self-mastery and autonomy at early ages as compared to Anglo and Black children. Weaning from the bottle, toilet training and self-dressing skills tend to be extended several months beyond the average mainstream childrearing norms.

Mexican American mothers value nurturing and perceive themselves as the main gratifiers of their children's needs. Usually it is an external event, such as the arrival of a new child or entry into school, rather than an internal readiness which shifts parents' expectations towards demanding more from their offspring (Falicov & Karrer, 1980).

When a child is hospitalized, the mother's need to offer comfort and protection to her child is strongly activated. She will cater to the child's wishes, indulging him with food, candy and affection. She will turn down lodging arrangements that may distance her from her child. Any suggestions that prompt her to leave the bedside to seek respite are to no avail. Separation anxiety in the mother is notorious regardless of the severity of the child's illness. In fact, insistence on separation from her child may trigger guilt reactions. The guilt is partly rooted in cultural and religious expectations. A woman's self-image is closely tied to her role as nurturer of her children, rather than as a spouse or individual. A mother's nurturing role is modeled after the Virgin Mary, a symbol of love and abnegation. Failure to live up to expectations of devotion to her children generates guilty feelings.

Hospitalization, particularly when it happens far away from

home, will separate the mother and ill child from the rest of the family. Almost always the mother chooses to protect the sick youngster and leave the other children behind. This split is a source of worry and ambivalence to parents, particularly when no suitable caregiving arrangements have been made. If the hospital visit is brief and not too far from home, the entire family may accompany the sick child. It is not uncommon for the school-aged siblings to miss school in order to remain and support the ailing one. Childrearing values prioritize cooperation among family members over individual achievement. In times of stress it is expected that the family will gather together and be cohesive. The sense of duty towards the family is valued beyond responsibilities towards meeting external obligations. This is often referred to as familismo (Hoppe & Heller, 1975). Spurred by this sense of obligation, the father usually accompanies mother and child to the hospital, although it is not expected that he partake in the child's care. That is the role of the mother. The father is usually there to offer support in times of crises and act as a mediator and buffer between his family and the hospital. Family roles are often markedly stereotyped and boundaries are not easily crossed. The less acculturated to the American mainstream, the more apparent is this behavior in families. Fathers are looked upon as the authority figure and expect respect from their wives. They also expect to be involved in the medical plans and decisions pertaining to the sick child. Failure to do so may be interpreted as an attempt to overstep boundaries by their spouses or a lack of respect by health providers. If a father does not feel competent in acting as mediator he may bring a support person to help out, particularly for translation purposes. Other times, an older child who has a better command of English will perform this task.

The interdependence among family members is strong and acts as a natural support system in times of stress. It extends to embrace compadres, relatives and godparents who may be closely involved in providing emotional, practical and financial assistance. This network plays a significant role in maintaining family stability. In situations where economic or legal constraints prevent a father from coming to the hospital, the network takes over. An older brother may take the place of the absent father. Other replacements are also in order: A "comadre" may fill the void left by a distant grandmother or take over the care of the children remaining at home while the family is in the hospital.

The G. family's experience is a good illustration.

> A.G., a three-year-old, was transported from Reno, Nevada for treatment of acute lymphocytic leukemia (ALL). She was accompanied by her parents who left their four other children behind, in care of a "comadre" who lived nearby. During the two week hospitalization period the couple remained faithfully next to A.G. spending the nights huddled in a narrow cot next to her bed. A.G. adamantly protested each time her mother left the room, while comfortably allowing Mr. G. to venture out. She often resisted the meals that her mother patiently spoon fed to her, accepting candy instead. As. A.G. improved Mrs. G. began to leave her bedside at naptime. Her anxiety shifted towards her children left behind. However, neither she nor her husband was ready to alter this arrangement. Albeit exhausted and uncomfortable, they refused to sleep in the parents' room, insisting that it would scare A.G. Mr. G., torn by the family split and work responsibilities in a restaurant, frequently questioned whether to stay. In the evenings, when A.G. was asleep they could call home to check on their children. Despite the upheaval, both parents knew that if they chose to leave A.G. behind they would break down. Their close presence was a necessary source of support.

Separation events that jeopardize family interdependence or judgmental attitudes by health professionals that label families as overprotective, anxious or intrusive, hamper adaptive skills necessary for coping at times of heightened vulnerability.

2. The Need for Easy Access to the Hospital

Families are very often faced with practical problems that impede access to the hospital. The lack of transportation, a phone or adequate child care arrangements are not uncommon among first generation Hispanics who are still uprooted from the mainstream socioeconomic system. A family may lack the financial means to purchase a car or may not qualify for a driver's license due to functional illiteracy or language barriers. Since families tend to have many children, child care can become a big concern. Who will take care of them if there is no money to pay someone and the family is not eligible for homemaker services? Should the father stay at home and assume the caregiving role, thereby jeopardizing his job and failing to earn the hourly wage that feeds the family? Should he accompany his wife and child to the hospital, neglecting both his job and the other children? Arrangements can be made by turning to the natural supports if available to the family. But recent immigrants often lack such resources and experience tremendous challenges to overcoming barriers to hospital accessibility. They may leave the children behind unsupervised by an adult, while both parents accompany the child at the hospital; or else the father will work, care for the children and in addition commute long hours for a brief hospital visit.

In the case of a 9-year-old child, admission for chemotherapy treatment disrupted the family's routine in many ways. M.S. was one of six children who had migrated to the U.S. recently with her mother and siblings to join her father. He was an undocumented immigrant worker in a chicken farm about 200 miles away from CHMC, working long hours for little pay. When M.S. was hospitalized he remained at work. He was paid by the hour and thus could not afford to stop. Since his wife accompanied the child to the hospital, the CCS worker agreed to pay for a homemaker to care for the children ranging in age between 2 and 11, while their father worked. However, the homemaker was unreliable and on those days when she did not come Mr. S. had to stay home. This family had no network to turn to for support. By the end of the month an angry Mr. S. worried over not having enough income to cover the rent and escalating telephone expenses incurred by his wife in the hospital. In despair Mrs. S. went back home leaving her child alone and depressed. Over the weekend Mr. S. came to pick her up, driving all night so that he could arrive home and not miss work the following day.

Separated families face difficulties contacting each other by phone. Unable to communicate in English, they often cannot express their needs to a switchboard operator or ward clerk. As a result, the call takes a long time to get through and not always reaches the appropriate party. The expenses increase alongside the frustration. Families complain that they don't have access to each other even by phone. Some hospitals lack sufficient lodging facilities for families, so that the option to visit with the entire family is not available either. As a result families end up being very isolated from the natural supports with increasing feelings of anxiety and depression.

3. The Need to Be Oriented to the Hospital

Delivery of care in a high-technology teaching hospital can be very confusing and threatening to families. The setting involves sophisticated equipment, collaboration with a team of medical and allied health providers and a quick tempo. For Hispanic families, particularly the undocumented immigrant, entry to this type of setting creates tremendous dissonance. Delivery of care is so different from the neighborhood health center, private practitioner, healer or home based care. It requires an array of skills necessary to function in a complex industrialized society: reading and writing; proficiency in English; assertiveness to ensure that one's needs are met; grasp of the billing system; basic concepts of biology and technology; a sense of the immediacy of time; a sense of how complex organizations function and of how mainstream society thinks and acts. As one parent visiting his infant in the Intensive Care Nursery described his experience: "Coming here is like entering a spaceship ready to be launched to the moon."

Obviously families cannot be educated in these skills throughout the course of hospitalization. But they can be supported through the cultural shock and be provided with basic tools to familiarize themselves with the hospital setting, routines and key resources. Brochures in Spanish, bilingual switchboard operators, guided tours and parent groups can be effective vehicles for bridging this gap.

4. The Need for Social Supports

When the natural support system is disturbed or fails to meet the demands brought forth by a crisis, some families become so overwhelmed by the complexity that they withdraw, becoming very passive or else stop visiting. Others respond by reaching out. They seek out health providers who can orient them to the setting, explain the diagnosis and health plans, relieve their anxiety, provide reassurance and comfort. Individuals naturally gravitate to those who express readiness to help, whether another patient's family or a staff member. Barriers are insurmountable, however, when health providers cannot communicate because of language limitations or because they are out of touch with the problems that families are undergoing. In a teaching hospital, communication gaps are also spurred by the discontinuity of care. In a setting where nurses shift duties which do not necessarily accommodate the same children and where medical students and house staff rotate, Hispanic patients encounter a variety of providers who have many questions but may offer few and often discrepant answers to their concerns. Under such circumstances it is difficult to develop trusting patient-provider relationships that allow for open access to medical information, clarification and reassurance. Families become very isolated, feel helpless and confused. At a time of increased vulnerability they are forced into a dependency with undermines their ability to grasp medical problems and reinforces the cultural, social and cognitive blocks already existing both in the family and the hospital systems.

5. The Need to Understand the Child's Diagnosis and Treatment

Usually diagnoses involving acute or chronic illnesses are not readily understood. It takes several opportunities for clarification before a family can incorporate the information. There is some evidence suggesting that working through a translator as opposed to communicating with the patient in his own language reduces the patient's trust in the physician and compliance with the treatment. It can also delay proper understanding of the medical problem and intervention plans. Several health professionals have commented that Hispanics place more emphasis on trust than on technology. Therefore explanations derived from an open, warm, clear conversation are more readily accepted than those based on pure facts or technical explanations (personal communication; Martinez, 1978).

Although a few families readily accept technology as a symbol of upward mobility, the majority are wary of sophisticated equipment.

Non-English speaking Hispanics need to be able to communicate with providers who can speak Spanish. They also need to review consent forms in Spanish and have the opportunity to go over these with proper help. Very often families are given consent forms to sign without adequate translation or explanation. This is another indication of the abdication of responsibility that families are thrust into, increasing their sense of helplessness and dependency on the medical system.

Some families express interest in descriptive information that they can keep. There is a dearth of brochures and health books in Spanish directed to the non-English speaking Hispanic to help them bridge the cultural and medical gap and encourage patient self-determination.

6. Need to Be Respected in a Non-judgemental Way

Hispanics share some cultural beliefs that are not readily accepted among other health professionals. Certain health beliefs conflict with Western medicine. For example, a reliance on herbal treatments as opposed to drugs for curing certain ailments; or drawing on superstition and magical or evil forces as a source of causation rather than on scientific facts.

A grossly underestimated cultural difference which often clashes with the mainstream culture is the attitude towards life and death. Hispanics, particularly those who are closer to nature and religion, have a tendency to accept death as the natural course of life. When death strikes or threatens to take a person away, one does not fight it, but succumbs to "God's will." This acceptance or surrender to "what is" conflicts with the basic tenets of science and the striving to save lives. Consequently a spontaneous acceptance of death is often met with resistance by the medical staff who subscribe to the power and efficacy of science and technology. Health professionals interpret this "fatalistic attitude" as defeatist, a symbol of "not caring," not valuing human life which clashes with the medical model that prescribes doing something to fight death. At other times it is interpreted as "ignorance" and "primitivism" rather than a coming to terms with the unknown and therefore with life itself.

This attitude of acceptance without struggle can also interfere with the expected compliance towards medical treatment or consent to treat. For example, a family can be hard pressed to accept the need for continuing painful treatment of a child with cancer if the chances of survival are low or if the pain outweighs the hope of survival.

These are delicate choices colored by philosophical, religious and cultural orientations that require tolerance and appreciation by health professionals. Another source of cultural variation lies in the area of food. Much has been written about the hot and cold approaches that some Hispanic cultures profess towards food and its relationship to disease (Clark, 1959; Acosta Johnson, 1979). From this perspective food ingredients are classified according to hot and cold properties and their effects on balancing the organism and curing disease. There is another dimension to food which so far has received little attention, yet is more widespread. For Hispanics food has a distinctive social connotation. It is an expression of identity and connectedness. Food denotes a person's regional-ethnic background and historical legacy which can be readily shared with peers in order to bring them closer together. Children are raised on ethnic food which excludes hamburgers and hot dogs. It is no wonder that they reject this food in the hospital. Parents respond to this apparent lack of appetite with anxiety and worry over the child's condition. The need for an ethnic menu that is consonant with the culture and the availability of facilities for self-cooking can significantly contribute towards family well-being. Cooking opportunities are most welcomed by mothers who through this vehicle can express their competence, please their children, regain some control and thereby enhance their self-esteem.

Respect for the Hispanic family also requires a recognition of the survival difficulties that first generation immigrants encounter. Many families are undocumented immigrants (MALDEF estimates that there are approximately 1.5 million undocumented immigrants in California) and live in constant fear of deportation. They feel particularly vulnerable in a complex, unfamiliar hospital which requires filling out forms and validation of documentation. Often families refrain from seeking or accepting help for fear of disclosing their status. They need strong reassurance to overcome this fear.

A lack of compliance with medical orders or treatment suggestions is not always based on inadequate communication. Sometimes families lack the adequate economic resources to afford the medication or treatment, but are afraid to disclose it because of legal repercussions, pride or shyness. Families often do not qualify for Medicaid and do not have another source of insurance to secure payment.

All these needs have to be incorporated in an assessment of Hispanic family functioning in a hospital setting. Nevertheless, by themselves assessments are not sufficient. Required is a concomitant institutional awareness of the role that the hospital plays in improving responsiveness to the health care needs of the families that it serves.

IMPROVING RESPONSIVENESS, REDUCING BARRIERS

Failure to respond to Hispanics in ways that are consonant with their cultural and social needs undermines their capacity to function in a hospital setting. Families are frequently placed in a double-bind situation in which they are expected to actively participate in their children's care and health plans while at the same time are forced into a dependent role which reinforces helpless behaviors, offering few mechanisms for redressing this situation.

Health professionals expect that families will actively cooperate with the medical team, consent to a treatment based on an understanding of the facts and comply with the treatment regimen. However, these expectations tend to be accompanied by institutional behaviors that deter Hispanic families from meeting such expectations. Often psychosocial needs are not recognized or not met. Consequently families experience barriers to proper utilization of hospital services and coping difficulties.

Families exposed to this double-bind situation stand the risk of under-functioning or over-functioning in the hospital setting. In the first case, families learn that the way to adapt to an unreceptive yet controlling environment (since it expects compliance) is to react to it rather than act upon it. This coping style is referred to as learned helplessness. Those who cope in this defensive manner become submissive, quiet and non-demanding. They express a sense of helplessness, futility and apathy that lowers their self-esteem and thwarts their motivation to act. They often exhibit depression and withdrawal during the hospital experience.

On the other hand, families who struggle against this dependency and want to maintain their autonomy show increased anxiety. They overfunction, persistently seeking out help and feeling frustrated or distressed when it is not forthcoming. They are susceptible to cues from providers encouraging active participation in their child's care while confronting personal or institutional obstacles that prevent them from doing so. Consider for example a mother who is encouraged by the nursery staff to regularly visit her premature infant. She understands the importance of bonding and is prepared to visit. As the child's stay in the hospital lingers, her access to transportation (i.e., availability of funds and a driver) begins to dwindle, she turns to health providers for help. When they have no solution to her transportation needs, she feels stranded, anxious and guilty. She owns expectations of good mothering, yet she cannot meet them. She may try to keep up with her baby's progress by phone contact. However, language barriers may undermine such attempts. She may call different providers, getting varying responses, all of which increase her level of anxiety and feelings of inadequacy opposite her baby and the nursery team.

Consider this other case in which a mother is requested to consent to a surgical intervention to be performed on her child. She agrees to sign the consent form without actually understanding the problem. She then tries to relay this information to her spouse without much success. They seek further clarification but by then the specialist and/or interpreter are not available. They anxiously try to locate a source of information. When they do, they find that the explanation is beyond their understanding. They persist on obtaining further clarification but are met with condescending or impatient remarks by health providers.

From an institutional perspective, both under- and over-functioning styles interfere with the smooth delivery of medical and patient care. This interference gets translated into increased referrals and utilization of social and mental health services; more medical team conferences per child; increased frustrations for families and health providers; and a higher risk of deterring Hispanics from further utilization of health services. The overall result is an increase in cost of services.

As long as these coping styles continue to be linked to individual weaknesses or deficiencies of Hispanics rather than stemming from a combination of family needs and institutional barriers, the issues will remain unresolved.

Health institutions need to promote the child and family's well-being by strengthening decision making skills in families and extending resources and opportunities to facilitate participation in health care. To the extent that families learn how to deal effectively with their problems, they experience more self-esteem (White, 1960). And to the extent that they learn how to make health promoting decisions, they experience a greater degree of control over their lives (Lenrow & Burch, 1981). For this learning to take place, a receptive atmosphere needs to develop in the hospital setting; one which addresses the culturally specific psychosocial needs described.

INTERVENTION STRATEGIES

1. Shifting the Definition of the Problem from a "Patient Problem" to an "Institution Problem"

This strategy aims at developing awareness among hospital administrators and health professionals of their responsibility in helping to create conditions that support family strengths. There is a growing recognition of the need for bilingual and bicultural staff in hospitals serving non-English speaking patients. Much remains to be done in terms of developing sensitivity among health providers to the cultural idiosyncracies of Hispanics. At Children's Hospital (CHMC) a Cross-Cultural Committee was established to focus on ways to develop cultural awareness in providers. It has organized workshops on specific cultural issues and ethnic pot-lucks aimed at sharing food, music and cultural heritages. It also has introduced multi-ethnic material in the orientation to new employees. There is an increased awareness by health providers and administrators of the value of these innovations designed to improve patient care.

2. Developing a Hospital Protocol for Hispanic Patients

This protocol includes a thorough medical and psychosocial history of the family. The information is obtained soon after admission and is reviewed periodically to assess changes in family functioning. The psychosocial intake includes the following information:

- County and region of origin; number of years in the U.S. Degree of acculturation to the American culture.
- Family structure and role distribution.
- Ease of access to the hospital in terms of: child care, lodging, transportation, telephone, financial resources.
- Availability and quality of supports, both within the family and in the community. Linkages with other health and social agencies.
- Proficiency in English.
- Understanding of child's condition. Cultural beliefs associated with it.
- Capacity to function in a complex hospital environment.
- Legal status (with proper reassurance of no incrimination if family is undocumented).
- Concurrent problems that the family encounters.

If this information suggests that the family is at risk of developing difficulties in adjusting to the hospitalization, a referral to social service or the appropriate department should be forwarded for proper follow-up.

The protocol ensures that each Hispanic family has the opportunity to establish a trusting relationship with at least one health professional who communicates in Spanish (if family is non-English speaking), advocates for the family's needs and bridges the gap between the home and the hospital, connecting the family to appropriate services.

The protocol also ensures that each family is provided with ample opportunities to understand the diagnosis and treatment plans. Consent forms must be available in Spanish and discussed in an open, supportive environment.

3. Developing a Hispanic Social Support Network

The need for social supports is predicated on the crisis intervention model which indicates that people facing crises and transitions have a need to share and compare their reactions and beliefs with others. It is likely that in crises precipitated by illness, existing social contacts are insufficient sources of support (personal communication at AMA meeting, Berkeley, July 1981). Therefore new network contacts need to be mobilized who have personal experiences with the problems encountered. This need is even more imperative for families who live far away from the hospital and who experience cultural and social dissonance in addition to the emotional and cognitive impact of illness.

Peers in social support networks serve important functions and there is accumulating evidence of the beneficial effects of support groups. Peers help to: (a) better understand the circumstances surrounding the life events; (b) exchange problem solving strategies; (c) support efforts towards change and (d) through social comparison they help reduce feelings of uniqueness regarding their problems and help establish new norms in the content of revised social identities (Gottlieb, 1981).

Evidence suggests that social supports reduce stress, increase connectedness (Syme, 1975), enhance coping skills (DiMatteo & Hays, 1981) and facilitate adaptation to a crisis (Gottlieb, 1981; Caplan & Killalea, 1976). Social supports also allow for an integration of the self. It has a synergistic effect whereby each individual feels helped, reassured as well as wanted, and as a result wants to reciprocate. The individual then becomes "at one" with himself and his environment, with his body, mind and spirit, thus experiencing an inner transformation (Ferguson, 1980).

The creation of a supportive network of Hispanics whose children have suffered life threatening, acute or chronic illnesses requiring hospitalization can enhance family functioning. The purpose of this network is to provide and obtain clarification and information, emotional support including active listening and the opportunity to vent feelings, reach out for physical contact, advice and concrete services, physical care, child care, lodging, transportation for running errands, financial assistance and any other resources that enable Hispanic families to overcome the temporary difficulties.

The advantage of this self-help network is that it brings together participants who have experienced similar life crises, and share a common language, cultural values and attitudes, thus increasing the opportunity for development of connectedness and receptivity. Nevertheless, it requires careful screening so that it is made up of people who can provide support and resources without fear of being drained.

Caution needs to be exercised when introducing this network to families in crisis. Some families could interpret this linkage as stigmatization. It can be particularly threatening when differences in social class backgrounds, extent of acculturation and the nature of the medical problem are not considered a priori. For this reason, an experienced Hispanic coordinator is more likely to be accepted by families who are invited to join the network.

The author postulates that the establishment of this network can help families to regain a sense of control and achieve better integration to the health system.

In sum, the recommendations that have been presented suggest that a commitment to enhance the well-being of Hispanic families can be cost effective. Prevention of coping disturbances means less crisis intervention and fewer professional services, particularly if it is built upon an increased level of understanding of the social-health needs of Hispanics and draws on self-help, active family participation and voluntary support networks. It may also yield organizational effectiveness in so far as it can bring about better cooperation from patients, improved physician family relationships and improved staff morale. Finally, it can foster consumer satisfaction with the health institution and promote its future use.

REFERENCES

Acosta Johnson, C. Infant diarrhea and folk medicine in South Texas. *Texas Medicine*, 1979, *75*(1), 69-73.

Budetti, P., Butler, J., & McManus, P., Federal health program reforms: Implications for child health care. *Health & Society*, 1982, *60*(1).

Caplan, G., & Killalea, M. (Eds.), *Support systems and mutual help: Multidisciplinary explorations*. New York: Grune & Stratton, 1976.

Clark, M. *Health in the Mexican-American culture: A community study.* Berkeley: University of California Press, 1959.

DiMatteo, R., & Hays, R. Social support and serious illness. In B. H. Gottlieb (Ed.), *Social networks and social support.* Beverly Hills: Sage Publications, 1981.

Falicov, C., & Karrer, B. Cultural variations in the family life cycle: The Mexican-American family. In E. Carter & M. McGoldrick (Eds.), *The family life cycle: A framework for family therapy.* New York: Gardner Press, 1980.

Ferguson, M. *The Aquarian conspiracy. Personal and social transformation in the 1980's.* Los Angeles: Tarcher, Houghton, Mifflin, 1980.

Gottlieb, B. H. Preventive interventions involving social networks and social support. In B. H. Gottlieb (Ed.), *Social networks and social support.* Beverly Hills: Sage Publications, 1981.

Hoppe, S., & Heller, P. Alienation, familism and the utilization of health services by Mexican Americans. *Job Health and Social Behavior,* 1975, *16*(3), 304-314.

Lenrow, P., & Burch, R. Mutual aid and professional services. Opposing or complementary? In B. H. Gottlieb (Ed.), *Social networks and social support.* Beverly Hills: Sage Publications, 1981.

MALDEF, 1977, According to the Mexican American Legal Defense Fund there were 1.5 Million Undocumented Immigrants in California in 1977.

Martinez, R. *Hispanic culture & health care: Fact fiction & folklore.* St. Louis: Mosby, 1978.

Personal communication: As expressed by a group of Hispanic health providers in a meeting with the American Medical Association, Health Education Division held at the University of California at Berkeley, July 1981.

Sandler, A., & Chan, L. Mexican American folk belief in a pediatric emergency room. *Medical Care,* 1978, *16*(9), 778-784.

Syme, L. Social and psychological risk factors in coronary heart disease. *Modern Concepts of Cardiovascular Disease,* 1975, *44*(4), 17-21.

U.S. HEW. Health status of minorities and low income groups. Health Resources Administration, Office of Health Resources Opportunity, 1977.

Factors Affecting Coping of Adolescents and Infants on a Reverse Isolation Unit

Margarita Kutsanellou-Meyer, CSW
Grace Hyslop Christ, CSW

SUMMARY. This paper describes factors that affect the coping processes of adolescents with aplastic anemia and infants with severe combined immunodeficiency disease treated on a reverse isolation unit. The adolescents demonstrated a rich diversity of coping styles depending on the interaction of a variety of factors. Special stresses to other family members, such as the reactions of the child donor, are also highlighted. For the infants, the dyadic relationship with the mothering figure, the feelings of the family about the fact of genetic transmission, and the impact of isolation on the infant's development are identified as important psychosocial variables in the infant's adjustment. A multidimensional perspective such as that provided within a systems framework, which encourages an appreciation of the interactive diversity of all factors, is presented as the most useful approach to interventions.

The treatment of such life-threatening diseases as leukemia, aplastic anemia, and severe combined immunodeficiency disease

At the time of writing Ms. Kutsanellou-Meyer was the staff social worker on the reverse isolation unit, Memorial Sloan-Kettering Cancer Center, 1275 York Avenue, New York, NY 10021. Mrs. Christ was Assistant Director, Department of Social Work, Memorial Sloan-Kettering Cancer Center, and doctoral candidate, Columbia University School of Social Work. Preparation of this paper was partially supported by United States Public Health Service Grant CA 19267. The authors gratefully acknowledge the encouragement and support of Dr. Richard O'Reilly, Director, Bone Marrow Transplant Unit, and Mrs. Evelyn Cooper, Director, Department of Social Work.
Reprinted from *Social Work in Health Care*, Volume 4(2), Winter 1978.

has greatly increased at least the short-term survival of many patients. The medical treatments used, however, are replete with extraordinary stress to patients, their families, and the medical and nursing staff. Bone marrow transplantation performed within the milieu of a reverse isolation unit is a treatment of this dimension.

Bone marrow transplant in the last decade has become the curative treatment of choice for aplastic anemia and severe combined immunodeficiency disease and has resulted in disease free remissions in up to 18% of patients with chemotherapeutic resistant leukemia (O'Reilly, 1978; O'Reilly, Pahwa, Dupont & Good, 1978; Thomas, Fefer, Buckner, & Storb, 1977).

Protected environments such as our reverse isolation unit have been increasingly used to decrease the incidence and severity of certain microbial infections particularly lethal to marrow transplant recipients immediately after radiation or chemotherapy. These radical medical treatments constitute an overt confrontation between a patient and his disease with an absolute recognition that his disease is lethal. Marrow transplantation is an extraordinarily aggressive approach that offers the potential of cure, but also a high likelihood of failure and death. Early failure and death complicates 30 to 50% of transplants in cases of aplastic anemia and leukemia. Recurrent leukemia may appear late in the transplant period of 20 to 30% of cases. A summary of the extraordinary stresses would include the reality of a lethal illness; immunosuppression, including in some instances chemotherapy and the prospect of total body irradiation in leukemia, isolation from normal body contact with others, and numerous uncomfortable and painful medical procedures. The enhancement of the survivor's coping capacities presents a new challenge to the mental health professional.

REVERSE ISOLATION UNIT

The reverse isolation unit at Memorial Sloan-Kettering Cancer Center was, prior to expansion, an intensive care facility equipped with four laminar flow isolation rooms designed to maintain a patient in a relatively germ-free environment. The rooms had no windows and were separated from the central nursing station by a large glass partition that contained an intercom system allowing verbal access between patient, family, and staff. A small corridor between rooms was utilized by staff or family to put on mask, hat, and boots before walking to the scrub area. Direct contact with the patient was possible only after a 10-minute scrub and the completion of sterile dressing, which consisted of two sets of gloves and a sterile gown. The procedure was obviously time consuming and limited the number of people entering the room. Although the diagnoses treated in a reverse isolation unit vary, as do the ages of the patients, what is common is the added stress of the isolation with its concomitant drastic reduction in normal emotional supports.

POPULATION

There are three different diagnostic groups admitted to this unit. The first consists of children born with severe combined immuno-deficiency disease, hereafter called SCID. These are genetically transmitted defects. The second group are patients diagnosed with aplastic anemia, an acquired disease in which there is a failure of production of normal blood cells by the bone marrow. These are primarily adolescents and young adults. Leukemia is the diagnosis of the third group. At the time of this report, only three patients with the diagnosis of leukemia had been treated on the unit during the period covered. Leukemics treated with bone marrow transplants have been discussed elsewhere (Brown & Kelly, 1976; Holland, Plumb, Yates, Harris, Tuttolomondo, Holmes, & Holland, 1977; Pfefferbaum, Lindamood, & Wiley, 1977).

PERTINENT LITERATURE

The available literature on psychosocial aspects of bone marrow transplantation and reverse isolation is sparse and derived from experiences with a small number of child and adolescent patients. Pfefferbaum et al. (1977) studied bone marrow transplantation in 19 children and adolescents. They correlated psychosocial factors of parent-child interaction with survival rates. No statistically significant correlation was made. The weakness of this study is that it focused on only one aspect of coping, namely, parent-child interaction, and related it to survival. We have been impressed that coping is affected by at least three groups of interacting variables: (a) stresses of different diagnoses, treatment, and disease course; (b) coping strategies as they are available to the patient at each developmental level and enhanced by his or her support system (i.e., family and nonfamily members); and (c) psychosocial interventions provided by medical and nonmedical staff. Because of the interaction of variables, statistically correlating an aspect of any one of these to survival rate could lead to insignificant findings.

Brown and Kelly (1976) described the psychosocial implications of the process in six adolescents and adults. Adaptive measures were employed by patients at various stages of bone marrow transplantation procedures. In general, our patient population differed in that all the 19 patients were either children or adolescents. The importance of the developmental level of the child in determining the impact of the stress and selection of coping strategies proved particularly important.

STRESSES ON PATIENTS WITH APLASTIC ANEMIA

Eleven patients, aged 2 to 22, were diagnosed with aplastic anemia (see Table 1). Their mean length of stay on the reverse isolation unit was 3.6 months. All but two patients had one bone marrow transplant, one had two, and another had three. Seven patients have been discharged and are doing well; two are still on the unit. The two 22-year-old patients, whose disease had a much longer history before treatment, died 8 months and 3 months after the bone marrow transplant.

The most severe psychosocial stress for these patients is the stark

Table 1

Patients on a Reverse Isolation Unit

Diagnosis	Age	0-2	5-8	14-16	22	23-40	Mean Length of Stay
SCID		8	-	-	-	-	19.7 months
Aplastic Anemia		1	2	6	2	-	3.6 months
Leukemia		-	-	-	-	3	3 months

isolation, particularly from normal body contact at the very time experimental treatment for their life-threatening illness is being undertaken. Holland et al. (1977) have emphasized that the lack of direct physical contact is the most distressing aspect of reverse isolation, producing a sense of loneliness and distance from others.

Children and adolescents find their initial entrance into the isolation rooms frightening in a way different from adults. Children are more distressed by the separation from people, objects, and activities important to them than by the possibility of death. One 13-year-old patient refused entrance into the room for several hours until he could be reassured that he was not being abandoned by his family. Families also have misconceptions and anxieties about the degree of isolation. Even though they learn that they will be able to enter the room, they are extremely apprehensive about the possibility of contaminating the patient.

We have observed a fairly typical sequence in the way a patient with aplastic anemia and the family react to bone marrow transplantation and isolation. A phase of optimism and hope, excitement, even euphoria, follows the family's hearing about the treatment. A cure has been found. As the time for admission draws close, the patient's and family's denial is broken down by repeated descriptions of the following facts and procedures. Immunosuppression to insure engraftment involves high dose chemotherapy which results in nausea, vomiting, loss of hair, and increased susceptibility to infection. This emphasizes the severity of the undertaking. In addition, patients are made aware of the possibility of graft versus host disease, that is, an immune reaction by the marrow graft against the patient's tissue resulting in severe skin reactions, hepatitis, diarrhea, and occasionally death. The high possibility of developing lethal pneumonia as a complication of the immunodeficiency induced and the graft versus hot disease process is also explained. Children, adolescents, and their families continue to express misconceptions about the transplant procedure itself although it has been carefully described to them by the physician and nursing staff prior to admission and during the initial period of treatment. For example, most express the belief that the treatment involves a surgical procedure removing a bone from the donor and transplanting it in the patient.

Heightened feelings of aloneness occur when the adult or adolescent patients enter the sterile room. They express awareness of the "no return" aspect of the procedure.

We have been impressed by one further stress that is developmentally specific to the adolescent. The loss of hair and other physical changes resulting from chemotherapy and medical procedures cause painful feelings of alteration in body image. This could be further complicated by the limitation in movement which is part of hospitalization. Several patients stated they felt that they looked quite different from their previous appearance and refused to look into mirrors.

SPECIAL STRESSES TO OTHER FAMILY MEMBERS

The psychological relationship of the donor to the patient may be another area of stress for patient, donor, and family. It has been observed that the adult donor has few strong psychological reactions to this procedure, especially when compared to the reactions of donors of organ transplants (Holland & Gerstenzang, Note 1). However, we have found that the child and adolescent donors often experience a variety of misconceptions and distressing emotional reactions. Careful attention to communication, such as giving concrete information on the facts about transplantation, is important for donor, patient, and family whether or not the patient survives.

The donor's awareness that if it were not for him or her the patient would die, can bring feelings of importance and pride, but also fear: What if the procedure is not successful? Will I be responsible for my sibling's death? Will I get the same disease? These are frequent questions and/or fantasies that may be expressed. There are also numerous idiosyncratic fears of possible damage to the donor: Will I be able to walk? Will I be able to continue involvement in sports? One 22-year-old donor worried that she would jeopardize her chances of having children. A Puerto Rican family expressed the concern that the 14-year-old donor's pain following the procedure was genital pain and that her sexuality had been compromised in some way. A 13-year-old patient questioned whether he would remain small like the 8-year-old donor since he now had his blood.

In addition to the emotional reaction of child donors, in three of the families other early adolescent siblings expressed anger and distress at being left out of such an important process. They resented that all the attention was focused on the patient and the donor. One 12-year-old burst into tears on the unit, saying that she felt neglected and left out because she was unable to participate in her sister's recovery.

We found that giving specific information and maintaining an openness to these kinds of misconceptions and reactions can be helpful. However, especially with children and adolescents, this is not sufficient. It is not always easy for patients and siblings to reveal these kinds of thoughts and feelings, whose suppression can have a destructive effect. Consequently, we have found that a more active exploration of thoughts and feelings about the illness and the treatment provides relief to the patient and siblings as well as important information to the staff.

COPING STRATEGIES OF THE ADOLESCENT PATIENT WITH APLASTIC ANEMIA

The physically ill adolescent struggles with needs to preserve independence, autonomy, identity, privacy, and approval of peers. We have been impressed with the rich diversity in adolescent patients' and their families' ways of adapting to this experience.

The adolescent's need to know the details of the disease and its treatment is a well-documented phenomenon. This mastery serves to protect against feelings of helplessness and fears of loss of control.

George, 16, exemplifies the use of control of the medical situation as both a defense and as a coping strategy. He quickly made efforts to take charge of his medical situation. He watched all indicators of his progress, such as blood count and bone marrow test results. He set goals for his improvement, for the change in his blood counts, as well as for the date of his discharge. At times he would allow a visitor into his room, at other times he would not. The staff were helped by the social worker to realize the value of the patient's control of his situation. This was particularly hard because it threatened their own need to be in charge of such a dangerous medical treatment. Tensions were created by the conflict between his view and our view of the timing of his discharge.

In marked contrast, John, a 14-year-old Greek patient, demonstrated very little need to control his treatment. His parents remained in Greece, communicating daily by telephone. In addition to attending school, John had worked in Greece on the family farm with his father. We surmised that he was not so threatened by the separation and the medical procedures because he had already achieved a level of independence. While in isolation, he was pleasant and cooperative, although not passive. He consoled himself by singing songs about his home and about separation from loved ones. He developed collaborative relationships with the staff that were mutually satisfying.

All of the adolescents attempted to maintain privacy by keeping the lights off in their rooms, making it difficult for staff and visitors to see them. The patients complained at length about the use of masks and gowns by staff and family, and often insisted that people stand outside the glass partition so they could observe their faces rather than the indistinct, masked figures. When feeling better, most of the adolescents insisted on wearing their adolescent garb instead of hospital clothing, enhancing the maintenance of previous identities.

The amount of contact that the adolescents maintained with peers varied. Where ongoing communication was possible, it became an important part of the adolescent's efforts to cope with both illness and isolation. When there are a number of adolescents on the unit, they spend much of their day on the telephone with each other discussing the details of the day's activities. The suggestion has been made that closed circuit television might be a way of providing group services to these patients. One 16-year-old boy ran up a $900 telephone bill during a 70-day stay in reverse isolation. He was athletically oriented and tended to rely heavily on peer acceptance for continued assurance of his worth and importance. In addition, his contact with peers shielded him from an overprotective mother whom he often refused to allow into his room.

Another moving example of peer support of the adolescent was provided by a patient in our pediatric oncology service. While he was undergoing chemotherapy and losing his hair, his three best friends accompanied him to the clinic, all with shaved heads. In this way they tried to protect him from being singled out as different from them in a crowd.

THE EFFECT OF THE FAMILY COPING STYLE ON THE ADOLESCENT PATIENT

We were impressed with the impact of the families' ways of handling independence and dependence on the adolescent patients' adjustment to illness and isolation.

George's mother had become overly involved with him over the past several years because of his illness. Her extreme anxiety about him and her overprotective behavior seemed at times to promote excessively independent behavior on George's part as a reaction. This counterphobic, sometimes dangerous behavior in response to an overprotective, guilt-ridden parent was also described by Agle and Mattsson (1976) in their work on hemophiliacs.

Vicky's family, on the other hand, had high expectations for her independent functioning. Both of her parents had worked outside the home for a number of years, and the children had become accustomed to accepting more responsibility. They visited Vicky regularly, but infrequently. Vicky easily substituted her need for her parents' attention with the nurses, welcoming them into her room and forming close attachments with them. She was also a very studious person and independently involved herself in painting and other creative activities.

Mary was one of nine children in a family that had recently moved to New York from Puerto Rico. The family moved because the father had been unable to find employment. They did not understand English well, nor did they comprehend the disease and its treatment. They thought that such a severe treatment meant that Mary would die, although this was not initially verbalized. From their perspective it was more important for them to put their energies into the survival of the rest of the family than Mary's (in their view) hopeless treatment. In addition, they feared that the 18-year-old donor would lose his job if he participated. The mother could not visit because she was phobic about the subway. The family withdrew from treatment for a period of time until the social worker was able to work with them and correct some of these misconceptions. It was also important for her to help them with their very real social and economic needs. Mary became passive and compliant on the unit, watching television most of the time and asking few questions. She expressed fears of leaving the protection of the room and returning to the care of the family whom she was not sure she could trust.

These are examples of three different ways that families responded to the disease and its treatment which further contribute to the diversity of the adolescent's coping style. This interactive diversity includes the specific disease, its progress and its treatment, the personality structure of the patient and his or her past history, the social and cultural characteristics of the family, and current situational and environmental factors. The social worker's role is to assess the relative importance of each of these and to select the most salient issues for intervention. The social worker's task is to enhance the family's natural coping abilities in this most unusual and stressful experience in order to optimize the patient's and the family's utilization of these stressful but potentially life-saving medical procedures.

STRESS ON PATIENTS AND FAMILIES WITH SEVERE COMBINED IMMUNODEFICIENCY DISEASE

Seven infants diagnosed with severe combined immunodeficiency were treated on the reverse isolation unit during this period (see Table 1). Five of these patients underwent fetal liver and thymus transplants. The other two had bone marrow transplants. The mean length of stay on the unit for these patients was 19.7 months.

Five of the infants lived and are doing well. Two of them died of infections at ages 2 and 2 1/2 years, underscoring the tremendous importance of the technique of isolation. What to a normal child is a mild infection is to these children a life-threatening illness.

In contrast to the diversity of adaptational responses observed in the adolescent patients and their families as described above, two common themes were highlighted by the infants in reverse isolation: (a) the impact on the family of the fact of genetic transmission of the disease; and (b) the importance of the developmentally specific dyadic relationship between the mother and the infant.

THE IMPACT OF GENETIC TRANSMISSION

There are multiple forms of SCID. Certain types are transmitted as a homozygous recessive disorder with a defective gene from both parents. There is also a sex-linked recessive form which is transmitted solely by the female parent. In our series of 8 patients, there were six males and two females. One of the males clearly had the sex-linked form of the disorder. The possibility of a sex-linked disorder was highly probable in two others.

The feelings about the genetic transmission of the disease are a most important stress on families of infants with SCID. Mattsson and Gross (1966) reported from their study of hemophiliac children and their families that "a crucial factor determining the common positive adaptive outcome seemed to be the mother's ability to master her guilt over having transmitted the illness' (p. 1355). Mattsson's studies on hemophiliacs are the only parallel investigations on the impact of genetic transmission.

We found that parents had more difficulty coping with the feelings about having transmitted the illness when they had another child or relative who had died of the same disease. In these cases the parents knew prior to conception of the second child that there were high risks involved for the child's health. In our series, four of the eight families of children with SCID had lost another child or sibling to the same illness.

Mrs. K. had two previous children die of this disease. It became clear to the social worker that much of her anxiety about Mark related to unresolved guilt, anger, and sadness about these deaths and that she subsequently displaced these feelings onto Mark.

This also agrees with Mattsson and Gross' (1966) finding that each of the mothers of the eight poorly adjusted hemophiliacs "identified her hemophiliac boy with a deceased relative (usually a hemophiliac) and saw her son as unrealistically vulnerable at all times" (p. 1355). It was also true for our families, however, that the fact of having previous children die of this disease alerted the parents to the symptomatology, making possible early diagnosis and treatment.

Initially, all of the fathers tended to be less involved with the medical treatment than the mothers were. In addition, three of the fathers viewed their wives as primarily responsible for the birth of a sick child and therefore withdrew emotionally and physically, leaving most of the decisions and care to the mother. This placed an added burden on these mothers who had already felt guilty for having insisted on bearing a child even though the chances of the child's being ill were high. Clearly, the role of the father, especially in relation to his adjustment to the fact of genetic transmission, was an important factor in the overall adaptation of the family to the presence of illness and its treatment.

THE IMPORTANCE OF THE DYADIC RELATIONSHIP BETWEEN MOTHER AND INFANT

Because of the developmentally specific needs of the infant, the dyadic relationship with the mother is most important. For all the mothers, caring for their infant in this environment was a difficult task. The lack of privacy and freedom to come and go is quite different from that which is possible in one's own home. The two mothers who had great difficulty in allotting sufficient time to the infant, and in using the time appropriately once there, were the mothers who were viewed as immature by the staff and who gave the most evidence of psychopathology. Compounding factors were present in the history of these two mothers. One had two children die of this illness, and the other had two siblings die of the same disease. In addition, neither of these mothers had emotional or physical support from their husbands. Two other mothers who had experienced deaths in their families from this illness and yet were better adapted to their infants and to the treatment situation presented an interesting contrast. These latter mothers had more emotional and physical support from their spouses than did the more poorly functioning mothers, and they seemed to have worked through their grief over previous losses and subsequent guilts more completely. In addition, they did not give evidence of prior psychopathology.

All of the mothers made use of intellectualization and cognitive mastery as primary coping mechanisms. Several of the mothers came from rural areas with less than a high school education. After a year or more on the unit they demonstrated an extraordinary amount of knowledge of the disease and its treatment and a greater sophistication and knowledge about the world in general. In addition, they revealed life goal changes for themselves, especially desires for higher education and more challenging employment. This increase in knowledge with a consequent raising of self-esteem proved a powerful coping mechanism. This also highlights the growth potential in good adaptation to crises.

REVERSE ISOLATION AND
THE DEVELOPING INFANT

Developing infants in the sensorimotor stage (Piaget) or the autistic, symbiotic, separation individuation stage (Mahler) have none of the intellectualizing defenses of older children, nor the ability to express themselves in play therapy as do the preschoolers. The infant has unique needs to see, touch, handle, and smell. In a reverse isolation unit there are mechanical barriers (i.e., gown, mask, hat, gloves) to the normal physical contact between mother and infant. Effects of deprivations of normal stimulation are imposed by the setting, by medical procedures, and in certain instances by the absence of the consistent integrating mothering figure.

There are two contradictory findings on the effects of long-term isolation of this kind on the developing infant. Simons, Kohle, Genscher and Dietrich (1973) identified a learning disorder and impairment of intellectual capacity in twins who were raised in isolation systems for 2.5 years. They attributed the mental retardation of both infants to the extended stay in isolation. Freedman, Montgomery, Wilson, Bealmer and South (1976), on the other hand, found that the cognitive and affective development of a child who had been in isolation for 52 months had proceeded along normal lines. They pointed out that the parents of the twins in Simons et al.'s study were known to be of limited intelligence and that the twin who was most limited in his functioning was the vulnerable child at birth with a number of early physical complications. They suggested that these factors could be contributing more to the twins' intellectual deficit than the impact of isolation.

Simons et al.'s isolator is described as a highly restrictive environment. On the other hand, Freedman et al. describe the environment of their patient as freer than most normal infant environments, with intensified stimulation and speech therapy. Therefore, Freedman et al. (1976) conclude that "the condition of reverse isolation when applied from birth through roughly the first four years is not per se incompatible with normal affective and intellectual development up to that point" (p. 603).

Our findings from the series of eight patients support Freedman et al.'s conclusion. This is being reported in greater detail by Tamaroff, Kutsanellou-Meyer, Christ, and Straker (Note 2). Several of the children developed transient self-stimulating behavior, such as rocking and head banging, as well as speech difficulties. These markedly improved, however, when appropriate stimulation was provided or when the child was discharged from the unit.

The most pathologic-appearing infant developed withdrawn behavior, echolalic speech, rocking, and head banging. However, the mother of this patient also presented the most disturbed mother-infant interaction.

Mrs. K. demonstrated severe anxiety and anger in her behavior with Mark in the isolator room. Mark reacted to his mother's tension by crying, rejecting her, and refusing to eat or take his medications. Even this child's symptoms markedly improved, however, when his physical state improved, which in turn greatly altered the mother's interaction. We speculated that the improved physical condition of the child allowed the mother to reinvest herself in the relationship. This was not possible when the infant's survival was so much in question because this mother had already lost two other children to the same disease. This was even more dramatically shown by the fathers who generally demonstrated a marked increase in their involvement with the infant once they learned that the transplant was successful.

It was our conclusion that it was not any one of these factors alone—isolation, medical treatments, severity of illness, quality and quantity of mother-infant interaction, genetic transmission, or paternal involvement and support—that prevented optimal adjustment. Rather, it was the interaction of a unique constellation of these stresses and factors affecting coping that presented unusual challenges for patients' and families' adaptive capacities and that contributed to a good or poor adjustment on the part of the infant. The social worker needs to understand this interactive diversity in order to select interventive strategies.

SUMMARY AND CONCLUSION

In this paper we have described factors that affect the coping processes of adolescents with aplastic anemia and infants with severe combined immunodeficiency disease treated on a reverse isolation unit. The adolescents demonstrated a rich diversity of coping styles depending on the interaction of a variety of factors. The specific developmental tasks of this age group, the interference to the resolution of these tasks presented by the illness and its treatment, and the various ways patients and families adapted to both were highlighted. We also explored special stresses to other family members such as the reactions of the child donor, which were observed to differ from adult donor reactions.

On the other hand, the infants' developmentally specific needs for intimacy with the mothering figure directed our focus with this group to that dyadic relationship. We explored the stresses on the relationship, especially the feelings of the family about the fact of genetic transmission of the disease. The differing opinions about the effects of reverse isolation on the development of the infant were presented. Our observations suggested that isolation per se is not incompatible with normal cognitive and affective development.

Patients and families undergoing this kind of stressful medical treatment can best be understood and helped from a multidimensional perspective such as that provided within a systems framework. The temptation to use a unidimensional or linear model is especially strong within a medical setting. However, it is inadequate to deal with the interactive diversity of the psychosocial aspects of this situation. The systems concepts of multidetermination and equifinality provide more useful guidelines for interventions. The relevant factors to this stressful medical treatment have been described. The principle of equifinality suggests that the social worker need not address all areas of stress, but rather can select the salient issues for each patient and family. Specific interventions utilized with patients, families, and staff will be discussed in a later paper (Christ, Kutsanellou-Meyer, & Monk, Note 3).

We were impressed that when it was possible to translate this unusual experience to patients and families in a way they could understand and integrate, successful adaptation was possible. Not only were they able to cope with the immediate stress, but in some instances they gave evidence of having achieved a new level of functioning.

REFERENCE NOTES

1. Holland, J., & Gerstenzang, M. *Bone marrow transplant in identical twins*. In preparation, 1978.

2. Tamaroff, M., Kutsanellou-Meyer, M., Christ, G. H., & Straker, N. *Observations of the developmental functioning of three children treated from birth in protected environments*. In preparation, 1978.

3. Christ, G. H., Kutsanellou-Meyer, M., & Monk, P. *Psychosocial interventive techniques on a reverse isolation unit*. In preparation, 1978.

REFERENCES

Agle, D., & Mattsson, A. Psychological complications of hemophilia. In M. Hilgartner (Ed.), *Hemophilia in children*. Littleton, Mass.: Publishing Sciences Group, 1976.

Brown, H., & Kelly, M. Stages of bone marrow transplantation: A psychiatric perspective. *Psychosomatic Medicine*, November-December 1976, *38*(6), 439-446.

Freedman, D., Montgomery, J., Wilson, R., Bealmer, P., & South, M. Further observations on the effect of reverse isolation from birth on cognitive and affective development. *Journal of the American Academy of Child Psychiatry*, Autumn 1976, *15*(4), 593-602.

Holland, J., Plumb, M., Yates, J., Harris, S., Tuttolomondo, A., Holmes, J., & Holland, J. Psychological response of patients with acute leukemia to germ-free environments. *American Journal of Psychiatry*, May 1977, *134*(5), 563-564.

Lipowski, Z. J. Physical illness, the individual and the coping processes. *Psychiatry in Medicine*, 1974, *1*, 91-102.

Mattsson, A., & Gross, S. Adaptational and defensive behavior in young hemophiliacs and their parents. *American Journal of Psychiatry*, 1966, *122*, 1349-1356.

O'Reilly, R. J. Immunodeficiency, severe combined. In A. R. Liss (Ed.), *Birth defects atlas and compendium (2nd ed.)*. New York: National Foundation, 1978.

O'Reilly, R. J., Pahwa, R., Dupont, B., & Good, R. A. Severe combined immunodeficiency: Transplantation approaches for patient lacking an HLA genotypically identical sibling. *Transplant Proceedings*, 1978, *10*(1), 187-199.

Pfefferbaum, B., Lindamood, M., & Wiley, F. Pediatric bone marrow transplantation: Psychosocial aspects. *American Journal of Psychiatry*, November 1977, *134*(11), 1299-1301.

Simons, C., Kohle, K., Genscher, U., & Dietrich, M. The impact of reverse isolation on early childhood development: Two and a half years of treatment in plastic isolation systems. *Psychotherapy Psychosomatics*, 1973, *22*, 300-309.

Thomas, E., Fefer, A., Buckner, C., & Storb, R. Current status of bone marrow transplantation for aplastic anemia and acute leukemia. *Blood*, May 1977, *4*(5), 671-681.

Trauma Centers:
A New Dimension
for Hospital Social Work

Jean M. Moonilal, LCSW, ACSW

SUMMARY. The development of the trauma center is one of the latest concepts in the delivery of emergency medical care. This paper proposes that social workers can play an important role in the initial management of trauma patients and their families. Through assessment, consultation, and direct intervention, social workers can provide a psychosocial component to trauma care. A prototype of a trauma center is discussed, along with case examples and implications for the role of social work.

Trauma centers are an exciting new development in the delivery of emergency medical care. For hospital-based social workers, particularly those assigned to emergency rooms and critical care units, familiarization with the relatively new technologies and systems of the trauma center is important if there is to be full understanding and impact on the delivery of comprehensive medical and psychosocial services to patients and their families. A review of the literature reveals that social workers are just now being introduced to the purpose and function of the trauma center, and that the unique contribution of social work to the initial management of trauma patients and their families is in the process of definition (Epperson, 1977). The purpose of this article, then, is twofold. It will introduce the reader to the development, scope and operation of the hospital

At the time of writing Ms. Moonilal was a Clinical Social Worker in the Emergency Department, University of California, Irvine, Medical Center, 101 City Drive South, Orange, CA 92668.
Reprinted from *Social Work in Health Care*, Volume 7(4), Summer 1982.

trauma center, and, secondly, it will speak to the innovative role of the trauma center social worker.

BACKGROUND

Trauma, generally defined as a physical injury caused by an external force, is one of the fastest growing specialties within the field of emergency medicine. Until recently, however, the systematic study and development of adequate emergency medical service systems (EMS) has been a largely neglected area of health care in this country. This lack of organized emergency care is particularly alarming when one considers that trauma is the third leading cause of death in the United States and the leading cause of death in persons under 45 years of age.

Studies conducted in different areas of the country have demonstrated that as many as one-third of all accident victims die needlessly as a result of their injuries, and as many as 80% of patients who die of shock might have been saved if specialized services had been available (National Academy of Sciences, 1966; West, Trunkey & Lim, 1979). In this age of medical sophistication, it is an unfortunate irony that patients are dying in emergency rooms, not necessarily as a result of their injuries, but because they have had the misfortune of being taken to hospitals that are incapable of saving them. Most consumers of emergency care are unaware of which hospital in their community is, for example, best able to deal with severe burns, an amputated limb, or multiple stab wounds. In cases where appropriate and timely intervention can mean life or death, the patient, more often than not, has been at the mercy of poorly organized and partialized emergency health care.

With the introduction of the Emergency Medical Services Systems Act of 1973 (PL 93-154), the Federal Government paved the way for the study, planning, establishment and improvement of local emergency medical service systems in order to significantly decrease death and disability rates (Harvey, 1975). Several states, including California, Maryland, and Illinois have already organized emergency services on a statewide basis and have designated trauma centers as the central part of this network. With the support of both the Federal Government and the medical profession, and with growing consumer demand for adequate emergency care, the systematic development of regional trauma centers would appear to be a nationwide trend (Montgomery, 1980).

TRAUMA CENTER

In most trauma centers, target patients are identified as those who sustain multiple, life-threatening injuries which result in shock, excessive blood loss, severe respiratory distress or cardiac arrest. Victims of multiple trauma are usually products of motor vehicle accidents, shootings, stabbings, or suicide attempts and are generally in shock, unconscious, or near death. Most arrive at the hospital with paramedics — a few are brought in by family or friends.

The highly specialized and calibrated system of emergency care found in the trauma center is designed to increase the survival rate and decrease disability for victims of substantial trauma. The term "trauma center" refers to a facility (typically, a large metropolitan hospital) which meets stringent criteria for specialized trauma care established by the American College of Surgeons, and which also has been so designated through regional health planning processes. In addition to basic life support services provided by the hospital emergency room, each trauma center is equipped with specialized resuscitation, surgical, and monitoring apparatus designed for immediate intervention and stabilization of the multiply injured patient. To be officially designated as a trauma center, each facility is required to comply with staffing and expertise standards, including 24-hour availability of trauma surgeons and anesthesiologists and of laboratory, radiology, and other diagnostic equipment, as well as round-the-clock availability of operating rooms and critical care units. Some trauma centers, such as the University of California, Irvine Medical Center, have the capacity to receive and treat patients suffering from severe burns or traumatic amputation of limbs and digits. In other large medical centers, notably the Medical College of Virginia and the Shock Trauma Center of Baltimore, Maryland, the concept of an integrated trauma service has expanded to include not only pre-hospital (paramedic) and emergency care, but an entire continuum of specialized staff and facilities to see the patient through the intensive, intermediate, and rehabilitative phases of treatment and recovery (Cowley & Scanlan, 1979; Maull & Haynes, 1977).

ROLE OF SOCIAL WORK

The social worker is a member of the trauma center team, along with trauma surgeons, anesthesiologists, and a trauma coordinator (typically, a nurse). He or she is often referred to as the team "psychotraumatologist," a title referring to a professional who specializes in the psychological aspects of trauma care. The tasks of the trauma center social worker are multiple and vary with each new case. This discussion will focus on the clinical aspects of trauma care. Clinical work includes initial assessment and consultation, crisis management, grief counseling and termination.

The social worker is often the first person the family meets upon their arrival at the hospital. Therapeutic tasks that require attention include informing the family of the news of the trauma, dealing with immediate questions and concerns, preparing the family for their initial encounter with the patient, and interfacing between them and the treatment team.

Being confronted with sudden and substantial physical trauma is a uniquely distressing experience for both patient and family. Not only is there no opportunity to prepare for the event, there seldom exist past experiences of a similar nature from which to derive effective coping mechanisms. Loss, either through mutilation, surgical intervention, or death, is generally inevitable, and irreversible. As Golden (1966) has observed, "perhaps nowhere else in his life does the physician enact his healing role amidst so much drama, tension, anguish, and consequence" (p. 5). Relatives, far removed from the frantic activity level being experienced by the patient, are silently and repeatedly challenged by the fears and fantasies which the traumatic event has ignited. This complex interplay of the external threat and internal "vulnerable state" is the focus of exploration and intervention (Golan, 1972).

Due to the serious condition of the patient and the need for immediate medical intervention, the social worker's initial focus is often on assisting friends and relatives through the crisis (Epperson, 1977). In the immediate aftermath of major trauma, the social worker functions as the primary hospital support system for families and as the interface between them and the treatment team. Solid crisis intervention skills are vital during this period if the family's strengths and coping skills are to be identified and reinforced. As in most crisis work, the therapeutic stance taken by the worker is an active and anticipatory one (Golan, 1972).

Assessment

Assessment is the basis for intervention. As Golan (1972) suggests, four areas of reaction merit exploration. These areas are: affective, perceptual-cognitive, behavioral, and biophysiological. Information about functioning in these different domains is obtained via direct questioning, personal observation, and collateral information. In order to intervene effectively, each individual's intellectual understanding of what has happened, emotional and somatic responses to the event, familiarity with medical crisis, and behavior must be evaluated. While the urgency of the situation does not allow the leisurely period of appraisal characteristic of other settings, the social worker skilled in crisis intervention uses whatever time and information is available to formulate a tentative clinical impression from which to proceed.

Informing the Family

It is the author's experience that if relatives are left detached and uninformed, they will respond by feeling helpless, disoriented, and resentful. One of the first tasks of the social worker dealing with major trauma, then, is to discern, as much as possible and in as little time as possible, the circumstances surrounding the trauma itself. The more information that can be obtained about the patient's condition and the mechanism of injury, the more one can anticipate how the family will respond to the initial news of trauma and what their concerns are likely to be. It is important to learn how seriously the patient has been injured and what his or her current condition is (i.e., stable, unstable, critical, expired, etc). What is the primary area of concern for the medical team? (Bleeding? Shock? Injury to major organs? Head trauma?) Was the trauma sustained in an accident, suicide attempt, argument, or during the commission of a crime? The social worker obtains this information from other members of the trauma team and may briefly interview "first responders" such as paramedic and ambulance drivers as well. Since it may be several minutes before a physician can leave the patient to speak with relatives, this time is utilized to secure a private place for the family to wait and to provide them with the facts surrounding the trauma. As the family may be in a state of shock, it is important to speak slowly and clearly, pausing when necessary to allow for integration of information and expression of feelings. The following is an example of an introductory statement:

> Mr. and Mrs. Smith, your son was brought to the emergency room by the paramedics after he was involved in a head-on traffic accident. The paramedics tell me that he was found unconscious at the scene of the accident. He has not yet regained consciousness. At this time, a team of specialized doctors are with him, trying to stabilize him and determine just where he has been hurt and how seriously. I will let the doctors know that you are here, and as soon as possible, I will have one of them come out and talk with you.

An informal clinical assessment concerning the family's dynamics, reactions, and coping styles is being formulated at the same time information about the patient is being shared with them. This assessment will enable the worker to determine how much and what kind of intervention is immediately required. A determination is made, for example, as to whether the patient and/or family has been through a similar crisis in the past, and whether or not they were directly or peripherally involved in the current traumatic incident. If other family members were involved, it is imperative to ascertain how much blame, if any, they assign to themselves, or others. If guilt is a predominant dynamic, it is explored early in the intervention. If the family is confused or needs clarification, this assessment is relayed to the medical team, and appropriate steps are taken to provide the family with the information needed to facilitate their understanding. It is most effective when the trauma surgeon and social worker function as a team, providing information and professional expertise in order that relatives and patients receive both technical and emotional care.

Dealing with Initial Reactions

Reactions to such "bad news" run the gamut of human emotions. Relatives express feelings of disbelief, anxiety, and grief. Regardless of the particular response expressed, an atmosphere of empathic understanding should be created in which feelings can be explored and clarified.

In one case, a mother, upon learning that her teenage son had been involved in a traffic collision, was relieved to know that he had not been at fault. Only when the issue of responsibility had been clarified was she fully able to redirect her concern from the event to the patient. Further questioning revealed that the patient had a history of vehicular carelessness, and that the mother lived with the constant anxiety that her son might be the cause of a serious accident. In another case, a wife became quite upset when she was told that her husband accidentally electrocuted himself on a high tension wire while billboard pasting. Immediately assuming that the accident was the result of the patient's perfectionistic working habits, the wife spent several minutes alternating between anxious tears and angry accusations. She was encouraged to express and come to terms with these conflicting emotions before she was allowed to speak to her husband.

In both of these cases, the social worker assessed the reactions to the news of trauma, intervened to facilitate the expression and initial management of conflictual feelings, and then consulted with the trauma surgeon in charge of the patient. This mutual consultation, while brief, has several important objectives. It advises the physician of the questions and interpersonal dynamics he or she will encounter when they meet the family. It also provides the social worker with updated information on the patient's condition and treatment plan. Finally, consultation allows the social worker and physician to coordinate their respective interventions in order to maximize the effectiveness of each.

Preparing the Family to See the Patient

Once the family has absorbed the initial shock of the trauma, they will typically request to see the patient. If at all possible, this wish is granted. Medical, rather than crisis intervention is rightly the priority of the trauma team; however, surgeons who have been sensitized to the emotional needs of their patients will advise the trauma social worker of lulls in activity that allow the patient and family time to spend with one another. It has been the author's experience that even a brief contact between patient and family is tremendously reassuring to all.

Before the family enters the treatment area, they are prepared for what they are about see. This is done in order to draw for the family a mental picture of what the patient will look like, and to desensitize them to this image. If the body has been altered in any way (e.g., color, lacerations, swelling, etc.) this fact is mentioned; the presence of medical equipment such as monitors, IV's, or intubation gear is carefully explained as well. Staff working with the patient are advised when the family is about to join the patient. Comments and behaviors which help staff to cope with their own anxiety in an emergent situation are not necessarily appropriate in the presence of highly distressed relatives, and are temporarily suspended. Trauma staff in the author's setting have become skilled in anticipating the anxieties and concerns of relatives specific to bedside treatment, and do what they can to accommodate and meet these needs. An intervention as simple as putting an arm around the shoulder of a distraught parent while treatment is being explained may do more than words to reassure the family.

Crisis Management

The literature on crisis theory identifies crisis situations as having four basic components: a hazardous event, a vulnerable state, a precipitating factor, and a state of active crisis. The first component, the hazardous event, is defined as "the initial blow or internal change that triggers the chain of reactions leading up to a state of disequilibrium" (Golan, 1972). When viewed from this perspective, the sudden, unanticipated personal disaster of a major medical trauma is the hazardous event that precipitates disequilibrium for significant individuals and the family unit of the trauma patient. In multi-system injuries, where more than one vital function or process is involved, physicians often have to treat first, then diagnose. This state of medical uncertainty is often accompanied by a parallel emotion of uncertainty for the relatives of trauma victims. Relatives may have to wait several hours before knowing precisely what injuries the patient has sustained, the severity of the trauma, and its implications. Often, just when families are beginning to adjust psychologically to what they believe is a complete picture of the patient's medical condition, the trauma surgeon will inform them of a new development or discovery that again throws them into a state of limbo. This emotional roller coaster may continue for several days, depleting the coping reserves of even the most functional of family members.

The trauma center social worker engages in purposeful interactions with relatives in order to maximize their ability to cope with the crisis. As Epperson (1977) has discussed, the social worker's ability to anticipate, understand and give therapeutic direction to the crisis reaction and concerns of family members helps to bring about successful "reconciliation" to what has happened. The primary goal throughout the early period of intervention is to keep the crisis clearly identified and in focus. By providing factual information about what has happened, what can be expected to happen and what role the family will have in the patient's treatment, relatives are given some structure in what is otherwise a totally unpredictable situation. At the same time, an acknowledgement is made of any ambiguity that may exist and of the difficulty inherent in dealing with uncertainty.

Faced with emotionally overwhelming and intellectually foreign information, relatives often immediately grasp the severity of the situation, but struggle for some time to integrate the specifics of the patient's condition. A recent example at UCI Trauma Center involved a family who had lost a son in a traffic accident the previous month. They were summoned to the hospital after being told that their daughter had been pulled from a flaming vehicle and was enroute to the trauma center. After some preparation of the parents by the social worker, the surgeon informed them that their daughter was in serious, but stable, condition. Their apparent understanding of this was gradually replaced by blankness and confusion. In this case and countless others like it, the social worker reassures the family that they are not "losing their minds" (a commonly expressed fear), but that they need time to adjust to the magnitude of the trauma. A concern of the social worker during this period is to remain sensitive to the emotional state of individual family members and to interpret their needs and behavior for trauma staff.

A secondary goal of intervention is to maximize the family's ability to help the patient. As Schnaper and Cowley (1976) have discovered, patients seen in trauma centers display a variety of emotional responses to their experience, but they almost universally report a struggle in dealing with feelings of helplessness, humiliation, and violation of body image. Most trauma center patients, unconscious when they are admitted, awake in a state of total confusion. As previously described, family members also have feelings of anxiety, uncertainty, and guilt. As much as possible, family members need to come to terms with their own crisis-related feelings. Successful resolution of these feelings will facilitate their ability to provide adequate emotional support to the patient who is experiencing physical and psychological turmoil.

An important aspect to consider when dealing with a significant medical crisis is that the trauma and its management represent abrupt loss as well as the threat of additional loss for the patient and family. What is lost immediately (not always at the conscious level) is one's belief in a certain degree of immunity from the disasters and misfortunes that beset others. This crust of denial, so essential for day to day functioning, is suddenly shattered when one is confronted with the reality of a loved one undergoing life-saving treatment. Statements such as, "It can't be true, tell me that this is a nightmare," or, "You can't be talking about my husband. Are you sure a mistake hasn't been made?" reveal the depth of denial that exists. Through effective listening and interpretation, the social worker can assist the family in facing this loss and gradually coming to terms with the reality of the situation. As in any crisis, one should not be forced to abandon denial until one is ready to do so.

A second type of loss, precipitated by the actual medical management of trauma, is loss of control over the opportunity to care for the patient oneself. The instinct to nurture one who is loved, and has been hurt, is suddenly thwarted. This situation gives rise to inevitable feelings of helplessness, dependency, and anger. The social worker can do several things in order to alleviate these feelings. A simple statement, such as, "Even though you know the doctors and nurses are doing all they can for your wife, it must be difficult to entrust her care to strangers," gives relatives permission to acknowledge and express ambivalent emotions, as well as the unrealistic fear that their anger might jeopardize staff's willingness to provide quality patient care. Helping the family formulate and express what psychosocial assistance is needed to deal with this predicament allows them to achieve some sense of control. One can ask, for example, what the nursing staff should know about the patient in order to better help that individual deal with the return of consciousness or the first critical days following surgery. An explanation can be given that this information will be shared with critical care staff so that they may care for the patient's emotional, as well as physical, trauma. As soon as possible, the family should be informed of the care plan for the patient, and they should be allowed to participate in some aspect of it. This will both reestablish them as important caretakers and prepare them for the patient's return home.

The final and perhaps most obvious loss, or threatened loss, particular to medical crisis is that to life, limb, or function. The following case illustrates the severity of loss with which some individuals are faced:

> Mark, 16, was rushed to the University Trauma Center following an accident in which he was dragged under a car for a mile. This gruesome accident cost the victim half of his face, his rectum, and larynx, and inflicted severe abrasion burns to most of his upper body. He spent seven hours in the operating room. Throughout Mark's ordeal, his parents were updated on their son's condition by no less than six medical specialists. Inundated with increasingly frightening information and attempting to cope with the emotional avalanche into which they had been thrown, the couple verbalized their two greatest fears—would their son survive, and if so, how badly would he be disfigured? The question of disfigurement proved to be a major theme for the first three days following the accident.

The parent's initial relief that their son had survived his injuries soon gave way to increasing anxiety regarding what he looked like under his dressings. Through special care and preparation of the parents by the social worker and trauma staff, they were gradually able to view Mark's injuries and begin the grieving process.

As the above case illustrates, the resolution of sudden, substantial loss is a major task which frequently faces the recipients of trauma center care. The teenager who is stabbed in the heart and dies in the Emergency Room, the parent of three children who is struck by a drunk driver and never regains consciousness, and the 20-year-old classical guitarist who loses a hand in an industrial accident, all represent the kinds of tragedy seen daily in the trauma center setting. When the loss encountered is one of limb or function, intervention is initiated as soon as possible with the patient. On an intrapsychic level, such a loss typically represents a narcissistic insult, or threat to the integrity of the patient's body image. Most patients readily verbalize feelings or depression, anger or fear, and are often relieved to be able to share these feelings openly (Golden, 1966).

Grief Counseling and Termination

When patients do not survive their injuries, the focus of social work intervention shifts from that of helping the family adjust to temporary medical uncertainty to management of the acute grief reaction. The social worker is routinely present when the physician delivers the news of death and engages in specific interventions so that the grief process might proceed normally. Relatives are allowed to ventilate strong emotions without fear of interruption or embarrassment. The use of sedatives is discouraged during this period, as it can blunt the initial grief reaction and retard the normal progression of the grief process (Dubin & Wolman, 1979). Friends and family members are encouraged to review their feelings toward, and relationships with, the deceased. As Dubin and Wolman note, such review prevents the family from somatization of their grief and from prolonged identification with the deceased. If the family feels that immediate spiritual support would be helpful, a clergy member of their choice is contacted and requested to come to the hospital.

Once initial reaction subsides, the family is given the option of viewing the body before it is sent to the morgue. Most family members feel strongly either that they would find it helpful to see the body, or would not. In either case, the decision made by each individual is respected. Often, relatives who have not outwardly expressed their grief will do so upon seeing and touching the body, as this experience validates for them the reality and finality of death. Before the family leaves the hospital, the physician discusses the issues of autopsy, organ donation, Coroner's involvement, and transfer of remains with them. The social worker helps the family to discuss these issues openly and make decisions about them. The social worker's final task is to assess the availability of supportive networks to the family and to encourage their utilization. The family is also advised that future help is available through access to the trauma social worker or community agencies if they should require professional assistance or intervention in the weeks or months to come.

CONCLUSION

The development and designation of hospital trauma centers brings with it the need for social workers who are specialized in the psychological aspects of trauma care. Functioning as an essential member of the trauma team, the social worker utilizes various roles and techniques in order to maximize the coping mechanisms and minimize psychiatric sequelae of the trauma patient and his or her family. By combining the skills of assessment, consultation, crisis management and grief counseling, the social worker helps to incorporate emotional, social, and cultural considerations into the overall care of the trauma patient. Many of the approaches and techniques described can be adopted by social workers in general emergency rooms, where crisis intervention is the primary treatment modality.

Improved paramedic programs and the development of specialized treatment centers cause more salvageable patients to come to the hospital now than ever before. Medical care by itself, no matter how superior it may be, is unable to provide for these patients in an optimum manner. It is anticipated that social workers will be called upon in ever increasing numbers to augment that care by providing immediate intervention to trauma patients and their families.

REFERENCES

Cowley, R.A., & Scanlan, E. University trauma center: Operation, design and staffing. *The American Surgeon*, 1979, *45*, 79-85.

Dubin, W.R., & Wolman, T. Evaluation and management of the grief reaction. *Pennsylvania Medicine*, 1979, *82*, 19-22.

Epperson, Margaret. Families in sudden crisis: Process and intervention in a critical care center. *Social Work in Health Care*, 1977, *2*(3), 265-273.

Golan, N. Social work intervention in medical crisis. *Hospital and Community Psychiatry*, 1972, *23*, 41-45.

Golden, J. S. Psychiatric management of acute trauma. In A. Nahum (ed.), *Early management of acute trauma*. St. Louis: The C. V. Mosby Co., 1966.

Harvey, J. C. The Emergency Medical Service Systems Act of 1973. *New England Journal of Medicine*, 1975, *292*, 529-530.

Maull, K. I., & Haynes, B. W. Jr. The integrated trauma service concept. *Journal of the American College of Emergency Physicians*, 1977, *6*, 497-499.

Montgomery, B. J. Emergency medical services: A new phase of development. *Journal of the American Medical Association*, 1980, *243*, 1017-1021.

National Academy of Sciences, Division of Medical Sciences, Committee on Trauma and Committee on Shock. *Accidental death and disability: The neglected disease of modern society*. Washington, D.C.: U.S. Department of HEW, 1966.

Schnaper, N., & Cowley, R. A. Overview: Psychiatric sequelae to multiple trauma. *The American Journal of Psychiatry*, 1976, *133*, 883-890.

West, J. G., Trunkey, D. D. & Lim, R. C. Systems of trauma care: A study of two counties. *Archives of Surgery*, 1979, *114*, 455-459.

The Intensive Care Unit: Social Work Intervention with the Families of Critically Ill Patients

Cindy Cook Williams, RN, MSW, ACSW
Donetta G. Rice, MSW, ACSW

SUMMARY. Hospital intensive care units can be a significant practice area for social workers. Nowhere are families in more obvious crises than when faced with the life-threatening illness of a significant other who may be unresponsive and dependent on a frightening array of highly technical equipment. Using the crisis model for their intervention, social workers can significantly lessen the trauma experienced by these families. Additionally, they can develop other supportive hospital resources such as family groups and volunteer services to help meet their needs.

With the expansion of scientific knowledge, changes in health care delivery are occurring more rapidly than ever before. Years ago private duty and recovery room nurses provided individualized care to the critically ill around the clock. Today this care has largely been replaced by hospital intensive care units. Patients with life-threatening diseases of the respiratory, cardiovascular, renal, and/or central nervous system are now able to receive constant observation and highly skilled nursing care in a concentrated location. This arti-

At the time of writing Ms. Williams was a social worker on the Intensive Care Units, Veterans Administration Hospital, 4435 Beacon Avenue South, Seattle, WA 98108. Much of her clinical practice in nursing took place on critical care units. Ms. Rice also practiced social work at the VA Hospital in Seattle, and was a clinical faculty member of the University of Washington School of Social Work.
Reprinted from *Social Work in Health Care*, Volume 2(4), Summer 1977.

cle describes how social workers can help the families of intensive care unit (ICU) patients with the traumatic effects of the experience.

CONTRASTING FEATURES OF ICU
AND GENERAL MEDICAL-SURGICAL UNITS

Intensive care units differ from general medical-surgical units in a number of ways. In the ICU each bedside area is set up with complex technical equipment necessary for continual monitoring of the patient's physical condition; lifesaving equipment is immediately available to meet each medical crisis. Patients are more closely observed by a higher ratio of nurses per patient. A general medical unit, as an example, can be staffed with one nurse for six patients while on the ICU one nurse may care for only two patients. In complex situations a one-to-one staffing pattern may occur. ICU nurses are highly experienced in dealing with medical emergencies; not all general duty nurses have the same experience or skill in dealing with these types of medical crises.

An immediate turning point in the patient's illness is usually expected on the ICU with a prognosis of either recovery or death. The technical equipment and constant nursing care enhance the likelihood of recovery through treatment on the ICU. When the patient's physical condition is stable he is usually moved to a general medical-surgical unit. Thus, intensive care units are further characterized by a shorter length of stay for patients. The close physical proximity of critically ill patients on the ICU often is markedly different from patient contact on other types of units. Continuous exposure to other seriously ill patients can provoke anxieties and fears for both the patient and his family members. As compared with the general wards, families of ICU patients observe a greater number of medical emergencies and deaths among neighboring patients.

IMPACT OF THE ICU ON FAMILY MEMBERS

In meeting acute medical crises, treatment can become highly mechanized and seem impersonal. It is not uncommon for patients to feel dehumanized and to be subjected to a complete lack of privacy. The family, of course, can easily observe this phenomenon on the ICU. They are assaulted by the impact of seeing their family member in this strange and impersonal environment, and by exposure to the suffering of others nearby. Hay and Oken vividly described the following reaction to the ICU:

> Initially, the greatest impact comes from the intricate machinery, with its flashing lights, buzzing and beeping monitor, gurgling suction pumps, and wheezing respirators. . . . Desperately ill, sick and injured human beings are hooked up to that machinery. And, in addition to mechanical stimuli, one can discern moaning, crying, screaming and the last gasps of life. Sights of blood, vomitus and excreta, exposed genitalia, mutilated wasted bodies, and unconscious and helpless people assault the sensibilities.[1]

The experience of seeing a family member comatose can be emotionally devastating, and it is not uncommon for some individuals to feel responsible for the patient's present condition. Statements reflecting guilt and fear are frequently expressed. Further emotional complications may arise when the patient is being sustained by technological means with little or no chance of recovery. The family, at times, is asked to participate in life-or-death decisions which can further exacerbate the crisis. Social work intervention based on the crisis model can assist families by lessening the trauma often inherent in the ICU hospitalization.

THE CRISIS MODEL

The potential loss of the patient through death is an ever-present reality on the ICU. Even with expert medical and nursing care, those patients who do survive may suffer long-lasting or permanent deficits in their physical and/or mental functioning. The threat of these potential losses significantly affects families of ICU patients. Customary role relationships and life goals of the family unit are in danger of upset because of the patient's altered physical condition. This disequilibrium in the family system constitutes a major crisis.

Individuals within a family may cope quite differently when confronted with the same crisis situation; and one family member's response to the course of events may directly influence how other members cope with the circumstances. Aguilera and Messick attribute individual differences in responses to the following factors: (a) the individual's perception of the stressful event; (b) the available support system; and (c) the coping mechanisms used to deal with the event.[2] Strengths and weaknesses in each of these areas have a significant impact on how effectively one regains equilibrium and resolves the crisis. Individuals who have a realistic perception of the crisis usually recognize the link between the precipitating event and feelings of stress. Problem solving can then be focused on reducing tension; successful resolution is subsequently more probable. The individual's support system, those resources currently available to assist with the crisis situation, can include other family members, friends, hospital staff, and community agencies. The more support an individual receives during a crisis, the better his chances for successful coping. Coping skills are those behaviors a person uses to resolve a problematic situation. Coping mechanisms used to deal with past crises may or may not be adequate for dealing with the current crisis.[3]

Social work assessment and intervention in these three areas can help families deal with the trauma experienced during the patient's ICU hospitalization. Evaluating the family's perceptions, coping skills, and situational supports lays the groundwork for appropriate intervention. Intervention is most often geared to strengthen areas with the most evident deficits. Using this crisis model, the ICU social worker can have a significant impact on the family's response to the circumstances and can promote their future functioning.

Perception of the Event

A family's perception of the crisis greatly influences cognitive, affective, and behavioral response to the situation.[4] How the family perceives the patient's physical status on the ICU can be incongruent with what is actually happening. One woman, for example, thought her husband was experiencing merely another bout of chest pain. Actually, however, the patient had had a cardiac arrest and was in critical condition. Although the woman had been told about the change in her husband's condition, high levels of anxiety prevented her from hearing and incorporating what was said. Detailed and complex verbal information is not always absorbed. The worker must not assume that explanations are always understood or remembered by family members. A wife who experienced the sudden traumatic death of her husband was able to make arrangements for the funeral with a minister and discuss the death with little display of emotion. One month later, however, she had no recollection of these conversations.

Social work intervention often involves strengthening and promoting communication lines between families and staff. Reinterpreting in laymen's terms the content of the physician's discussion about the patient's condition can be helpful. Periodically relaying information about the patient's physical status to the waiting family forges a supportive linkage. Family members are less likely then to let their imaginations fill in gaps of knowledge. If the patient is dying, they can begin to let in some awareness of the approaching death and are afforded some opportunity for anticipatory grieving. The social worker can also prevent and correct misconceptions about the patient's physical condition, as in the following case example:

> The wife of a patient who was being treated on the ICU following an automobile accident had been reassured by the physician that her husband's condition was stable. Suddenly a group of five men in white coats rushed up the hall and entered the unit. Upon watching this occurrence, the wife's response was, "Oh no, I knew he'd go downhill! It must be his heart again!" In reality the physicians were busy on rounds and had hurriedly entered the ICU to assist with a minor technical procedure. The social worker investigated the situation and relayed the actual purpose of the visit to the patient's wife. Her apprehension noticeably decreased, and she was also reassured that her husband, too, was receiving close medical attention.

The family's perception of the patient's course of medical treatment can be clarified by information giving.[5] A simple word of explanation about the use of intravenous feedings may serve to dispel unfounded fears and reduce anxiety. Although the equipment and medical procedures are commonplace to staff, they often are strange and unknown to the family. As their advocate, the social worker needs to alert the medical and nursing staff of the family's need for explanations. A conference that includes the family and staff is an effective way to facilitate the sharing of such pertinent information.

The social worker can also make sure the members of the family are allowed to see the patient when the medical situation becomes critical. If the patient is surrounded by medical and nursing staff during an emergency, it is understandable that the family simply cannot walk in. If at all possible following emergency procedures, however, it is beneficial for selected family members to see the patient. They may need to express a multiplicity of feelings or bring up unfinished business. Others look for reassurance that all measures are being taken to preserve the patient's life.[6]

Situational Support

Modern day strains accompany life-and-death issues in our society. We live in a highly mobile culture. Young families rarely live with their parents or grandparents. A network of nearby friends, relatives, and close neighbors is not always available during a time of crisis to provide the support that was often available in the past.[7]

The spouse of the ICU patient can often be found waiting alone in the lounge area. Mobilizing situational support for the family is essential. Asking them who has been helpful when problems were experienced in the past provides clues to determine whom the social worker or functioning member of the family can call on for immediate support. Direct observation of visitors can also reveal which individuals are most supportive to the family. Of those persons present, which individuals are spoken to most often concerning specific decisions and/or concerns? Another valuable source of situational support is the hospital staff. A staff member or trained volunteer can stay with the family during the crisis period, and the social worker is often in the best position to alert the staff/volunteer of this need. Staying with the family and allowing them to ventilate their feelings can be reassuring.

Mobilizing the support of community resources is often necessary. Practical concerns, such as housing, may present problems with which the social worker can help. Some families do not reside within the immediate catchment area of the hospital, and the worker can help them plan to use short-term housing resources near the hospital. Frequently referrals are needed for immediate or long-term financial assistance. Many families are not prepared for medical emergencies, and financial difficulties add enormously to the feelings of anxiety.

Coping Mechanisms

A crisis often brings back thoughts and feelings about similar situations in the past. Families of ICU patients frequently discuss life-threatening illnesses of other important people in their lives. How they responded to these past crises is often predictive of how they will cope with the present circumstances. An individual's coping style, according to Kiely, will most likely reflect personality characteristics typical of previous functioning.[8]

Some family members react to the illness of a significant other with much hostility and anger. Their fear for the life of the patient can easily be projected onto the medical and nursing staff. They may see staff paying more attention to another patient and assume their family member is being neglected. A soiled bedsheet may represent poor nursing care to them.[9] The open expression of anger and hostility by families can be extremely difficult for staff. The social worker can be instrumental in discussing the psychodynamics of the situation with the ICU staff. As they better understand the family's response, staff may be more tolerant and able to allow expression of these types of feelings. Attempts to defend the staff's actions to the angry family, however, may escalate their expressions of hostility. It is not an issue of taking sides; the family must be allowed to react in a manner that is characteristic for them.

Another common defense mechanism used by family members is rationalizing feelings of guilt. A wife may search the events before hospitalization for her failure to do right by her husband. Other family members may use denial as a way of dealing with the crisis, as in the following case:

One husband repeatedly emphasized that he was able to deal with his wife's illness without difficulty. He would comment to family, friends, and staff, "I'm fine. Things are under control. It's not getting to me." Close family members, however, reported that he was not sleeping at night, would pace the halls, and ate very little. With help the husband was able to express his fear and anxiety.

Family members' reactions to the death of the patient vary. Some individuals react by weeping, moaning, clinging to staff, or pacing the halls. Others panic, cry, and shout. These people, in one way or another, are able to express their grief. A box of tissues, a cold wet washrag, and a darkened private room are often helpful. The tissues give the individual an "OK" to cry openly and express feelings of grief. Some people respond to human touch—a hug or hand on one's shoulder. Others wish to be left alone. The approach for the social worker is simply to be there, to be sensitive to the family's needs and allow them to express their feelings in their own way.

When a patient does die, hospital staff frequently prescribe tranquilizing medication for family members. Sedating a screaming, crying, or hysterical person to quiet him down is not always indicated. Administering sedating drugs may be a way that staff cope with their feelings of helplessness in the situation. It is wise to question whether it is the client's or the staff's crisis that is being treated with drugs. Whenever possible it is preferable to provide human support rather than chemical masking of the traumatic reaction.

Family members experiencing shock and disbelief may need assistance with decision making. Issues such as the choice of funeral home, what to do with the patient's personal effects, or permission for an autopsy may arise.

One family had difficulty deciding when and how to notify the elderly mother of a patient who had died unexpectedly. The woman had a long history of cardiac problems, and the family feared for her physical health. After discussion with the social worker, the family decided to confer with the family physician; those individuals closest to the mother then approached her with the unfortunate news.

Establishment of Hospital Services
for the Families of ICU Patients

The physical layout of hospitals is primarily geared to meet the medical needs of patients. Little attention is given to the space needs of family members. Nowhere is the lack of adequate space more pivotal than with the families of ICU patients.

Families can frequently be found hovering outside the ICU doors, as most want to stay as close to the patient as possible. In most hospitals the alternative is to wait in the lobby or a room some distance away from the unit. To humanize our health care institutions, more attention needs to be paid to providing physical space and privacy for families during this time of crisis. Health planners should consider these needs when designing and constructing new hospitals. Kübler-Ross recommended that hospitals establish a nearby "screaming room" where families can wait in privacy and in an atmosphere that would be more conducive to the family's open ventilation of feelings about their circumstances. A room with a couch, comfortable chairs, a telephone, clock, and perhaps a coffee or coke machine would provide the family a refuge away from busy corridors, the traditional cold, remote waiting rooms, and the stares of others.[10]

In addition, a core of workers is needed who can stay with families and provide emotional support. Availability of workers on a twenty-four-hour basis is essential; family needs are not limited to specific shifts. The workers might include social workers, chaplains, nurses, and trained volunteers. Family members of former ICU patients can form a nucleus for a pool of volunteers.[11]

Group meetings with the families of ICU patients are another helpful service that should be offered. Participants in the group can share their fears and concerns, as well as find psychological support knowing that their emotional responses are being experienced by others as well. Camaraderie often develops between group members, and it is not unusual for them to maintain supportive contact with each other outside the hospital. Many are also able to extend their support to other family members and friends.

A twenty-three-year-old female was brought to the emergency room in cardiopulmonary arrest. She responded to emergency medical procedures and was subsequently placed in the ICU. The patient's mother came from the East Coast to be with her. After the shock of seeing her daughter in acute crisis had worn off, she continued to stay near the unit twelve to fourteen hours a day and made continued demands for information from the staff. Since the cause of her daughter's condition was in doubt, there was relatively little specific information for staff to provide. As the mother's frustration and anger grew, her complaints about the care increased. She was asked to join a group composed of family members, staff, and patients. During the group meetings she was able to cry and openly express her fears and anger. As the weeks passed, the mother made friends with other families, and a mutual support system developed. Staff contacts decreased, and she needed to spend less time at the hospital. The daughter's oxygen deprivation at the time of crisis caused brain damage, and she needed an intensive retraining program prior to discharge. The mother continued to use the group for problem solving until her daughter was released.

CONCLUSION

Family members are often aghast at the sight of their relative being cared for in the hectic, mechanical, and impersonal environment of an ICU. Seeing a patient comatose with tubes in his orifices can be frightening. When critically ill patients die they leave families with heartbreaking adjustments to make. As their advocate, the social worker can provide needed intervention at the scene of the crisis. His assessment of and help with the family's perception of the circumstances, their coping mechanisms, and the situational supports available to them are an integral component of the team's effort in caring for the patient. Social work intervention can lessen the trauma inherent in a patient's ICU hospitalization and significantly improve the family's functioning in the crisis.

REFERENCES

1. Donald Hay and Donald Oken, "The Psychological Stresses of Intensive Care Unit Nursing," *Psychosomatic Medicine* 34 (1972):110.

2. Donna C. Aguilera and Janice M. Messick, *Crisis Intervention: Theory and Methodology* (Saint Louis: C.V. Mosby Co., 1974), p. 63.

3. Ibid., p. 64.

4. Kathleen Obier and L. Julian Haywood, "Enhancing Therapeutic Communication with Acutely Ill Patients," *Heart and Lung* 2 (1973):50.

5. Carolyn Bascom Bilodeau, "The Nurse and Her Reactions to Critical Care Nursing," *Heart and Lung* 2 (1973):358-63.

6. Elisabeth Kübler-Ross, "Crisis Management of Dying Persons and Their Families," in *Emergency Psychiatric Care: The Management of Mental Health Crises*, ed. H. L. P. Resnik and Harvey L. Ruben (Bowie, Md.: Charles Press Publishers, 1975), p. 150.

7. Ibid., p. 145.

8. William F. Kiely, "Psychiatric Aspects of Critical Care," *Critical Care Medicine* 2 (1974):140.

9. Hay and Oken, "Psychological Stresses," p. 112.

10. Kübler-Ross, "Crisis Management," p. 154.

11. Ibid.

Social Work and Primary Health Care: An Integrative Approach

Joan R. Brochstein, MSW, MPH
George L. Adams, MD
Michael P. Tristan, MD, MPH
Charles C. Cheney, PhD

SUMMARY. An interinstitutional, interagency Consortium has been formed in Houston to develop an innovative service model and provide interdisciplinary primary care/mental health training. The Houston Consortium Program integrates mental health professionals and trainees into the primary care framework of a neighborhood center serving a low-income, predominantly Mexican-American population. The introduction of mental health, psychosocial, and cross-cultural perspectives to complement the long-standing physiological concerns of health professionals fosters an holistic approach to patient care. The social workers' full participation as members of primary care teams builds upon their traditional training to provide them the experience and skills required to function effectively in the expanded coordinative capacity of health/mental health manager as defined by the President's Commission on Mental Health. It is anticipated that Consortium Program can serve as a heuristic model in the development of a nationwide pattern of comprehensive care.

At the time of writing the authors were from the Departments of Psychiatry, Community Medicine, and Pediatrics, Baylor College of Medicine, Texas Medical Center, Houston, TX 77030. A preliminary version of this paper was presented in a session entitled "Social Work in Primary Care" at the 106th Annual Meeting of the American Public Health Association, Los Angeles, CA, on October 15-19, 1978. This work has been supported by NIMH Grant #1 T21 14863-02.

Reprinted from *Social Work in Health Care*, Volume 5(1), Fall 1979.

INTRODUCTION

Recent decades have witnessed the achievement of impressive advances in American medical science and the development of technologically complex and sophisticated health care specialties (Coggeshall, 1965; Millis, 1971). This period has also been marked by a concurrent national trend toward fragmentation, high cost, and inaccessibility of health care services (Regional Workshops on Health Manpower Distribution, 1975).

A major focus on efforts to address this situation is primary care medicine, which has been defined as entailing the individual physician or primary care team providing "first contact" care, assuming longitudinal responsibility, and serving "integrationist' functions vis-à-vis the broader health care system for the patient and his or her family (Alpert & Charney, 1974). Examples of the current thrust to significantly augment the manpower pool in the primary care fields of family practice, general pediatrics, and general internal medicine, include the following: establishment of the Board of Family Practice in 1969; passage of federal legislation in 1971 to finance family practice training; promulgation of recommendations on manpower and training in 1978 by the Institute of Medicine Committee on Primary Care; and passage of the Health Professions Educational Assistance Act of 1976, which sets the goal of providing 50% residency training positions in the primary care professions by 1980 (Coordinating Council of Medical Education, 1975; Institute of Medicine, 1978; Health Professions Educational Assistance Act, 1976).

Similarly, the community mental health movement has since its inception in the early 1960s sought to establish programs which provide community-oriented prevention, early detection and treatment of illness, and rehabilitation and supportive care for the chronically ill (Musto, 1977). Although performance may have fallen short of these objectives, the President's Commission on Mental Health has recently reaffirmed the commitment to effectively address such national mental health issues as community-based prevention and aftercare — especially for such traditionally underserved segments of the population as children, the elderly, and minority groups — through the interlinking of existing public sector health and mental health service resources (Holland, 1977; President's Commission on Mental Health, 1978).

The developments in primary care and community mental health bear crucial importance for the discipline of social work in terms of both service delivery and professional training. In recent years, employment among social workers in the health care field has undergone rapid increases, with the number of practitioners rising from 11,700 in 1960 to 29,800 in 1970 (Bracht, 1974; DHEW, 1971). A 1975 report of the National Association of Social Workers notes that close to one-third of its members currently practice in health care settings (16.6%) or mental health organizations (14.4%) (NASW, 1975). Moreover, it has been predicted that within the next two decades health and mental health service systems will employ more than 50% of all practicing social workers (Shulman, 1977). The profession of social work has long advocated the provision of holistic, comprehensive services to clients and has come to increasingly recognize and apply the principles of general systems theory in working at the interface of human service systems (Raymond, 1977; Gordon, 1969). The integrationist aspects of the primary care and community mental health movements are therefore of special significance to social workers (Lurie, 1977). The question remains, however, as to how these developing health care systems will incorporate the particular knowledge and skills which social work has offer, and conversely, how social workers will prepare themselves to practice effectively within the health/mental health care fields.

Following an overview of the relationship of primary care and mental health, this paper provides an outline of an experimental primary care mental health program and a discussion of its potential relevance to future social work training and practice.

PRIMARY CARE AND MENTAL HEALTH

It has been estimated that primary care providers devote as much as 70% of their time to their patients' emotional difficulties, the spectrum of psychological problems which they encounter ranging from the stresses of modern life, to the emotional concomitants of physical illness, to the severe psychotic disorders (Borus, 1976).

Yet the available mental health expertise required to effectively deal with these problems is often limited. Seldom are mental health professionals incorporated into primary care settings; interagency referral mechanisms between primary care and mental health care systems are usually intricate and obstacle-ridden, if they exist at all (Borus et al., 1975); and physicians and other primary caregivers generally do not possess the skills necessary to handle the psychological factors of patient care (Wise et al., 1974).

The delivery of community mental health services is characterized by difficulties ranging from the complexity of establishing and maintaining effective preventive care to issues of interagency coordination in the hospitalization and aftercare of the mentally ill, including the reintegration of returning patients into their families and communities (Borus et al., 1975; Scherl & English, 1969). Moreover, the failure of mental health centers to make services appropriate to the specific sociocultural characteristics of consumer populations can seriously impede the provision of care to minority groups (Kline, 1969; Phillipus, 1971).

The capacity of primary care settings and neighborhood mental health care centers to provide optimal mental health services is often constrained by limitations in the training experiences of their staff members (Wise et al., 1974). In the course of their training, physicians and other primary care providers generally receive little psychological education that is relevant and applicable to primary care delivery; health and mental health professionals do not tend to acquire either a first hand knowledge of primary care delivery or flexibility in interpreting the respective roles and functions of their various disciplines (Goldberg et al., 1976; Lazerson, 1976; Banta & Fox, 1972; Brenneis & Laub, 1973; Morrison et al., 1973). Furthermore, the standard training of both primary care providers and mental health professions is seldom focused on meeting community-oriented service needs. That is, their education does not equip them with the psychosocial and cross-cultural perspectives required to readily comprehend and appropriately address problems they may encounter in the context of providing neighborhood-based primary care and mental health care services to underprivileged minority populations (Garcia, 1971; Karno & Edgerton, 1969).

The inability of primary care and mental health systems to adequately provide comprehensive services to patients is a profound dilemma in health care today. The Houston Consortium Program is an attempt to address this problem, to train caregivers of a variety of professional disciplines to provide full-scale, quality patient care. Social workers, with their background in treating the client in a holistic and humanistic manner, play a central role in this process. The Houston Consortium Program represents an experimental effort designed to integrate social work practice with primary care/mental health service and training (Adams et al., 1978).

An Integrative Approach

The Houston Primary Care Mental Health Training Consortium comprises three educational institutions and two service agencies: The University of Houston Graduate School of Social Work; The University of Texas School of Nursing at Houston; The Baylor College of Medicine (Departments of Psychiatry, Community Medicine, Internal Medicine, and Pediatrics); The Harris County Hospital District, a public agency which delivers care to the mentally indigent; and the Mental Health and Mental Retardation Authority of Harris County, a public provider of mental health services.

The Consortium Training Program has the following objectives:

1. To educate mental health trainees in the delivery of mental health services, both as fully integrated members of primary care teams and as members of secondary mental health teams providing consultation and backup services in primary care settings;
2. To enable primary health care professionals and trainees to acquire mental health skills which will help them to better serve their patients;
3. To develop teaming and interdisciplinary working skills in the delivery of health and mental services in primary care settings; and
4. To provide health and mental health caregivers with psychosocial and cross-cultural perspectives in the delivery of care to minority populations.

Initiated in July, 1977 at Casa de Amigos Neighborhood Health Center, the Program is located in a large Mexican-American *barrio* in north central Houston. This facility is a multi-service neighborhood center which contains components of the Harris County Hospital District, the Mental Health and Mental Retardation Authority of Harris County, and the Houston Public Health Department. It serves a catchment area including more than 400,000 persons. Adjacent to the facility is a community center which houses a variety of human service, educational, and cultural enrichment activities. This training site was chosen for the following reasons: its mission is to provide comprehensive services to meet the needs of the low-income, predominantly Mexican-American population of the surrounding community; it has both primary care and mental health service programs; primary care is delivered through teams composed of physicians' extenders, nurses, and nutritionists; and two of the Consortium's participating educational institutions were previously using the facility for training purposes.

The Program's trainees include graduate social work, psychiatric nursing, and clinical psychology students; residents in psychiatry, pediatrics, internal medicine, and the prototype primary care; and medical students. An interdisciplinary, bilingual, bicultural core faculty renders direct and indirect services and provides supervision and didactic instruction to all trainees. In addition, they provide continuing education and inservice training to the neighborhood center's primary care and community mental health personnel and work on a consultation basis with local social service organizations.

The structure of the Consortium Program encompasses two primary care teams, one for pediatric and one for adult services, and a secondary mental health care team. Together with primary care residents and medical students, graduate social work and nursing trainees are integrated into the primary care teams to provide mental health assessment, to render mental health services for patients, and to link the two teams in addressing family mental health problems. The majority of services for patients who present with emotional or psychosocial difficulties are provided by social work and nursing students. Clinical psychology interns and psychiatric residents comprise the secondary team within the framework of the neighborhood center's mental health unit to provide consultation, liaison, and backup services for the primary care teams; deliver preventive and aftercare services to the mental unit's psychiatric patients; and render consultation and education to community organizations. Interdisciplinary collaboration occurs routinely within each team, as well as between the adult and pediatric primary care teams and between the primary and secondary teams. The latter generally occurs when nurses and social workers are presented with a patient whose emotional problems are too complex to be handled on the primary care team level; in such cases secondary team psychologists and psychiatrists are available to either work directly with the patient or provide consultation to the primary care team member who is working with the patient.

In the course of providing health and mental health services to patients in the primary care setting, trainees acquire a wide range of practical skills in their respective disciplines as well as knowledge of the many aspects of primary care medicine. Mental health trainees develop both basic mental health skills and those specialized skills which enable them to provide direct and indirect services within the primary care framework. Skills acquired by primary care trainees include the ability to distinguish normal from abnormal behavior; to evaluate psychological difficulties in their patients; and to design and implement treatment plans for patients and their families with mental health or psychosocial problems. The Consortium Program enables all trainees to acquire skills in recognizing and handling cross-cultural and psychosocial aspects of physical and emotional illness, in working competently on interdisciplinary teams, and in utilizing the resources of the surrounding community for the benefit of their patients. In addition to their minimum of three days per week of practicum experience at the field training site, all trainees pursue coursework at their respective home institutions and participate in weekly Consortium seminars and case conferences at Baylor College of Medicine.

In the Consortium Program, social work trainees, in close collaboration with graduate nursing students, are involved in all aspects of patient care and bear long term responsibility for the patient. At each level of care—primary, secondary, and tertiary—the social worker plays a significant role. He or she is actively involved in screening, assessment, and treatment planning processes for new patients, and has an important part in the early detection and prevention of individual and family difficulties. On the secondary level, the social worker participates in treatment through such activities as crisis intervention and short-term, goal-oriented psychotherapy. Finally, social workers are involved in rehabilitative efforts, helping patients reintegrate into a life of social and job functioning. When the social worker is not directly involved in providing secondary and tertiary care, he or she takes on longitudinal responsibilities, acting in a liaison capacity to other providers.

The experience of training under the Consortium format is a unique opportunity for the social work trainee. Unlike most ambulatory care settings, the Consortium Program accords social work students authority in decision-making processes; the assessments and recommendations of social workers, and of other non-medical professionals, are judiciously considered in team decisions regarding diagnosis and treatment. With the participation of mental health trainees in patient staffings, close attention is paid to issues of patient care not normally considered by primary care providers. Thus, social workers focus on the patient in the context of his family and neighborhood and help to engender an awareness among team members of psychological, cultural, socioeconomic, and other influences on the patient's health.

In addition to their clinical participation in the Program, social workers play a vital role in developing and maintaining connections between the many components of the Consortium. Drawing on their skill in working with systems, social workers are involved in in-house coordination among the public health, hospital district, and community mental health programs; in primary care interteam connections (e.g., in working with family problems, social workers will provide ongoing communication between the pediatric and adult teams); and in community consultation. In the latter endeavor, social workers have developed intensive working alliances with neighborhood schools, drug abuse programs, and geriatric organizations in the surrounding community. The efforts of social workers in the management of specific cases have led them to do valuable work in bridging the various systems operating overtly and covertly in the community. Improved patient care is becoming evident as barriers to communication gradually dissolve.

DISCUSSION

A clear challenge confronting social work practitioners in the Houston Consortium Program and, indeed, in the health care arena nationally, is how to utilize their strengths and knowledge in such a way as to enhance the quality of care which patients receive in health and mental health service systems. With the rapidly changing nature of health care delivery and with the increasing participation of social workers in medical settings, the opportunity to influence the course of patient care is open to the social work professions as it has not been in the past. The comprehensive approach to care so familiar to the social worker is also being implemented by the primary caregivers; the rich experience of social workers in this area should be tapped as development in the field occurs.

Essentially, the participation of the social worker in health care delivery systems is not new. But despite the fact that social workers have been involved in multidisciplinary working relationships for many years, they have not functioned as an integral part of the health care process; their role has generally been circumscribed and limited to that of helper or enabler to other health professionals (Kane, 1976; Rusnack, 1977). Prior to the launching of the Consortium Program, for example, social workers at Casa de Amigos were delegated responsibilities which might be considered typical of the standard social work role. That is, social workers provided intake, liaison, and referral services, functioning essentially as aides to other professionals at the site. They were not integral members of the health care system and did not participate actively in the decision-making processes regarding patient care. They ultimately had little impact on the quality of care delivered to the consumer.

In the Houston Consortium model, an effort has been made to draw on the strengths and knowledge of social workers, to utilize their talents fully within the context of providing services to patients and training those of other disciplines in social work approaches to patient care. Unlike the previous system which operated at Casa de Amigos, the participation of social workers is crucial to the functioning of the primary care teams and the health care delivery process in general. The traditional social work role has been redefined and expanded so that the social worker has substantial influence on the course of patient care and on the training experiences of all who participate in the Program.

It seems apparent that social workers may have a vital role to play in guiding primary care providers toward a holistic perspective in the formulation of their patients' difficulties. In addressing the whole of a patient's problems, the social worker takes a very different stance from that of traditional medicine. Health providers have generally been taught to take a specific and highly focused approach to treatment, working exclusively with a patient's physical problems. Such a perspective is contrary to the demands of the primary care setting, where a broader, more inclusive approach is needed if patients are to receive comprehensive care.

A considerable portion of the skills which providers must master if they are to function effectively in a primary care setting are skills and strengths which are within the purview of social work. Comprehensive care entails consideration of the many facets of a client's life which impinge on his health. Social workers, with their real-world orientation, are well practiced in this approach to care; assessing a client with full regard for his life circumstances is a cornerstone of social work practice. The social worker's expertise in psychosocial, cross-cultural, and socioeconomic perspectives as well as community dynamics and agency resources should be shared with all providers, regardless of discipline, as such issues must be fully considered in the assessment and management of patients.

The profession's orientation toward holistic human services, coupled with an increasing utilization of general systems approaches, provides social workers with a strong foundation for taking a leading role in the training experiences of multidisciplinary primary care providers and in the coordination of health and mental health delivery systems. With their broad, humanistic view and the new skills learned through participation in a training model such as the one described herein, social workers can function as managers in integrating multiple aspects of patient care. The possibility of assuming such a role represents a serious challenge for social work educators: if social workers are to function effectively in complex health care systems and, indeed, if they are to play a central role in ensuring comprehensive care for patients, training experiences must be designed which will prepare social workers to accept these new and difficult responsibilities. By training social work students to work competently within the evolving health and mental care systems, social workers can affect the skills and attitudes developed by those of other disciplines as well as ultimately having influence on the quality of care delivered to patients.

CONCLUSION

Efforts to redress the fragmentation and inaccessibility of the nation's health/mental health resources have in recent years included the parallel development of the primary care and community mental health movements. Moreover, the President's Commission on Mental Health in 1978 called for the coordination of public sector health and mental health service systems in order to make them more responsive to the needs of the consumer. In the same spirit, the Houston Consortium Program has been established to provide comprehensive care to patients through the inter-linking of health and mental health care systems, as well as to generate a pool of highly trained providers through interdisciplinary primary care mental health training. In the Consortium Program, the traditional adjunctive status of the social worker has been supplanted by a stronger, more active role: in terms of both systems management and clinical care, the social worker fulfills important service and training functions.

With the current trend of health and mental health care moving toward greater coordination and integration, the Consortium Program can serve as a viable model for the achievement of comprehensive service delivery and training. A synthesis of social work's holistic, systems orientation and of the new capabilities acquired through a model such as this can equip social workers to effectively assume the responsibilities of case management as defined by the President's Commission on Mental Health (1978:24):

> Strategies focused solely on organizations are not enough. A human link is required. A case manager can provide this link and assist in assuring continuity of care and a coordinated program of services. Case management is an expediting service. The case manager should be sensitive to the disabled person's needs, knowledgeable about government and private agencies that provide housing, income maintenance, mental health, and social services, and should be in close touch with the community's formal and informal support systems.

Through such a pivotal management role, social work can make a significant contribution to a revitalized nationwide integrated pattern of health and mental health care delivery.

REFERENCES

Adams, G.L., Brochstein, J.R., Cheney, C.C., Friese, J.H., & Tristan, M.P. A primary care/mental health training and service model. *American Journal of Psychiatry*, 1978, *135*, 121-123.

Alpert, J.J., & Charney, E. *The education of physicians for primary care* (DHEW Publication No. (HRA) 74-3113). Washington, D.C.: U.S. Government Printing Office, 1974.

Banta, D.A., & Fox, R.C. Role strains of a health care team in a poverty community. *Social Science and Medicine*, 1972, *6*, 697-722.

Borus, J.F. Neighborhood health centers as providers of primary mental health care. *New England Journal of Medicine*, 1976, *275*, 140-145.

Borus, J.F., Janowitch, L.A., & Kieffer, F. The coordination of mental health services at the community level. *American Journal of Psychiatry*, 1975, *132*, 1177-1181.

Bracht, N.F. Health Care: The largest human services system. *Social Work*, 1974, *19*, 538.

Brenneis, C.B., & Laub, D. Current strains for mental health trainees. *American Journal of Psychiatry*, 1973, *130*, 41-45.

Coggeshall, L.T. *Planning for medical progress through education*. Evanston, IL: Association of American Medical Colleges, 1965.

Coordinating Council on Medical Education. *Physician manpower and distribution: The primary care physician*. Chicago, IL: CCMA, 1975.

Department of Health, Education and Welfare, *Health Resources Document*. Washington, D.C.: U.S. Government Printing Office, 1971.

Garcia, A. The Chicano and social work. *Social Casework*, 1971, *52*, 174-178.

Goldberg, R.L., Haas, M.R., Eaton, J., & Grubbs, J.H. Psychiatry and the primary care physician. *Journal of the American Medical Association*, 1976, *133*, 964-966.

Gordon, W.E. Basic constructs for an integrative and generative conception of social work. In G. Hearn (Editor), *The general systems approach: Contribution toward a holistic conception of social work*. New York: National Association of Social Workers, 1969.

Health Professional Educational Assistance Act of 1976. (S. 3239) H.R. 5546, as amended.

Holland, B.C. An evaluation of the criticisms of the community mental health movement. In W.E. Barton & C.J. Sanborn (Editors), *An assessment of the community mental health movement*. Lexington, MA: Lexington Books, 1977.

Institute of Medicine, *Manpower policy for primary health care* (National Academy of Sciences Publication No. 2764). Washington, D.C.: U.S. Government Printing Office, 1978.

Kane, R.A. Interprofessional education and social work: A survey. *Social Work in Health Care*, 1976, *2*, 2.

Karno, M. & Edgerton, R.B. Perceptions of mental illness in a Mexican American community. *Archives of General Psychiatry*, 1969, *20*, 233-238.

Kline, L.Y. Some factors in the psychiatric treatment of Spanish Americans. *American Journal of Psychiatry*, 1969, *125*, 1674-1681.

Lazerson, A.M. The psychiatrist in primary medical care training: A solution to the mind-body dichotomy? *American Journal of Psychiatry*, 1976, *133*, 964-966.

Lurie, A. Social work in health care in the next ten years. *Social Work in Health Care*, 1977, *2*, 4.

National Association of Social Workers. *Manpower data bank frequency distributors* (NASW Publication No. 4). Washington, D.C.: NASW, 1975.

Millis, J. *A rational public policy for medical education and its financing.* New York: National Fund for Medical Education, 1971.

Morrison, A.P., Shore, M.F., & Grobman, J. On the stresses of community psychiatry and helping residents to survive them. *American Journal of Psychiatry*, 1973, *130*, 1237-1241.

Musto, D.F. The community mental health movement in historical perspective. In W.E. Barton & C.J. Sanborn (Editors), *An Assessment of the Community Mental Health Movement.* Lexington, MA: Lexington Books, 1977.

Phillipus, M. Successful and unsuccessful approaches to mental health services for an urban hispanic population. *American Journal of Public Health*, 1971, *61*, 820-830.

President's Commission on Mental Health. *Report to the President of the President's Commission on Mental Health, Vol. 1.* Washington, D.C.: U.S. Government Printing Office, 1978.

Raymond, F.D. Social work education for health care practice. *Social Work in Health Care*, 1977, *2*, 4.

Regional Workshops on Health Manpower Distribution. *Report on national health 1974-1975.* New York: National Health Council, 1975.

Rusnack, B. Planned change: Interdisciplinary education for health care. *Journal of Education for Social Work*, 1977, *13*, 104-111.

Scherl, D.J. & English, J.T. Community mental health and comprehensive health service programs for the poor. *American Journal of Psychiatry*, 1969, *125*, 1666-1674.

Shulman, L. Social work education for health care practice: Response to Professor Raymond. *Social Work in Health Care*, 1977, *2*, 4.

Wise, H., Beckhand, R., Rubin, I. & Kyte, H.L. *Making health teams work.* Cambridge, MA: Ballinger, 1974.

Commentary

These articles demonstrate that medical specialization breeds social work specialization in the design of social work programs for patient populations treated by an increasing number of physician specialists (*Health and Social Work*, 1981). Yet these diverse programs connect with each other.

Skilled, rapid assessment of clients' needs and resources, rapid tempo of work, extended work schedules, and intensive teamwork characteristic of emergency room social work (Farber, 1978, and Groner, 1978) are to a considerable degree applicable to social work in other health care programs, for example, in trauma centers and critical care surgery units where the factors of crises and time are characteristic. These functions may also be considered, tested, and extended to quite different services and settings. For example, pediatric high-risk teams, concerned with the prevention and detection of child abuse and neglect require the same emphasis on rapid assessment, flexibility of staff's work schedules, and close collaborative teamwork. In neonatal intensive care units, in addition to providing services to the anxious parents of the infant, social workers can help support other staff members who experience high levels of stress as they provide exacting technological care to premature and weak infants whose future is uncertain (Mahan, Krueger, and Schreiner, 1982).

Likewise, as health care services are delivered through prepaid HMO plans and home health care programs, patients' needs for psychosocial evaluation and treatment services will be adequately met only if social workers are successful in evolving strategies to participate actively in the development of such programs (Greene, Kruse, and Arthur, 1985).

Changing demography and life-prolonging advances in medical technology have combined to create new populations of chronically ill patients with as yet incurable conditions such as Alzheimer's disease, amyotrophic lateral sclerosis, renal failure, and cancer, among others. Formerly fatal illnesses are transformed into chronic illnesses, even in the case of the young (Ross, 1982). These and other populations require complex supports to sustain them through major and enduring difficulties in managing the routines of daily life. They need basic social as well as medical care.

The emotional stress and need for support experienced by staff caring for cancer patients have been documented (Davidson, 1985). It has been observed that professionals in these settings seem readier for collaborative teamwork, probably because the nature of the stresses that accompany the treatment or conditions such as amyotrophic lateral sclerosis, for example, make the members of the care team more receptive to the support and contribution of their colleagues, both for themselves and for the patient and family. Incurable, progressive illness tends to foster closer teamwork.

REFERENCES

Davidson, Kay W. "Social Work with Cancer Patients: Stresses and Coping Patterns," *Social Work in Health Care 10*(4) Summer 1985, pp. 73–82.

Farber, John M. "Emergency Department Social Work: A Program Description and Analysis," *Social Work in Health Care 4*(1), Fall 1978, pp. 7–18.

Greene, Gilbert, Kruse, Katherine A., and Arthurs, Ruth J. "Family Practice Social Work: A New Area of Specialization," *Social Work in Health Care 10*(3), Spring 1985, pp. 53–73.

Groner, Edith. "Delivery of Clinical Social Work Services in the Emergency Room: A Description of an Existing Program," *Social Work in Health Care 4*(1), Fall 1978, pp. 19–29.

Health and Social Work 6(1), November 1981. Supplement on "Specialization and Specialty Interests."

Mahan, Carol K., and Schreiner, Richard L. "Management of Perinatal Death: The Role of the Social Worker in the Newborn ICU," *Social Work in Health Care 6*(3), Spring 1981, pp. 69–76.

Nason, Frances, and DelBanco, Thomas L. "Soft Services: A Major, Cost-Effective Component of Primary Medical Care," *Social Work in Health Care 1*(3), Spring of 1976, pp. 297–308.

Ross, Judith. "The Role of the Social Worker with Long-Term Survivors of Pediatric Cancer and Their Families," *Social Work in Health Care 7*(4), Summer 1982, pp. 1–13.

Additional Readings

Barstow, Linda. "Working with Cancer Patients in Radiation Therapy," *Health and Social Work* 7(1), February 1982, pp. 35–40.

Becerra, Rosina M. "Knowledge and Use of Child Health Services by Chinese Americans," *Health and Social Work* 6(3), August 1981, pp. 29–38.

Bell, Cynthia, and Gorman, Laurel M. "The HMOs: New Models for Practice," *Social Work in Health Care* 1(3), Spring 1976, pp. 325–335.

Demby, Annette. "Preventive Intervention in an HMO: The Social Worker's Role in a Marital Separation Program," *Social Work in Health Care* 5(4), Summer 1980, pp. 351–360.

Dillard, Robert G.; Auerbach, Kathleen G., and Showalter, Anne H. "A Parents' Program in the Intensive Care Nursery: Its Relationship to Maternal Attitudes and Expectations," *Social Work in Health Care* 5(3), Spring 1980, pp. 245–251.

Dunkel, Joan, and Hatfield, Shellie. "Countertransference Issues in Working with Persons with AIDS," *Social Work* 31(2), March-April 1986, pp. 114–117.

Epperson, Margaret M. "Families in Sudden Crisis: Process and Intervention in a Critical Care Center," *Social Work in Health Care* 2(3), Spring 1977, pp. 265–273.

Furlong, Regina M., and Black, Rita Beck. "Pregnancy Termination for Genetic Indications: The Impact on Families," *Social Work in Health Care* 10(1), Fall 1984, pp. 17–34.

Gentry, Martha E. "Early Detection and Treatment: Social Worker and Pediatricians in Private Practice," *Social Work in Health Care* 3(1), Fall 1977, pp. 49–59.

Guendelman, Sylvia. "At Risk: Health Needs of Hispanic Children," *Health and Social Work* 10(3), Summer 1985, pp. 183–190.

Hancock, Emily. "Crisis Intervention in a Newborn Nursery," *Social Work in Health Care 1*(4), Summer 1976, pp. 421–432.

Hedblom, Janice E., Hubbard, Felicity A., and Andersen, Arnold. "Anorexia Nervosa: A Multidisciplinary Treatment Program for Patient and Family," *Social Work in Health Care 7*(1), Fall 1981, pp. 67–83.

Hess, Howard. "Social Work Clinical Practice in Family Medicine Centers: The Need for a Practice Model," *Journal of Education for Social Work 21*(1), Winter 1985, pp. 56–65.

Hookey, Peter. "The Establishment of Social Worker Participation in Rural Primary Health Care," *Social Work in Health Care 3*(1), Fall 1977, pp. 87–99.

Koocher, Gerald. "Adjustment and Coping Strategies Among the Caretakers of Cancer Patients," *Social Work in Health Care 5*(2), Winter 1979, pp. 145–150.

Lang, Priscilla A., and Mitrowski, Christine A. "Supportive and Concrete Services for Teenage Oncology Patients," *Health and Social Work 6*(4), November 1981, pp. 42–45.

Lorenzo, May Kwan, and Adler, David A. "Mental Health Services for Chinese in a Community Health Center," *Social Casework 65*(10), December 1984, pp. 600–609.

Mahan, Carol K., Rosueger, Joan C., and Schreiner, Richard L. "The Family and Neonatal Intensive Care," *Social Work in Health Care 7*(4), Summer 1982, pp. 67–78.

Marples, Margot. "Helping Family Members Cope with a Senile Relative," *Social Casework 67*(8), October 1986, pp. 490–498.

Miller, Rosalind. Primary Health Care: More Than Medicine. Englewood Cliffs, N.J.: Prentice-Hall, 1983.

Milner, Clara Joan. "Compassionate Care for the Dying Person," *Health and Social Work 5*(2), May 1980, pp. 5–10.

Mintz, Nancy. "A Descriptive Approach to Bulimia," *Health and Social Work 10*(2), Spring 1985, pp. 113–119.

Needleman, Sima K. "Infertility and In Vitro Fertilization: The Social Worker's Role," *Health and Social Work 12*(2), Spring 1987, pp. 135–143.

Pines, Ayala, and Maslach, Christina. "Characteristics of Staff Burnout in Mental Health Settings," *Hospital and Community Psychiatry 29*, 1978, pp. 233–237.

Rosin, A.J., Abramowitz, L., Diamond, J., and Jesselson, P. "Environmental Management of Senile Dementia," *Social Work in Health Care 11*(1), Fall 1985, pp. 33–43.

Sands, Roberta G. "Social Work with Victims of Huntington's Disease," *Social Work in Health Care 9*(4), Summer 1985, pp. 63–71.

Saunders, Ronna. "Bulimia: An Expanded Definition," *Social Casework 10*(66), December 1985, pp. 603–610.

Schild, Sylvia. "Social Work with Genetic Problems," *Health and Social Work 2*(1), February 1977, pp. 59–77.

Schild, Sylvia, and Black, Rita Beck. *Social Work and Genetics: A Guide for Practice.* New York: The Haworth Press, 1984.

Shapiro-Steinberg, Lois, and Neamatalla, Georgeanne Stiglitz. "Counseling for Women Requesting Sterilization: A Comprehensive Program Designed to Insure Informed Consent," *Social Work in Health Care 5*(2), Winter 1979, pp. 151–163.

Taylor-Brown, Susan, Johnson, Kay Hannon, Hunter Kathryn, and Rockwitz, Ruth J. "Stress Identification for Social Workers in Health Care: A Preventive Approach to Burn-Out," *Social Work in Health Care 7*(2), Winter 1981, pp. 91–100.

Twersky, Reva K., and Deisher, Joseph B. "Social Workers in a Family Practice Residency Network," *Social Work in Health Care 6*(3), Spring 1981, pp. 13–23.

Wasow, Mona. "Support Groups for Family Caregivers of Patients with Alzheimer's Disease," *Social Work 31*(2), March-April 1986, pp. 93–97.

Weiss, Joan O. "Psychosocial Stress in Genetic Disorders: A Guide for Social Workers," *Social Work in Health Care 6*(4), Summer 1981, pp. 17–31.

Wilk, Ruth J. "The Haitian Refugee: Concerns for Health Care Providers," *Social Work in Health Care 11*(2), Winter 1985-6, pp. 61–74.

Wright, Janet M. "Fetal Alcohol Syndrome: The Social Work Connection," *Health and Social Work 6*(1), February 1981, pp. 5–10.

PART 8
PREPARATION FOR SOCIAL WORK
IN HEALTH CARE

Introduction

How should social workers be prepared for the complex roles and functions of practice in health care settings? How is a fine educational balance maintained between what is core and relatively unchanging in social work's knowledge, skills, and practice wisdom and the pressing need to prepare students and beginning workers for the pace and challenges of practice as it evolves in a rapidly changing environment? Earlier chapters of this book have noted the impact on patients and institutions alike of changes in technology, demography, and fiscal planning that require rapid and creative responses from social work practitioners. Discussions between practitioners and teachers about education and training of social workers frequently ring with concerns that schools are behind the times, out of touch with current practice, and still teaching old methods for new tasks.

Administrators of social work departments and field instructors share the goal of educating students in the base generic knowledge as they at the same time integrate specialized knowledge and skills. Today's social workers in health, facing challenges such as AIDS, homelessness, and shortened hospital stays, must know, as never before, how to assess their clients' needs with speed and accuracy.

To make a rapid assessment, however, requires prior knowledge of the process of study and assessment, which is often compressed as curricula content enlarges.

Schools need to develop solid concentrations in health care social work practice to support what is taught in the field, and the field needs to contribute to the academic content its knowledge of practice. Active collaboration can be developed through agency representation on committees at school, joint curricula building, including practitioners as faculty and guest lecturers, and faculty liaison and consultation to agencies.

As schools and field collaborate to carve out effective ways to prepare social workers for the many roles and functions of current practice, new teaching models are evolving.

Experienced practitioners as well as students and beginning MSWs need continuing educational vehicles to maintain, update, and upgrade their competencies in an ever-changing and challenging environment where concerns about staff "burnout," a pressing issue of the past decade, are heightened. Professional social work supervision is a major structure used in preparation, development, and support of competent, responsible, and autonomous practitioners.

In the articles selected to illuminate these issues, Kane's overview demonstrates the relatively low significance attached to the preparation for the vital professional function of collaboration and makes a firm case for social work educators to place greater emphasis on the skills and processes of interprofessional teamwork. The article provides a good base for comparisons with later developments in education for collaborative roles in the health field.

Bennett and Grob's article explores territory virtually uncharted in professional literature as the authors consider the learning tasks of social workers entering practice in health care settings. They delineate the specifics of the practice competencies that need to be mastered and identify appropriate teaching methods and content. Their work is based on their experience with beginning practitioners but it is applicable to continuing education for more experienced workers as well as to graduate students. Performance evaluations have a number of professional and administrative uses, but in this work they are examined to identify a sequence of learning needs, teaching content and desired outcomes. The authors emphasize the concept of mutuality in the evaluation and teaching processes and the goals of fostering worker autonomy and self-responsibility.

Walsh's article is important not only for its clear conceptualization of field work learning opportunities for students in health care settings, but also for its application of generic concepts to field teaching and learning in the psychiatric emergency room. Typifying today's practice in health care, the setting is fast paced and demands students' rapid acquisition of theoretical knowledge, methods, skills, and adaptations to the special characteristics of emergency care. A sequence of learning opportunities is provided to enable students to gain incremental abilities to take independent responsibility for assessment, treatment, and rapid decision making. Students need to be able to learn rapidly, to adapt with flexibility, to respond equally to pressure, to apply new learning to practice, and to exercise good judgment in seeking supervisory guidance. Walsh's suggestion that students may be taught to recommend and monitor psychotropic drugs is controversial, and may be evaluated within the context of other discussions of that topic (Matorin and DeChillo, 1984; Gerhart and Brooks, 1983; Miller, Wiedman, and Linn, 1980). The competencies achieved in the emergency psychiatric setting are those needed in every area of health care today, and although some educators have considered it a setting too stressful for students, Walsh illustrates its fine potential for preparing social workers for practice.

Interprofessional Education and Social Work: A Survey

Rosalie A. Kane, DSW

SUMMARY. In 1974, the author surveyed all graduate schools of social work to determine how team concepts were being introduced to master's degree level students. A 76% response rate was achieved; 31% of the schools offered joint courses with other professional schools, 17% offered courses on teamwork itself within the school of social work, 10% had virtually no content on interprofessional collaboration, and the majority attempted to introduce this content through the practicum and the overall curriculum, especially health courses. These modalities are further described along with advantages and disadvantages of various approaches.

The interprofessional team has become a standard feature in the delivery of professional services. Social workers have been involved in the interprofessional health team since the turn of the century,[1] and now advanced teamwork skills are considered mandatory for practice in hospitals.[2] Social workers have also been regularly included on the large interprofessional rehabilitation team,[3] where facility in team relationships has become necessary for effective functioning.[4]

Teams are flourishing in mental health, ranging from the old child guidance team, of which social work is a charter member, to the modern community of mental health teams with their four basic professions of psychiatry, psychology, social work, and nursing.[5]

At the time of writing Dr. Kane was Associate Professor, University of Utah Graduate School of Social Work, Salt Lake City, UT 84112.

Reprinted from *Social Work in Health Care*, Volume 2(2), Winter 1976-77.

Specialized health fields, an admixture of health and mental health, such as geriatrics[6] or mental retardation,[7] are fast developing the interprofessional team modality as an essential tool of practice.

Continuing the catalogue, interprofessional teams are manifest in the juvenile court,[8] in corrections,[9,10] and in schools, especially in learning disability programs.[11,12] They are now coming into prominence as vehicles for urban planning, health planning, and a variety of indirect services.[13,14]

The challenge to the social work profession in forging a role on the team is magnified because so many professions have boundaries that overlap their own. The psychologist, the psychiatrist, and, more recently, the psychiatric nurse perform therapeutic and community services similar to social work. The occupational and recreational therapists may work closely with both the group worker and the caseworker. The public health nurse, the health educator, and even the home economist may utilize much of the social worker's expertise. Clergymen, rehabilitation counselors, guidance counselors, schoolteachers and school psychologists, planners, and administrators have at various times interfaced with social work function. As various groups have expanded the boundaries of their roles, many professionals have added a psychological dimension to their self-definitions; one now reads of "psychodietetics"[15] or "psychoreligious counseling."[16] At the same time, other professions such as nursing[17] and occupational therapy[18] have begun emphasizing knowledge of community agencies as part of the expertise their groups bring to the team. Perhaps no profession as much as social work enjoys so large a cast of collaborators with similarities of interest and role.

EDUCATION
FOR INTERPROFESSIONAL PRACTICE

Translating a conviction about the necessity for teamwork skills into a social work curriculum raises a host of ideological and practical problems. It is debated whether such content is best conveyed through courses offered in separate professional schools, through interdisciplinary ventures with students and faculty from a number of professional disciplines, or through a continuing education approach involving more seasoned professional practitioners. Some authorities advocate all of these modalities.

Before learning experiences can be designed, educational objectives are required. Again the social work educator is faced with a dilemma. Does social work practice in interprofessional contexts lend itself to a generic course with a single set of objectives? Or is social work practice so related to particular settings that it must be taught in specific contexts such as health, education, corrections, or a myriad of others? Several volumes of the 1959 curriculum study on social work education, particularly those on group work, rehabilitation, and corrections, highlighted the need for interprofessional skills in their particular fields.[3,19,20] Other commentators have suggested a generic base in team skills, taught within one's own professional school before the student mingles with students of other disciplines.[21]

Lately it has been suggested that the MSW level of practice should be characterized by teamwork in emerging fields.[22] In forecasting future practice to lay a rational groundwork for curriculum building, moreover, Andrew[23] reports that "participation in interprofessional treatment teams" and "participation in interdisciplinary planning" both figured highly in the experts' projections of master's degree level social work in 1985. The present paper reports on a survey of MSW programs to determine what schools of social work are now doing to meet the present and future need for teamwork skills.

METHOD

The population surveyed consisted of 84 MSW programs in the United States and Canada listed by the Council on Social Work Education as accredited schools or schools in the process of becoming accredited.

The questionnaire was designed to be brief (a single page) and for the most part contained objective questions. By use of a checklist, respondents indicated the existence of content for interprofessional teamwork in the classroom and in the practicum, and the degree of emphasis placed on such content. They also indicated which courses in the curriculum, if any, incorporated teamwork concepts, and the timing of such content over the 2-year program.

The questionnaire differentiated two approaches to interprofessional education: (a) courses for social workers within a school of social work that deal with the nature of collaboration; and (b) collaborative courses offered with another discipline on a mutually significant subject or field, or on teamwork processes themselves. While these latter courses would not always focus on teamwork per se, they would permit students from different disciplines to mingle and communicate with each other.

The questionnaire was circulated in the late spring of 1974; about 3 weeks after the initial mailing, a reminder was sent along with a time-saving card for the use of schools with no content at all related to the topic. As a result of the first two mailings, 63% of the programs surveyed responded. A third solicitation was made in the fall of 1974 to those schools that had not replied in the spring, bringing the total of respondents to 76%.

FINDINGS

Tables 1 and 2 illustrate the presence of teamwork concepts in the practicum and in the general classroom curriculum. As Table 1 indicates, 50% of the respondents declared a strong emphasis on

TABLE 1

*Interprofessional Teamwork
Emphasis in Practicum*

Amount of Emphasis	Number of Schools	Percentage
Strong emphasis	32	50.0
Slight emphasis	22	34.4
Other	2	3.1
None	8	12.5
Total	64	100.0

TABLE 2
Interprofessional Teamwork
Concepts in Overall Curriculum

Amount of Emphasis	Number of Schools	Percentage
Strong emphasis	12	18.8
Slight emphasis	33	51.6
None	19	29.6
Total	64	100.0

teamwork in the practicum component of their programs, 34% declared a slight emphasis in the practicum, and 13% stated that no content on teamwork had been deliberately introduced in the practicum. Three percent stated that the degree of emphasis on teams in fieldwork depended on the particular setting involved.

Since the fieldwork sequence is traditionally the place where it has been assumed that students would develop a competence in teamwork, the fact that half the respondents reported a strong emphasis here was not surprising. However, the fact that almost half reported a slight emphasis or none at all was rather unexpected.

Table 2 reports the presence of teamwork concepts in the classroom curriculum. Fifty-two percent of the group stated that the subject was emphasized slightly throughout the curriculum as a whole, 19% reported strong emphasis, and 30% indicated that no theme regarding teamwork appeared in the curriculum.

Additionally, respondents checked curriculum areas in which they tended to introduce teamwork concepts. Thirty-eight schools designated practice electives in special fields, 39 practice courses, 23 administration courses, and 15 policy courses; schools could, and did, check off more than one area for this question.

Seven schools replied that they had no content around teamwork either in field or class, and nine additional schools had no content other than a slight emphasis in the curriculum. The majority of schools indicating teamwork content permitted it to fall equally in the 1st or 2nd year. Eleven percent placed the content primarily in the 1st year, 6% in the 2nd, 69% in both years, 9% in neither year, and 4.7% could not address the questions because their patterns differed from the traditional 2-year program.

As Figure 1 illustrates, 31% of the schools offered joint courses with other professional schools, and 17% offered courses on teamwork per se in the school of social work. Six schools, or 9% of the respondents, offered both of these modalities, while 60% offered neither pattern.

The nine schools offering courses on teamwork processes placed them in the following curriculum areas: three schools, as general electives; three as practice electives; two, as an elective on the health team; and one, as a behavior elective.

Several schools illustrated the variety of organizational thrusts possible by providing additional information about their intraschool electives on teamwork processes. Since all schools did not do so, this information cannot be quantified, but some of the patterns in use can be enumerated. One course focused on manpower arrangements, asking students to develop a viable model for collaboration in their particular field of practice. Several courses were structured around the different professions with whom social workers collaborate, with the reading list divided according to collaborating professions such as law, medicine, nursing, divinity, and so on. One

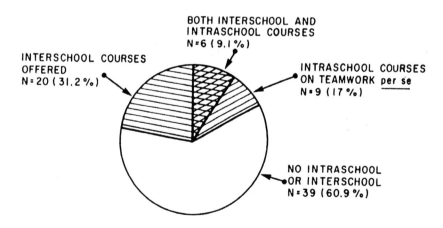

FIGURE 1. Intraschool and interschool courses.

course emphasized the sociology of the various professions, examining the socialization processes and the various status concerns of the different disciplines. Another offering was subdivided into four topical areas, namely, the organization, the work group, the participants, and the skills. The several courses devoted to teamwork in health tended to highlight descriptive accounts of role conflict in health and mental health settings.

The 20 schools reporting electives offered jointly with other professional disciplines accounted for at least 39 collaborative courses. Table 3 shows the frequencies of the various collaborative alliances. Health schools were involved in the largest number of joint courses, and law schools were second. These courses shown on the table under the heading "large-scale interprofessional effort" refer to courses planned with a large number of disciplines; in this category one school mentioned five cooperating schools, one mentioned six, and one mentioned nine. As an example, the most ambitious effort involved physical therapy, occupational therapy, rehabilitation counseling, speech pathology, psychiatric nursing, nursing education, leisure education, and gerontology, as well as social work. Beginning as a course on "Interdisciplinary Collaboration in Social Work," it evolved into an experimental offering with an emphasis on the common skills needed by all professionals to engage in the collaborative process. According to the report, content was drawn from activity directed at patient care, program development, policy change, and relevant research.

The right-hand column of Table 3 lists the subject areas mentioned for the interprofessionally sponsored courses. Not all respondents provided this detail so the list is suggestive rather than exhaustive. Some respondents supplied additional detail about the organization of the courses from which it was learned that some courses attempted to equalize the numbers of students from the participating disciplines and to form student teams. One such example was a course on urban and social planning that sent student teams into local communities to study needs from the physical and social perspective.

The outlines volunteered listed a number of objectives for interprofessional courses. These objectives have been culled and, with duplications eliminated, are listed below:

1. To identify trends and dilemmas in social work manpower.
2. To explicate team models that have developed in the field and examine them critically.
3. To develop for personal professional use a viable model of teamwork.
4. To expose graduate students from several disciplines to interdisciplinary team approaches.
5. To identify what is common and unique to various professions.
6. To expand students' knowledge of and capacity to use collaboration as a technique of intervention.

DISCUSSION

No patterns distinguished the nonresponding from the responding schools. All parts of the country were represented: Urban and rural schools were present in the same proportion as they are in the population. The early returns tended to include most of the respondents who reported vigorous programming in interprofessional teamwork. Only a few replying to the second mailing reported any substantial emphasis on teamwork, and the positive returns dwindled further with the third mailing. It seems plausible that the nonrespondents resemble the late respondents and that the findings more likely overstate than understate the proportion of schools of social work engaged in some form of interprofessional education. About a third of the responding schools were offering courses on teamwork principles or collaborating with other professional schools on joint courses. A small group of schools (9%) were doing both.

Despite this activity, the survey also indicated that the majority of schools were giving little attention to the subject matter. When the questionnaire was devised, it seemed likely that all schools would claim at least a slight emphasis on teamwork in the practicum and a slight emphasis throughout the curriculum. A "slight emphasis" seemed to be a minimal expectation, yet some schools did not even claim this much involvement. Seven schools had no emphasis at all, and 9 additional schools claimed only a slight emphasis in the curriculum and no emphasis in the practicum. Thus 16 schools had virtually no content in the area.

TABLE 3
Joint Courses with Social Work and Other Professional Schools

Name of Cooperating Disciplines	Number of Schools
Health Schools	16
Medicine (4)	
Nursing (2)	
Public Health (2)	
Combinations (8)	
Law schools	8
Large-scale interprofessional effort	3
Urban planning	2
Education	2
Engineering	1
Psychology	1
Business	1
Public communication	1
Public administration	1
Architecture and design	1
Law, psychiatry	1
Medicine, theology	1

NOTE: Subject matter of the interprofessional courses:

Teamwork processes	Mental development
Health planning	Mental health in children
Issues in health care	Family law
Medical social work	Correctional law
Death and dying	Juveniles and the law
Mental retardation	Use of media
Alcoholism	Organizational analysis
Family planning	Interviewing skills
Gerontology	

The great majority of respondents felt that the teamwork content was equally appropriate for 1st- or 2nd-year students; there no longer seems to be a philosophy of sequencing that exposes the student to a social work setting in the 1st year and an interprofessional or "secondary" setting in the 2nd year.

Teamwork content appeared in a wide variety of niches in MSW curricula. A number of respondents utilized courses on consultation that were part of administration offerings to discuss collaboration with other professionals; since collaboration and consultation are quite distinct processes with different assumptions, this combination is interesting. The administration sequence in general seemed a hospitable home for content on teamwork. Perhaps, as one respondent commented, this affinity occurs because administration students are expected to analyze the systems in which social workers are employed. It was interesting to note that one course on teamwork even occurred in the human behavior sequence. If such a course emphasized the role behavior of professional groups, this placement seems justifiable. Most schools introduced content in teamwork in practice courses, focusing on the practice skills needed to collaborate effectively.

The breakdown of offerings shows an association between teamwork and health-related courses. Thirty-eight schools introduced some teamwork concepts in electives on social work in health settings. A number of the courses on teamwork per se were centered around the health team, and the majority of the joint courses involved collaboration with one or more health schools. This result is not surprising in view of the long history of collaboration in the health field, the close interdependence of the health professions, and the current impetus toward interprofessional education in health schools across the country.

More striking than the predominance of health-related courses on the team was the variety of other directions that have been taken in interprofessional education involving social work. These include the use of media with a school of communications, attitudes toward death with a theology school and a medical school, and program analysis in cooperation with a school of public administration. Social work educators have forged a great variety of collaborative alliances.

Responsiveness to demands of practice does indeed suggest the current need for an emphasis on interprofessional teamwork in social work education. The question remains as to whether the social work response should be separate for all the fields in which social workers are employed or be cast in a generic framework, or whether both these approaches are needed.

The form such content takes must grow out of a conviction about the behaviors that constitute competent teamwork. A conference on interprofessional education for medicine and social work debated whether the objectives should be to develop shared abilities or rather a mutual appreciation.[24] The preference of the group was toward "combined understanding, but separate talents" as an objective of interprofessional educational efforts. The final form, too, must be compatible with the philosophy of social work education and permit identification with the social work profession. A social work educator who has strongly advocated interdisciplinary education puts the dilemma well: "All professional schools have the same curriculum problems; namely to limit the content so that the school has sufficient opportunity to learn what is distinct and essential to the practice for which he is preparing and, at the same time, to broaden his base of learning so that he perceives what is related significantly to his practice."[25]

The survey reported here shows that MSW programs are beginning to approach that task.

REFERENCES

1. Cabot, Richard. *Social Work: Essays on the Meeting Ground of Doctor and Social Work*. Boston: Houghton Mifflin, 1919.

2. Phillips, Beatrice; McCulloch, J. Wallace; Brown, Malcolm; and Hambro, Naomi. "Social Work and Medical Practice." *Hospitals 45* (1971):76-79.

3. Horwitz, John. *Education for Social Work in the Rehabilitation of the Handicapped*. New York: Council on Education for Social Work, 1959.

4. Ellwood, Paul. "Can We Afford So Many Rehabilitation Professions?" *Journal of Rehabilitation 34* (1968):47-52.

5. Smith, Neilson. "Interprofessional Training for Community Mental Health." *Journal of Education for Social Work 10*(1974):106-13.

6. Brody, Elaine; Cole, Charlotte; and Moss, Miriam. "Individualizing Therapy for the Mentally Impaired Aged." *Social Casework 54* (1973):453-61.

7. Stone, Nellie. "Effecting Interdisciplinary Coordination in Clinical Services to the Mentally Retarded." *American Journal of Orthopsychiatry 40* (1970):835-40.

8. Brennan, William, and Khinduka, Shanti. "Role Expectations of Social

Workers and Lawyers in the Juvenile Court." *Crime and Delinquency 17* (1971):191-201.

9. Conrad, J.P. "The Interdisciplinarian at Home and Abroad." *Prison Journal 44* (1964):7-13.

10. Hogan, Charles, and Campbell, Charles. "Team Classification in Federal Institutions." *Federal Probation 32* (1968):30-35.

11. Anderson, Robert. "School Social Work: The Promise of a Team Model." *Child Welfare 53* (1974):524-30.

12. Chrisopholos, Florence. "Multidisciplinary Paradigm." *Journal of Learning Disabilities 3* (1970):167-68.

13. Ardell, Donald. "Urban Planning/Health Planning Interrelationships." *American Journal of Public Health 59* (1969):2051-55.

14. Smith, James. "Study Seeks to Help Form Future of Rural Towns." *Lutheran Social Welfare Quarterly 11* (1971):54-57.

15. Manning, Mary Louise. "The Psychodynamics of Dietetics." *Nursing Outlook 13* (1965):57-59.

16. Peterson, Dennis. "The Broadening Role of the Hospital Chaplain." *Hospitals 42* (1968):58-60.

17. De Young, Carol. "Nursing's Contribution in Family Crisis Treatment." *Nursing Outlook 16* (1968):60-62.

18. Wanatabe, Sandra. "The Developing Role of Occupational Therapy in Psychiatric Home Service." *American Journal of Occupational Therapy 21* (1967): 353-56.

19. Murphy, Marjory. *The Social Group Work Method in Social Work Education.* New York: Council on Education for Social Work, 1959.

20. Studt, Eliot. *Education for Social Workers in the Correctional Field.* New York: Council on Education for Social Work, 1959.

21. Dana, Bess, and Sheps, Cecil. "Trends and Issues in Interprofessional Education." *Journal of Education for Social Work 4* (1968): 35-41.

22. Vigilante, Joseph. "Social Work Education Matures to the Undergraduate Level." *Social Work 19* (1974):638-46.

23. Andrew, Gwen. "Forecasting Social Work Practice as a Base for Curriculum Development." *Journal of Education for Social Work 10* (1974):3-8.

24. Rehr, Helen, ed. *Medicine and Social Work,* New York: Prodist, 1974.

25. White, Grace. "Preparation of Social Workers for Interprofessional and Interagency Collaboration." *Education for Social Work, 1960 Proceedings.* New York: Council on Education for Social Work, 1960.

The Social Worker
New to Health Care:
Basic Learning Tasks

Claire Johnson Bennett, MSW
Gail Green Grob, MSW

SUMMARY. The authors review twelve evaluations of MSW social workers new to an acute care hospital and discuss the evaluative
findings in a context of problems, teaching content and learning
gains. Specific practice problems are matched with specific teaching
content and learning carry-over. The positives of structure and mutuality in the evaluation process are emphasized as aids for the
worker in achieving practice effectiveness and in strengthening the
worker's capacity for professional self-direction.

In an article concerning expectations of the entry level MSW in a
hospital setting, Grace Fields states that

> when we look at the transition spot where the student is reclas-
> sified the practitioner we are looking at a place of critical deci-
> sion-making in the professional process — the quality and
> quantity of service provision becomes the responsibility of an-
> other group of gatekeepers at the point of agency employment.
> (Fields, 1980)

Claire Bennett and Gail Grob at the time this article was written were both
Preceptors in the Medical/Surgical Units of the Department of Social Work Services at The Mount Sinai Hospital, One Gustave L. Levy Place, New York, NY
10029.

Reprinted from *Social Work in Health Care*, Volume 8(2), Winter 1982.

This article is written by two such gatekeepers who are preceptors in the Medical/Surgical units at a large urban medical center in New York City. It is addressed to practitioners, supervisors and directors involved in the orientation, teaching and evaluation of the newly hired MSW in a health care setting. The purposes of the paper are (1) to explicate the frequently encountered learning needs of the entry level workers and (2) to provide supervisors with guidelines which facilitate the workers' job performance and professional growth. Our particular thrust is specificity — that is, we have delineated specific practice problems and have correlated these problems with specific teaching interventions. We have also described the learning gains that can be carried over and integrated into skilled, refined practice. The data used for this paper consist of evaluations of 12 MSWs, 8 recent graduates and 4 social workers new to a health setting with experience ranging from 3–7 years. We have devised a problem/teaching content/learning gains outline for evaluation material on practice. We conclude with recommendations made for future professional development and suggestions for implementation.

DEPARTMENTAL EDUCATIONAL PHILOSOPHY

Basic to our discussion and review is the awareness that our efforts take place in an organizational setting with a management philosophy and approach which emphasizes patient-focused supervision and professional accountability. In discussing the principles underlying continuing education in the Department of Social Work Services, Rosenberg (1979) describes the triadic relationship of continuing education, peer review and the self-directed worker. The single most important goal of continuing education within the department is to produce responsible and accountable self-directed workers. The departmental peer review system, the structured method of chart notations and review is "one step toward the achievement of a long range goal — written documentation that reflects quality practice" (Young, 1979). The peer review instrument identifies the essential practice components as entry, assessment, contract, intervention, collaboration, and outcome. The departmental evaluation guidelines for the new worker and the post-probationary worker incorporate these basic practice components, thus offering a conceptual structure to workers and preceptors. The management information system within the department aims for quantitative accountability, as well.

THE PROBATIONARY EVALUATION

The probationary evaluative phase provides an opportunity for joint assessment by worker and preceptor. The new candidate is encouraged to weigh professional interests and goals in relation to the setting and the demands of the specific assignment. From a broader view of health systems and the goals and missions of the department, the preceptor weighs the worker's capacity for generic and creative practice.

Two essentials of the probationary evaluation we wish to highlight are (1) the mutuality of the evaluation process and (2) the continuity of the process which begins from the first day of employment.

To insure a method of evaluation which encompasses practice expectations and accountability, an evaluation outline for the six-month probationary period has been developed within the Department of Social Work Services. This outline is given to each worker by the preceptor at an appropriate time within the first month of hiring and prepares the new worker for a written evaluation based on multiple departmental sources. The formal evaluation process starts in the fourth or fifth month when the worker selects five cases which illustrate diversity of problems, population and practice skills. Preceptor and worker independently review the cases using the peer review instrument. This is followed by joint discussion with the focus on practice patterns, strengths, and problems.

Content for evaluation is also derived from observation of patient/family interviews, group meetings, and tapes. Workers are asked to analyze data from management information systems, for example, the ratio of their direct and supportive services; case activity; patterns in collaboration. Service delivery and program development are also considered. From all this material, the preceptor produces a report which reflects the individual performance strengths and learning patterns and includes recommendations for future development of knowledge and skills.

REVIEW OF PRACTICE COMPONENTS

I. Entry

The ratings on entry in most of the reviews is excellent, meaning that the worker had documented date, purpose, and source of referral well. Usually, there is no problem with delayed or late intervention. We think this absence of difficulty reflects the teaching that starts from the beginning with new workers who must learn the concepts of accountability and social risk screening that are paramount emphases within the department. Initiative in casefinding and early entry are practice expectations that are supported by a system which provides workers with a tool for screening within a select patient population (Rehr, 1979).

II. Assessment

Doremus' (1976) formulation of the "Four R rule" for assessment offers a convenient, alliterative checklist for the new worker. It emphasizes roles, reactions, relationships and resources. Golan (1978), who places physical illness in the situational crisis category, stresses several key concepts in the exploration phase: (1) beginning with the precipitating factor; (2) sensitivity to subject reactions — affect, feelings expressed; (3) attention to past crises and losses, and coping mechanisms used; (4) current role responsibilities; (5) problem areas for which client or patient expresses a need for help, leading to agreement with worker as focus for future contract; (6) plans for resource contacts.

Some frequently encountered problem areas in assessment are listed in Table I. We have highlighted the corresponding teaching content and learning gains. These are to be seen as illustrative and not definitive.

In a broad range, these problems encompass such areas as insufficient factual data, narrow focus on the immediate problem, and significant omissions in personality strengths, feeling areas, and family support potential.

TABLE I

PROBLEM	TEACHING CONTENT	LEARNING GAINS
Worker does not include sufficient factual data in assessments.	Such information is important in a setting where comprehensive services from entry to post hospital phase are provided. A psychosocial approach must include social data such as, housing, diet, cooking facilities, shopping, money, neighbors. Inexperienced workers tend to ignore or dismiss resource needs as secondary.	Worker views patient from individualized, realistic situation and weighs impact of illness accordingly. Values interplay of reality and dynamics.
Assessments are too narrowly focused on the current crisis and loss.	Worker can start to predict strengths and vulnerabilities through a longitudinal perspective which requires expanding exploration to previous problems, crises and coping patterns.	Worker learns purpose in broader exploration. The resultant data base makes contract and treatment plan more accurate.

TABLE I (continued)

PROBLEM	TEACHING CONTENT	LEARNING GAINS
Worker does not describe ego strengths and coping mechanisms specifically.	Ego strengths and defenses are assessed in relation to patient's reality, that is, to the extent they are functional or dysfunctional to adaptation. Identify avoidance mechanisms such as denial, isolation, and repression and their impact on patient's appraisal of illness and ability to use medical care.	Knowledge of adaptive behavior mechanisms enables worker to see the legitimate functions of defenses.
Worker does not assess impact of illness on the family system.	Secure information on who comprises family, quality of relationships, coping mechanisms, sociocultural factors and patterns. Observe family interactions in the hospital and shifts in roles, particularly in dependency area. Involve the family in the process of assessment. Assess	Worker learns to view family as a system and the impact of illness on this system. In reviewing the developmental stages in the life cycle of family members, the worker recognizes the necessity of a family-oriented assessment and treatment plan and its therapeutic value

PROBLEM	TEACHING CONTENT	LEARNING GAINS
	the interpersonal relationships, strengths and weaknesses in family and support systems.	for patient and family.
Worker is hesitant to explore feelings, particularly hurt and anger.	This problem is often related to nature of uninvited entry which leads to worker's insecurity in role. Worker first explores own feelings of vulnerability and helplessness and can then proceed to accept need for eliciting feelings in order to complete the psychological part of the psychosocial assessment. The understanding of anger as part of loss and mourning, i.e., a sequential emotion in adaptation is emphasized. Anger needs expression and in crises of hospitalization and	Worker becomes freer to risk; freer to elicit feeling and to make connections with current situation. Gains skill in timing empathy, support and pursuit of feelings.

TABLE I (continued)

PROBLEM	TEACHING CONTENT	LEARNING GAINS
	illness anger has many forms and outlets. Anger may obscure the more painful feelings of sadness and loss.	
Worker does not explore functional changes imposed by illness.	A sense of patient's prior life style, (i.e., roles, values, sense of responsibility for self and family) helps in assessing the impact of illness. Is this the first physical crisis or one of a long chain of hospitalizations for a chronic condition? (prior coping) Teach task and role concepts (what are day-to-day tasks at work and home; ecological view in larger environment). Identify tasks in hospital to maximize patient/family ego	Worker obtains expanded picture of person-in-situation. Sees patient involved in other systems and gets sense of how he functions and what supports are available in family and community.

PROBLEM	TEACHING CONTENT	LEARNING GAINS
	strengths. With knowledge and facts of medical diagnosis and functional implications, worker can help patient anticipate and accept change in functioning while preserving psychosocial assets.	

III. Contracting

Most social work practice in an acute care hospital is short-term and problem-focused. The new worker must learn, in addition to entry and assessment skills, the conceptual and practice value of contracting.

The literature on contracting underscores its value in clarifying target problems for client and practitioner and evaluating outcome (Maluccio and Marlow, 1975; Seabury, 1976), and in providing boundaries around problems, thus reducing the workers bewilderment and frustration (Epstein, 1980). Studies on the effectiveness of casework confirm the linkage between contract and successful outcome (Wood, 1978). So contracting for the new worker becomes a practice skill, a safeguard against confusion and futility, and a useful tool in measuring outcome.

Table II contains specific problems encountered in the contracting area in the evaluations reviewed. In summary, these problems show difficulty in explicit contracting and contracting that is either too global or too narrow.

---

*More experienced workers must retain the concept of contracting, but certain therapeutic approaches may warrant less explicit contracting.

TABLE II

PROBLEM	TEACHING CONTENT	LEARNING GAINS
Contracts are implicit rather than explicit.* There is confusion between plan and contract.	Including patient and family in problem identification and in establishing therapeutic priorities encourages mutuality in the helping process.	Worker achieves clearer treatment focus. Increases opportunities for worker/patient satisfaction.
Worker overwhelmed by emotional impact of severe physical illness and has difficulty partializing stresses into workable treatment plan.	Contracting helps partialize areas of patient stress, simultaneously utilizing ego strengths to maximize coping.	Views client from strength rather than medical model of pathology.
Tends to set global or overly ambitious goals.	Goals need to be realistic with consideration given to the patient's physical, psychological capacities and social resources. Time is a critical factor in hospital settings linked to brief stays. Thus, new worker sets	Contracting minimizes worker's frustration. Aids in conceptualizing change and outcome.

PROBLEM	TEACHING CONTENT	LEARNING GAINS
	small, achievable, sequential goals and partializes problems into component parts.	
Contracts are narrowly focused on emotional reactions to hospitalization to the exclusion of pertinent reality needs.	Contracts should reflect a comprehensive ongoing assessment of patient needs. The inner and outer needs evident in psychosocial approach are emphasized.	Learns that role clarity means expanding beyond "Therapeutic" to biopsychosocial perspective.

IV. Intervention

Theories of case work practice have consistently recognized that assessment (study, diagnosis) and intervention (treatment) go hand in hand. The crisis model clearly validates this approach. The use of short-term treatment in a health care setting necessitates an integration of assessment and interventive skills as a tandem process. For purposes of clarity the authors have identified learning needs in each of these areas with the acknowledgement that there is a simultaneous aspect of both assessment and intervention.

Table III illustrates specific examples of problems in practice in the area of intervention.

Most of the problems in intervention cluster around feeling areas, that is, the worker is hesitant in exploring feelings because of personal reactions to the stress of illness and to the expression of painful feelings of loss. The tendency to overreact to patient's fragility and vulnerability was noted. In addition, some situations calling for assertive or directive techniques proved to be problematical.

TABLE III

PROBLEM	TEACHING CONTENT	LEARNING GAINS
Worker's response is constricted, negatively affecting empathy and the quality of the therapeutic alliance.	Worker needs to be aware of own reactions and understand that this inhibition affects patient's and family's ability to share feelings.	Acknowledgement of own feelings enhances ability to establish rapid therapeutic alliances.
Worker is defended against awareness of own counterreaction.	Use case material to illustrate the worker's need to avoid patient's expression of feelings. Hold worker to necessity of getting in touch with subjective attitudes and feelings to assess what is being avoided and why. Formulating dynamics and exploring the meaning of behavior renders emotional content less threatening.	Worker's capacity to empathize with and accept patient's increases.
Worker views patient and family as separate systems.	Broader perspective identifies the patient as an integral part of the family. Focus on the impact of illness	Family is more available to patient, a positive which reestablished balance in the

PROBLEM	TEACHING CONTENT	LEARNING GAINS
	as it affects relationships, roles, family economics and equilibrium of the family unit. Maximizing communication between patient and significant others strengthens the supportive network.	family and helps to insure a greater compliance with the social health plan.
Limited understanding of ethnic, cultural, social and religious differences.	View patient as teacher. Read literature.	Increases skills in accurate empathy with a heterogeneous population.
Difficulty in responding to non-verbalized feelings.	Focus on clues in non-verbal, language, voice tone, affect, attitude and behavior.	Develops a broader understanding of patient and family responses.
Narrow view of patients as fragile and vulnerable.	Try to understand source of patient's vulnerability. Then proceed to reinforce worker's ability to assess and utilize patient's ego strengths and coping capacities.	Focus on tasks maximizes functional capacities.
Worker is hesitant to be directive and assertive in ways	Highlight theory from brief therapy and crisis work	Positive impact of helping moves patient and family

TABLE III (continued)

PROBLEM	TEACHING CONTENT	LEARNING GAINS
that could facilitate the therapeutic process.	which emphasizes worker activities and validates worker's role as facilitator. As an example, worker in the discharge role provides alternate choices, commensurate with patient's medical and social needs, while identifying realities and constraints in each option.	into a phase of appropriate decision-making.

V. Collaboration

In a multidisciplinary setting, the social worker becomes a team member who must be clear about his or her position on that team (role clarity); must develop skill in eliciting relevant information from other team members; and must be able to communicate and incorporate psychosocial content into the team efforts of problem-solving and treatment planning.

Mailick and Jordon (1977) summarize the diverse tasks of collaboration in describing the complexity of the process.

> The classic importance of assessment in social work tradition is emphasized in the collaborative process. The nature of the assessment, however, is complex. It requires an ecological approach, encompassing the organization context, the nature of the task, the time perspective, and professional orientation of

the collaborative approaches to be used selectively in effectively meeting patient, organizational and professional goals.

Table IV cites problems encountered by workers in collaborative efforts. These examples reflect the workers' difficulty in cooperative ventures with other professionals who appear to be insensitive to the stresses of illness, or unduly harsh in their judgments of patients and families. Role strains and insecurities are noted, particularly as they affect treatment focus, sound planning and the workers' individual comfort in day-to-day interdisciplinary activities.

TABLE IV

PROBLEM	TEACHING CONTENT	LEARNING GAINS
Worker thinks physician's note regarding patient's personality is judgmental. Worker responds with a contradictory note.	The chart is not the place for collaborative disputes. The worker learns to share perceptions of patient's personality with M.D., highlighting relevant sources of stress and coping problems. Identifies areas of patient strengths. Worker remains focused on the patient.	Worker increases skills in communicating relevant information to other disciplines. Patient-problem-plan focus for team efforts is maintained and strengthened.
Worker believes nursing and medical staff insensitive and abrupt to the effects of harsh medical treatment and crisis	Teach worker to consider the stress on medical caretakers and their need for defenses; to use opportunities	Worker can empathically identify with the pressure and stress felt by the collaborative group.

TABLE IV (continued)

PROBLEM	TEACHING CONTENT	LEARNING GAINS
of dying for patient and family.	for case discussion to help nurses and collaborative staff deal with their own feelings around stress and dying. Include collaborative staff in developing care plan sensitive to patient and family needs.	Worker is instrumental in preserving caretakers' sensitivity.
Worker becomes overwhelmed with the severity of illness. Feels helpless, futile and becomes overly dependent on the physician for perspective and direction.	Overemphasis on medical treatment and activity can obscure psychosocial needs. Worker becomes aware of own responses and defenses in working with critically ill patients.	Working as a colleague with medical team is necessary in order to maintain bio-psychosocial perspective and approach. Social work contribution to that perspective is integral.
Worker is caught between conflicting opinions of physicians regarding patient's aftercare needs.	Worker first identifies the primary physician, learns how to focus questions. Utilizes information from other disciplines who are involved with patient on a	Worker gains an understanding of the complex nature of planning in a health care setting. Worker has helped the collaborative group to respect and respond to

PROBLEM	TEACHING CONTENT	LEARNING GAINS
	daily basis. Combine this information with worker's own assessment of patient's strengths, wishes and needs.	patient's right for self-determination and choice.
On a service with an active psychiatric liaison program, the worker feels insecure or competitive and adapts too narrow a treatment focus or duplicates the psychiatrist's efforts.	Some overlap in collaborative efforts is inevitable in a complex system. The social worker's social and psychological assessment with a problem-contract focus has a broader base for helping and interventions.	The coordination of multidiscipline interventions enables the worker to avoid unproductive competition.
Worker underutilizes or is overwhelmed by institutional resources.	Knowledge of organizational structure helps worker to negotiate services on the patient's behalf.	Worker has learned to mobilize services on a selective basis.
New worker feels "left out" by a team reacting to change of social workers.	Group dynamics used to explain group feelings of anger and distrust at the loss of the old and the uncertainty about the new.	Worker learns consistent patient-focused efforts result in team respect and acceptance.

VI. Outcome

Outcome is a relatively new entity to be measured routinely in social work practice. A problem-outcome classification (Berkman-Rehr, 1978) has been used in our department for several years and has strengthened the concept into everyday practice. New workers have a tendency to underestimate the value of their interventions in the face of death and severe functional loss. By reviewing their problem-focused contracts and goal-related intervention in a systematic way, they can evaluate outcome within more realistic boundaries. Since outcome was not incorporated in Peer Review instrument at time of evaluation reviews, we do not have data on specific practice problems for this category.

ADDITIONAL EVALUATION CRITERIA

Other areas considered in the evaluation process are productivity, the teacher-learner relationship and goals for future performance.

Productivity

Departmental expectations for quantitative productivity are closely defined. Normative quantitative expectations related to the provision of direct and supportive services are reviewed individually to account for variables in caseload and assignment. These reviews enable the worker to assess whether they are meeting productive standards, to identify patterns in practice, and to select service delivery areas for future attention. Some examples of practice patterns illustrated through a statistical review showed a few workers had considerable fluctuations in direct services; some had relatively small numbers of family interviews; some needed to make a greater effort to increase case openings and the size of their active caseload. One worker acknowledged she was not crediting herself for most of her collaborative contacts and another became aware of the need to involve physicians and nurses in conference with patients/families.

TEACHER-LEARNER RELATIONSHIPS

During the first six-month period the supervisory relationship provides the core for the educative, supportive and administrative help and direction required by the new worker. To this one-to-one relationship the department adds an experience for mutual support from and learning with peers via the new workers' group which lasts generally from four to six months. Since this group is led by another "preceptor" and includes colleagues who share a range of experiences, learning needs and reactions, there is an early exposure to different styles of learning and teaching. The preceptor title captures the expanded role of a supervisory relationship which identifies learning needs and appropriately refers on to other sources of expertise.

The first six months is by no means a problem free time which results magically in a perfect prescription for self-development. While the preceptor and worker strive to achieve a capacity for planned self-direction and ultimate autonomous practice, both are mindful of the sequential phases in integration of learning and knowledge, as well as the forces of anxiety and associated regression.

Evaluation reviews show that certain themes emerge within the teacher-learner transaction. For example, experienced workers can accept intellectually the demands of evaluation, but with time become anxious or resentful at the process which they find unnecessary in the face of being "proven." Workers new to health care can resent the manifold accountability facets of hospital, teams, other disciplines, social work department, peer review systems, etc. The recent graduate can be more accepting of her dependency but may be quite overwhelmed with quantitative expectations. For all workers, the emotional impact of illness calls for an outlet that is sympathetic and supportive, but ultimately channeled toward a professional performance which ensures appropriate empathy and enabling skill.

The accountability expectations provide objective guidelines for a contract between the worker and the preceptor in which both become active partners in the evaluation process. These expectations help the worker test out an interest in the setting. They also help the preceptor avoid polarities of permissiveness or defensiveness and enable an early assessment of practice strengths and weaknesses so that obvious failure is discerned well before the six-month evaluation, usually at mid-point. A definite challenge for the preceptor is the worker experiencing difficulty in an erratic pattern. In this instance, the preceptor targets areas for attention, giving priority to serious practice gaps, and examines the worker's capacity for growth in these areas during the crucial three months remaining. The evaluations used in this paper were those of workers who passed the probationary period successfully.

GOALS FOR FUTURE PERFORMANCE

The final phase of the evaluation summarizes findings and looks to the workers' job performance. Singling out areas for development in practice skills confirms the mutuality in problem identification and problem resolution. The preceptor gives a positive message for going beyond the one-to-one and for considering other educational opportunities within a framework of accountability.

As might be predicted, the most frequent recommendations focused on the areas in which practice was analyzed. Assessment, contracting and intervention were most often targeted as needing ongoing development, with explicit recommendations and ways to implement these recommendations. For example, workers with lesser experience with families were encouraged to seek open-preceptorship with a family therapy specialist. Collaboration skills seemed quite steady with most workers but program development prompted recommendations for expanded use of group modality. With this, education opportunities via continuing education seminars, open-preceptorship or consultation were examined. A plan for continued work with an administrative preceptor was made in each situation with a variation based on practice strengths and weaknesses. Group supervision was a choice for several experienced workers with an assured availability for problem-case consultation. Bimonthly conferences for systems, accountability and productivity considerations were usually agreed upon.

CONCLUSION

We began with a quotation from Fields' cogent article which focused on the expectations for a new worker in the health care setting. We have extended this focus to the six-month probationary period and elucidated specifics of practice and teaching aimed at solidifying the skills of a group of workers new to a hospital setting. This review of worker training and development provides a guide which highlights some predictable learning tasks for workers new to health care and which identifies a variety of teaching approaches geared to these tasks.

REFERENCES

Doremus, Bertha. "The Four R's: Social Diagnosis in Health Care," *Health and Social Work*, Vol. 1, No. 4, Nov. 1976, pp. 121-139.

Epstein, Laura. *Helping People: The Task-Centered Approach*, C.V. Mosby Co., St. Louis, 1980, pp. 127-176.

Fields, Grace. "What Does a Director of a Hospital Social Work Department Expect of a Beginning MSW?" *Social Work in Health Services, An Academic Practice Partnership*, edited by Phyllis Caroff and Mildred Mailick, Prodist, New York, 1980, pp. 155-166.

Golan, Naomi. *Treatment in Crisis Situations*. The Free Press, New York, 1978, pp. 84-88.

Mailick, Mildred D. and Jordon, Pearl. "A Multimodel Approach to Collaborative Practice in Health Settings," *Social Work in Health Care*, Vol. 2, No. 4, Summer, 1977, p. 453.

Maluccio, A. and Marlow, W. *"The Case for the Contract,"* in B. Compton and B. Galaway (eds.) *Social Work Processes*. Homewood, Illinois: The Dorsey Press, 1975.

Rehr, Helen. "Looking to the Future." *Professional Accountability for Social Work Practice*. Helen Rehr, ed., Prodist, New York, 1979, p. 153.

Rehr, Helen and Berkman, Barbara. "Social Work Undertakes Its Own Audit." *Social Work in Health Care*, Vol. 3, March 1978, pp. 273-286.

Rosenberg, Gary. "Continuing Education and the Self-Directed Worker." *Professional Accountability for Social Work Practice*. Helen Rehr, ed., Prodist, New York, 1979, pp. 155-166.

Seabury, B.A. "The Contract: Uses, Abuses and Limitations." *Social Work*, Vol. 21, January, 1976, pp. 16-21.

Wood, Katherine M. "Casework Effectiveness: A New Look at the Research Evidence." *Social Work*, Vol. 23, No. 6, Nov. 1978, pp. 437-458.

Young, Alma T. "The Chart Notation." *Professional Accountability for Social Work Practice*. Helen Rehr, ed., Prodist, New York, 1979, pp. 62-73.

The Psychiatric Emergency Service as a Setting for Social Work Training

Susan F. Walsh, PhD

SUMMARY. The psychiatric emergency service can provide rich training opportunities for social work students. It is a site where they can learn to function in clinically autonomous, independent roles as primary care providers who are responsible for the evaluation, treatment, and disposition of psychiatric emergencies. Assuming responsibility for evaluating and intervening with a wide variety of people in acute distress prepares the student to enter professional practice with self-confidence. The abundant educational opportunities available on the psychiatric emergency service are discussed, teaching strategies to facilitate learning are suggested, and the unique professional growth experiences which derive from training are identified.

The number of patients who seek psychiatric care in hospital emergency rooms has increased dramatically in recent years and the psychiatric emergency service has now become a major portal of entry to the mental health system (Gerson & Bassuk, 1980). Increased utilization has led to innovations in the staffing of psychiatric emergency services: the traditional model of a lone psychiatric resident-on-call is being replaced by new models which emphasize interdisciplinary collaboration. These shifts have opened the psychiatric emergency service as a significant domain for clinical social workers (Bartolucci & Drayer, 1973; Grumet & Trachtman, 1976; Hillard, O'Shanick & Houpt, 1982; Sheridan & Teplin, 1982).

At the time of writing Dr. Walsh was Associate, Department of Psychiatry and Behavioral Sciences, Northwestern University Medical School, Chicago, Illinois and Lecturer, School of Social Service Administration, University of Chicago.
Reprinted from *Social Work in Health Care*, Volume 11(1), Fall 1985.

Increasingly, social workers now function in clinically autonomous, independent roles as primary care providers who are responsible for the evaluation, treatment, and disposition of psychiatric emergencies (Groner, 1978; Grumet & Trachtman, 1976). On psychiatric emergency services that offer brief, crisis-oriented followup treatment to patients, social workers provide this treatment (Bell, 1978). In addition, social workers teach and supervise psychiatry residents, psychology interns, nursing students and social work students who are learning to deliver emergency psychiatric services (Spitz, 1976; Steele, 1972).

Social workers have made substantial contributions to the delivery of psychiatric emergency services. For example, assigning to and housing a clinical social worker in the emergency room has been found to increase significantly emergency room physicians' recognition of psychiatric symptoms and referrals for psychiatric evaluation (Sheridan & Teplin, 1982). Because social workers know and regularly use the resources of the family and other support systems to sustain patients in the community, they recommend the admission of psychiatric emergency patients to the hospital less frequently than other disciplines (Mendel & Rappaport, 1969; Streiner, Goodman & Woodward, 1975).

For the most part, social workers have had to develop the specialized array of knowledge and skills necessary for practice in psychiatric emergency services after they have completed their social work training. Yet, the psychiatric emergency service is a valuable field training site for clinical social work students, a resource which can be tapped for professional social work education. This paper describes the learning opportunities available for social work students in the psychiatric emergency service, discusses supervisory and teaching structures which can facilitate learning, and identifies the benefits which can be derived from this educational experience.

LEARNING OPPORTUNITIES

Learning experiences on the psychiatric emergency service are abundant in major areas: in making diagnoses, in brief treatment including the use of environmental resources, in interviewing, in patient management, and in interdisciplinary collaboration. It is a single setting where the social work student can systematically build and practice skills in many clinical areas.

Diagnosis

Diagnostic assessment and decision-making are primary goals on the psychiatric emergency service (Lazare, 1976). Within a limited time span, the clinician is required to conduct a clinical evaluation and decide which intervention plan is likely to be most helpful to the patient. The plan that emerges, whether it be hospital admission, a therapeutic intervention, or the use of the alliance to promote follow-through on a referral, is determined on the basis of a diagnostic interview.

The psychiatric emergency service provides the social work student with opportunities to learn and integrate a variety of diagnostic approaches. In assessing mental disorders, the student learns to focus on the presenting problem or chief complaint: to describe mental functioning comprehensively and incisively through the use of a sophisticated mental status examination; to become skilled at taking a psychiatric history; to assess ego functioning; and, to apply systematically the DSM III multiaxial evaluation and classification system. Using an ecological perspective, the student learns to focus on the relationship between the individual's inner and outer environments in the examination of the events that have led to the current crisis and request for help. Assessing the patient's symptoms, history, current life situation, and cultural, ethnic, and socioeconomic milieu, helps the student learn to identify not only the forces which are contributing to the patient's predicament but also those which have potential therapeutic value.

Psychopathology

The wide range of diagnostic problems encountered on the psychiatric emergency service provides an unparalleled opportunity for the student to learn psychopathology. Special emphasis is placed on the assessment of clinical conditions which constitute serious psychiatric emergencies: evaluation of risk for suicide, homicide, or violence; assessment of severe impairments in thinking, perception, judgment, affect, and behavior; and, the recognition and identification of factors which differentiate functional from organic disorders

(Hanke, 1984; Hipple & Hipple, 1983; Slaby, Lieb & Tancredi, 1981; Soreff, 1981). Exposure to the family perspective and the broader social context of the patient's problems enhances the student's learning (Perlmutter & Jones, 1985).

Crisis Intervention

Frequently, psychiatric emergencies arise from unmanageable psychosocial stressors. An individual's customary methods of problem-solving may be taxed by stresses such as interpersonal conflict, chronic illness, financial difficulties, marital separation, divorce, or retirement. Traumatic events such as an accident, a death in the family, rape, or other violent assault may also overwhelm an individual's coping mechanisms. Among vulnerable individuals, crises may exacerbate the symptoms of a preexisting mental disorder or precipitate a stress disorder.

Crisis intervention, a brief treatment approach comprising one or more sessions, has steadily gained acceptance and application among mental health professionals who practice with psychiatric emergencies and is the emergency treatment of choice for patients with symptoms engendered by stress and trauma. Crisis theory, extended and elaborated in the crisis intervention practice model, provides the cognitive framework to understand the problem and to develop an intervention strategy.

Briefly stated, the theory posits that an individual in crisis is experiencing an acute state of emotional incapacitation and turmoil in which affective, cognitive, and behavioral dysfunction occurs. The state of crisis is understood to ensue from a sequence of stressful events that cannot be handled by the individual with usual expedience and effectiveness. Crisis theory also holds that the individual in a state of crisis is especially accessible to outside influence; an individual whose own coping mechanisms are not working is more willing to take seriously the help that others offer. On the psychiatric emergency service, the primary goal of crisis intervention is to help the patient return as quickly as possible to at least a precrisis level of psychosocial functioning. Assessment of the patient's specific intrapsychic, interpersonal and social functioning, with special attention to why and how the precrisis equilibrium was upset, enables the clinician to identify and employ the necessary measures to accomplish this goal. Most interventions focus on the restoration of equilibrium between the individual's internal and external environments (Caplan, 1964; Golan, 1978; Hankoff & Robbins, 1969; Jacobson, et al., 1965; Langsley & Kaplan, 1968; Lindemann, 1944; Parad, 1965; Paul, 1966; Rapoport, 1970).

On the psychiatric emergency service, the student routinely practices crisis intervention. The student learns approaches which aim to reduce anxiety, defuse stress or solve problems through the use of supportive techniques, as well as approaches which aim to help the patient relinquish maladaptive behavior and improve functioning. For example, a 72-year-old man from out of town was brought to the emergency room by his wife when he became confused and belligerent during a vacation trip. Evaluation revealed a mild organic brain syndrome in an individual who had been behaviorally stable at home. The precipitant for the decompensation was the patient's being away from a familiar environment. Crisis treatment aimed to help the wife recognize the reason for the decompensation and to return home. Follow-up revealed that the period of decompensation was remedied by recognition and removal of the precipitating stress.

Interviewing Skills

The need for rapid and relatively comprehensive assessment of the psychiatric emergency patient requires that the clinician be able to establish rapport and conduct an interview that will elicit quickly the data upon which the assessment will be based. The student learns not only empathic listening skills that encourage the patient to "tell his story" and express feelings, but also a style of interviewing which is structured, direct, active, and focused. By asking pertinent questions, giving feedback, and refocusing nongermane monologues, the student practices sorting relevant from irrelevant information in order to reach the crucial therapeutic decisions which must be made on the basis of the emergency evaluation.

In conducting the assessment interview, the student learns to focus on a series of general questions: What is the patient's presenting problem? What is the history of the problem from the patient's perspective? How is the problem affecting the patient and others? Has the problem occurred before? Why has the patient come for help now? Are there recent changes or stresses in the patient's life? Does the patient use medication, drugs, or alcohol? What does the patient want or expect from the psychiatric emergency service? The answers to these questions provide a framework for further exploration as the interview proceeds, distinguish acute from chronic problems, identify factors that contribute to the problem situation, and furnish useful information for planning an effective emergency intervention.

Environmental Resources

Because formulating and carrying out a treatment plan is an integral part of providing psychiatric emergency services, the student has numerous opportunities to identify and utilize environmental resources on behalf of patients. These may include the patient's informal social support networks as well as the services of formal organizations and institutions. Planning and effecting an intervention which involves diverse individuals and organizations provides the occasion for the student to conceptualize the goals of the treatment plan, to provide case management services, and to deal with the feelings of those who are involved in positions of situational support or as providers of future services. In this way, the student learns about the strengths and weaknesses of various health and social welfare organizations and systems and also develops clinical skills as the plan is implemented.

Patient Management

Clinicians on the psychiatric emergency service frequently evaluate seriously disturbed patients who are acting out in violent ways and need to be controlled, as well as individuals who have high potential for disruptive or violent behavior. Most field placement settings offer infrequent opportunities to develop the clinical skills necessary to assess and manage dangerous patients, although these skills are often needed in clinical practice (Star, 1984). In this setting, responsibility for the initial evaluation and direct treatment of individuals who are loud, abusive, agitated, threatening, panicked, or even combative, provides the student opportunities to develop the skills needed to address calmly potentially dangerous clinical issues.

The student learns to assess impulse control and to recognize the signs of potential dangerous behavior. When signs of potential violence are evident, the student learns to comment and ask the patient to discuss these signs. When the patient's loss of inner controls appears to be escalating, the student learns how to provide external structure and set limits aimed at protecting the patient from dangerous impulses. The student also learns how restraints, seclusion and medication can be employed to help the actively violent patient regain self-control. In addition to these patient management techniques, the student learns to use specific measures to maintain a sense of personal safety and control while responding to the patient's disturbed emotional state (Hanke, 1984; Hipple & Hipple, 1983).

Interdisciplinary Collaboration

On many psychiatric emergency services, the role distinctions between medical and nonmedical personnel have been virtually erased, with all clinicians performing similar functions (Spitz, 1976). Social work practice involves conferring, cooperating, and consulting with colleagues from medicine, psychiatry, nursing, and/or psychology to develop plans to meet patients' needs, solve problems, and carry out clinical tasks.

Because the psychiatric emergency service is a collaborative work environment, social work students have many opportunities to develop a capacity for mutuality with colleagues form other disciplines. As a member of an interdisciplinary team, the student can develop facilitating attitudes and communication skills, as well as respect and empathic responsiveness to the perspectives, interests, and concerns of colleagues.

TEACHING AND SUPERVISION

Although the psychiatric emergency service provides multiple opportunities for learning major aspects of clinical social work practice, special demands are placed on the field instructor for supervision and teaching. The characteristics of the setting, patients' presenting problems and the nature of the clinical interventions that experienced professionals have found useful in addressing psychiatric emergencies call for both unique case-based supervisory methods and the development of interdisciplinary training experiences.

Case Supervision

A contemporary apprentice model of supervision (Wijnberg & Schwartz, 1977) provides intensive and comprehensive case-based instruction and is well-suited to the psychiatric emergency service. This model of supervision emphasizes the use of modeling techniques, stresses learning by doing, and facilitates the student's gradual advancement toward clinical autonomy. As this approach to supervision is used, the student and field instructor are both present at the time of the first clinical contact with the patient. During these joint interviews, the student progressively assumes clinical responsibility. Initially, for example, the field instructor may assume complete responsibility for evaluation, intervention, and treatment planning, while the student listens, observes and learns through post-interview discussion. Next, the student may contribute to the interview, get in touch and talk with significant others, assist with referrals, and write the chart note. As experience and knowledge are accrued, the student begins to participate equally as a cotherapist with the field instructor. Eventually, when the student and field instructor agree that the student is ready, the student accepts primary responsibility for the case, while the field instructor observes and provides consultation when needed. After this joint interviewing phase, the student begins to evaluate, treat, and plan for patients independently, conferring with the field instructor during a break in the evaluation interview or directly afterwards. Evidence suggests that "on-the-spot" supervision results in superior learning (Doyle, Foreman & Wales, 1977).

A field placement on the psychiatric emergency service can be demanding for a myriad of reasons. For example, involuntary patients, seriously regressed patients and substance abusers, groups seen frequently in this setting, present multiple, complex clinical challenges. Hostile or disruptive patients or those who are not considered by emergency room staff to be "true" emergencies may engender antagonism in the milieu. Few adequate treatment resources may be available for some patients and referral relationships with other institutions and agencies may be frustrating. The need for immediate decision-making can add pressure to an already difficult clinical process. However, if field placements are sufficiently structured, they can offer optimal learning opportunities. The apprentice model of supervision provides sufficient support to moderate the stresses inherent in the field placement, since the student assumes increasing clinical responsibility only as skills and confidence are acquired.

Interdisciplinary Training

Field-based education is enhanced when the social work student participates in interdisciplinary training experiences. Joint interviewing and informal case collaboration with professionals and trainees from allied disciplines enable the student to learn from others, to hear alternative conceptualizations of the same case, and to give and receive feedback from colleagues. These experiences promote a spirit of camaraderie and facilitate team functioning.

Participation with trainees from allied disciplines in formal seminars taught by an interdisciplinary team of instructors offers the social work student another rich opportunity to learn specific aspects of practice with psychiatric emergencies. Diagnosis, psychopathology, crisis intervention theory and methodology, interviewing techniques, the use of community resources, and principles of patient management can be taught effectively in a structured, didactic forum.

Learning is optimal when the teaching content of interdisciplinary seminars focuses on both those aspects of practice in which the clinical roles and functions of the various disciplines overlap, and also includes the development of knowledge and skills which have traditionally been the province of a single discipline. For example, all trainees need to be taught how to conduct a mental status examination. Teaching content focused on the nature of the mental status examination, its applicability in the evaluation process, and the use that can be made of the data that come from the examination prepares the student to organize data and formulate major treatment planning decisions. Also, because psychotropic drugs are often indicated in the management of psychiatric emergencies (Ketai, 1975), interdisciplinary seminars provide an ideal forum for the social work student to learn about this dimension of practice. As social workers assume increasing responsibility for recommending and monitoring psychotropic drugs, specialized knowledge to carry out these functions is essential (Miller, Wiedeman & Linn, 1980). The student can be taught the indications and contraindications for drug treatment; the properties, therapeutic dosages, and effects of various drugs; considerations in drug selection; and, the principles of acute management through rapid tranquilization.

TRAINING BENEFITS

Learning experiences on the psychiatric emergency service expose the student to broad dimensions of life and death — acute psychosis, chronic mental illness, alcoholism, drug overdoses, homelessness, rape, family violence, suicide and homicide. The disabling stresses of unemployment, poverty, urban crowding, the disintegration of family structure, and social alienation are readily apparent. The relationship between health policy and practice quickly becomes clear as clinical issues associated with health care funding, deinstitutionalization, and patient rights emerge and service gaps and fragmentation in the health care system constrain service options.

The setting offers the student specific learning experiences that generalize well to a wide variety of clinical settings. The diagnostic skills mastered are applicable in almost all clinical social work practice arenas. Judgments, decisions, and interventions often have immediate and drastic real-life consequences and may even involve temporarily usurping the patient's right to self-determination. These decisions prepare the student to assume and discharge professional responsibility and authority. The acquisition of crisis intervention skills grounds the student in therapeutic strategies which are the treatment of choice for many who use social work help. Interdisciplinary training, especially as it focuses on areas which have traditionally been the domain of other disciplines, enables the student to acquire specialized knowledge and skills that prepare for the assumption of expanded clinical responsibilities.

Growth experiences emerge from the knowledge that one has learned to handle oneself effectively in a crisis. Emergencies arise in all clinical settings. Evaluating and assuming responsibility for a wide variety of people in acute subjective distress provides sufficient comparative experiences to enable the student to learn what constitutes a real emergency and to acquire both depth and perspective in assessment and treatment planning. Maturity develops when the student is able to recognize and respect the sense of urgency on the part of the patient and still synthesize his own clinical perceptions and judgments. In addition, the student gains realistic self-confidence and assurance as the ability is acquired to handle competently urgent clinical situations.

CONCLUSION

Professional social workers want and need to acquire the capability for clinically autonomous practice as soon as possible. A field placement on the psychiatric emergency service prepares the clinical social worker to assume weighty responsibilities with a reasonable degree of comfort and assurance. The setting, by nature of its rigorous demands, offers training experiences which accelerate the process of knowledge and skill building and enables the student to enter professional practice with an enhanced ability to deal with people in a responsible role.

REFERENCES

Bartolucci, G. & Drayer, C. (1973). An overview of crisis intervention in the emergency rooms of general hospitals. *American Journal of Psychiatry, 130*(9), 953-960.

Bell, C. (1978). The role of psychiatric emergency services in aiding community alternatives to hospitalization in an inner-city population. *Journal of the National Medical Association, 70*(12), 931-935.

Caplan, G. (1964). *Principles of Preventive Psychiatry.* New York: Basic Books.

Doyle, W., Foreman, M. & Wales, E. (1977). Effects of supervision in the training of non-professional crisis intervention counselors. *Journal of Counseling Psychology, 24*(1), 72-78.

Gerson, S. & Bassuck, E. (1980). Psychiatric emergencies: An overview. *American Journal of Psychiatry, 137*(1), 1-11.

Golan, N. (1978). *Treatment in Crisis Situations*. New York: The Free Press.

Groner, E. (1978). Delivery of clinical social work services in the emergency room: A description of an existing program. *Social Work in Health Care 4*(1), 19-29.

Grumet, G.W. & Trachtman, D.L. (1976). Psychiatric social workers in the emergency department. *Health and Social Work 1*(3), 113-131.

Hanke, N. (1984). *Handbook of Emergency Psychiatry*. Lexington, Massachusetts: The Collamore Press.

Hankoff, L. & Robbins, L. (1969). *Emergency Psychiatric Treatment*. Springfield, Illinois: Charles C Thomas.

Hillard, J., O'Shanick, G. & Houpt, J. (1982). Residency training in the psychiatric emergency room. *American Journal of Psychiatry, 139*(2), 236-238.

Hipple, J. L. & Hipple, L. B. (1983). *Diagnosis and Management of Psychological Emergencies*. Springfield, Illinois: Charles C Thomas.

Jacobson, G., Wilner, D., Morley, W., Schneider, S., Strickler, M., & Sommer, G. (1965). The scope and practice of an early-access brief treatment psychiatric center. *American Journal of Psychiatry, 121*(12), 1176-1182.

Ketai, R. (1975). Psychotropic drugs in the management of psychiatric emergencies. *Postgraduate Medicine, 58*(4), 87-93.

Langsley, D. & Kaplan, D. (1968). *The Treatment of Families in Crisis*. New York: Grune & Stratton.

Lazare, T. (1976). The psychiatric examination in the walk-in clinic. *Archives of General Psychiatry, 33*, 96-102.

Lindemann, E. (1944). Symptomatology and management of acute grief. *American Journal of Psychiatry, 101*(2), 141-148. Reprinted in E. Lindemann. *Beyond Grief* (59-78), 1978, New York: Jason Aronson.

Mendel, W. & Rappaport, S. (1969). Determinants of the decision for psychiatric hospitalization. *Archives of General Psychiatry, 20*, 321-328.

Miller, R., Wiedeman, G. & Linn, L. (1980). Prescribing psychotropic drugs: Whose responsibility? *Social Work in Health Care, 6*(1), 51-61.

Parad, H. (Ed.). (1965). *Crisis Intervention: Selected Readings*. New York: Family Service Association of America.

Paul, L. (1966). Treatment techniques in a walk-in clinic. *Hospital and Community Psychiatry, 17*, 49-51.

Perlmutter, R. A. & Jones, J. E. (1985). Assessment of families in psychiatric emergencies. *American Journal of Orthopsychiatry, 55*(1), 130-139.

Rapoport, L. (1970). Crisis intervention as a mode of brief treatment. In R. Roberts & R. Nee (Eds.). *Theories of Social Casework* (267-311). Chicago: University of Chicago Press.

Sheridan, E. & Teplin, L. (1982). Evolution of an emergency room psychiatric staffing. *American Journal of Orthopsychiatry, 52*(1), 172-175.

Slaby, A., Lieb, J. & Tancredi, L. (1981). *Handbook of Psychiatric Emergencies*. Garden City, New York: Medical Examination Publishing Co.

Soreff, S. (1981). *Management of the Psychiatric Emergency*. New York: John Wiley.

Spitz, L. (1976). The evolution of a psychiatric emergency crisis intervention service in a medical emergency room setting. *Comprehensive Psychiatry*, *17*(1), 99-113.

Star, B. (1984). Patient violence/therapist safety. *Social Work*, *29*(3), 225-230.

Steele, T. (1972). Psychiatric emergency services: Their relationship to residency training and supervision. *Social Psychiatry*, *7*, 75-81.

Streiner, D., Goodman, J. & Woodward, C. (1975). Correlates of the hospitalization decision: A replicative study. *Canadian Journal of Public Health*, *66*, 411-418.

Wijnberg, M. & Schwartz, M. (1977). Models of student supervision: The apprentice, growth, and role systems models. *Journal of Education for Social Work*, *13*(3), 107-113.

Commentary

As schools struggle to update curricula, revise approaches, and integrate new ideas, they retain core, enduring social work knowledge and skills, including those specifically applicable to health care settings. Attempting to incorporate new approaches, schools also keep in mind Bracht's (1983) observation that "Illness will continue to disrupt families in characteristically painful ways." Frequently, discussions between "town and gown" about education for the profession demonstrate that both partners have congruent goals in the educational effort. What remains to be achieved, however, is agreement on how the educational partnership can best provide maximum generic/special skills within the realities of limited time and resources (Fields, 1980).

There has always been consensus that the school's academic curricula and the field's teaching curricula need to be better integrated and that this goal is best achieved through structures established to institutionalize the concept of partnership in the educational effort (Caroff and Mailick, 1980; and Caroff, 1977). A recent study found increasing use of such models as task supervision, assignment of students to more than one area of practice, multimethod assignments, the development of interagency consortia for shared didactic teaching, and students' peer learning and teaching. In face of limited resources, faculty and field teachers are actively seeking new models to facilitate students' rapid learning of complex content (Marshack, Davidson, and Mizrahi, 1987).

REFERENCES

Bracht, Neil. "Preparing New Generations of Social Workers for Practice in Health Settings," *Social Work in Health Care* 8(3), Spring 1983, pp. 29–47.

Caroff, Phyllis. "A Study of School-Agency Collaboration in Social Work in Health Curriculum Building," *Social Work in Health Care* 2(3), Spring 1977, pp. 329–339.

Caroff, Phyllis, and Mailick, Mildred (Eds.), *Social Work in Health Services: An Academic Practice Partnership*. New York: Prodist, 1980.

Fields, Grace. "What Does a Director of a Hospital Social Work Department Expect of a Beginning MSW?" in Phyllis Caroff and Mildred Mailick (Eds.), *Social Work in Health Services: An Academic Practice Partnership*. New York: Prodist, 1980, pp. 155–166.

Gerhart, Ursula, and Brooks, Alexander. "The Social Work Practitioner and Antipsychotic Medications," *Social Work 28*(6), November-December 1983, pp. 454–460.

Marshack, Elaine, Davidson, Kay, and Mizrahi, Terry. "Preparation of Social Workers for a Changing Health Care Environment," *Health and Social Work 13*(3), Summer 1988, pp. 226-233.

Matorin, Susan, and DeChillo, Neal. "Psychopharmacology: Guidelines for Social Workers," *Social Casework 65*(10), December 1984, pp. 579–589.

Miller, Rosalind S., Wiedeman, George H., and Linn, Louis. "Prescribing Psychotropic Drugs: Whose Responsibility?" *Social Work in Health Care 6*(1), Fall 1980, pp. 51–61.

Additional Readings

Bartlett, Harriett M. "Responsibilities of Social Work Practitioners and Educators Toward Building a Strong Profession," *Social Service Review, 33*(4), December 1960, pp. 379–391.

Bassoff, Betty Zippin. "Interdisciplinary Education for Health Professionals: Issues and Directions," *Social Work in Health Care* 2(2), Winter 1976-77, pp. 219–228.

Bassoff, Betty Zippin, and Ludwig, Stephen. "Interdisciplinary Education for Health Care Professionals," *Health and Social Work* 4(2), May 1979, pp. 58–71.

Berkman, Barbara. "Knowledge Base Needs for Effective Social Work Practice in Health," *Journal of Education for Social Work* 17(2), Spring 1981, pp. 85–90.

———. "Adapting Course Content to Meet the Needs of Social Work Practice in Health Care," *Journal of Education for Social Work 21*(3), Fall 1985, pp. 43–51.

Berkman, Barbara, and Carlton, Thomas Owen. *The Development of Health Social Work Curricula: Patterns and Progress in Three Programs of Social Work Education.* Boston, Mass.: MGH Institute of Health Professions, 1985.

Caroff, Phyllis, and Mailick, Mildred D. "Health Concentrations in Schools of Social Work: The State of the Art," *Health and Social Work 10*(1), Winter 1985, pp. 5–14.

Dana, Bess. "Social Work in the University Medical Center," *The Johns Hopkins Medical Journal 124*(5), May 1969, pp. 227–282.

Dinerman, Miriam, Schlesinger, Elfriede G., and Wood, Katherine M. "Social Work Roles in Health Care: An Educational Framework," *Health and Social Work 5*(4), November 1980, pp. 13–20.

Falck, Hans S. "Interdisciplinary Education and its Implications for Social Work Practice," *Journal of Education for Social Work* *13*(2), 1977, pp. 30–37.

Hookey, Peter. "Education for Social Work in Health Care Organizations," *Social Work in Health Care* *1*(3), Spring 1976, pp. 337–345.

Lane, Helen J. "Toward the Preparation of Social Work Specialists in Health Care," *Health and Social Work* *7*(3), August 1982, pp. 230–234.

Moore, Kathleen. "Training Social Workers to Work with the Terminally Ill," *Health and Social Work* *9*(4), Fall 1984, pp. 268–273.

Olson, Miriam Meltzer. "Beyond Specialization: Social Work Education and Practice for Health Care and Family Life," *Journal of Social Work Education* *22*(2), Spring-Summer 1986, pp. 30–37.

Perretz, Edgar A. "Social Work Education for the Field of Health: A Report of Findings from a Survey of Curricula," *Social Work in Health Care* *1*(3), Spring 1976, pp. 357–365.

Rauch, Julia B. "Helping Students to Begin Hospital Field Placements: An Active Learning Approach," *Social Work in Health Care* *9*(3), Spring 1984, pp. 63–75.

Rauch, Julia B., and Schreiber, Hanita. "Discharge Planning as a Teaching Mechanism," *Health and Social Work* *10*(3), Summer 1985, pp. 208–216.

Raymond, Frank B. "Social Work Education for Health Care Practice," *Social Work in Health Care* *2*(4), Summer 1977, pp. 429–438.

Rehr, Helen, and Caroff, Phyllis. *A New Model in Academic-Practice Partnership: Multi-Instructor and Institutional Collaboration in Social Work*. Lexington, Mass.: Ginn Press, 1986.

Rehr, Helen, and Rosenberg, Gary. "Today's Education for Today's Health Care Social Work Practice," *Clinical Social Work* *5*(4), Winter 1977, pp. 342–350.

Robinovitch, Arlene E., and Nash, Kermit B. "Issues for Hospitals in Educating Social Work Students for Social Work Practice in Health Care Settings," *Social Work in Health Care* *9*(2), Winter 1983, pp. 97–105.

Rusnack, Betty. "Planned Change: Interdisciplinary Education for Health Care," *Journal of Education for Social Work 13*(1), Winter 1977, pp. 104–111.

Swack, Lois G. "Education and Practice: Their Responsibility to Complement Each Other," *Health and Social Work 5*(1), February 1980, pp. 64–70.

PART 9
AN EXPANDED ROLE
FOR SOCIAL WORK

Introduction

Throughout their professional history social workers in health care have experienced competition by other professionals for functions integral to the psychological components of patient care. When these occur, social workers may gear their efforts toward the maintenance of existing roles and thus have little time and energy for innovation. The positive side of this professional competition is the growing importance assigned to a biopsychosocial view of health and health care. In a climate of increased awareness of the social needs of patients, social workers have flourished in settings such as HMOs, primary care services, and federally funded and regulated programs such as renal dialysis. As new medical technologies proliferate and psychosocial consequences for patients ensue, social workers in health care have new opportunities.

The four articles selected for this section depict additional knowledge needs.

Rosenberg's article provides a clear overview of theory and practice as the profession seeks sharper definitions, greater accountability, and firmer ownership of critical roles and functions. Rosenberg reviews developing ideas on changing contexts for social work practice in the health care field. He considers expanding roles and functions along with anticipated struggles and conflicts, as, for example, in relation to value dilemmas that arise when social workers work in for-profit health care organizations. Rosenberg notes the challenges and difficulties to be faced and predicts an expanded role for social workers in health care settings.

In Vera's article on rape crisis intervention, social work's role is clearly defined and shown to be effective as it makes its unique contribution to care in emergency medical services. The social work role in the physical and psychological sequelae of assaultive traumas is identified in the context of the multiple functions of professionals who work together in the emergency room. The "new and challenging area of practice" that Vera maps out expands our conception of social work's role in health and mental health care and has wide application for programs in the next era of our development.

Research by Jansson and Simmons sheds new light on the functions and roles of social workers in hospital settings. The authors explored the organizational factors that promote or impede the development of social work departments. Their study determined that an expanded role for social work is most likely to occur when the hospital administration is supportive of the department's goals. They emphasize that social workers need to know and understand the sociology of health care organizations in order to negotiate effectively and expand their roles in these complex structures.

Clarke, Neuwirth, and Bernstein's article spells out the broader role that can be carried by social workers in a medical group practice. Here social workers function as principal service providers to clients, as educators of physicians in the psychosocial components of health care, and as consultants to other members of the health care team. Each aspect of the expanded role is analyzed and illustrated with practice examples. The authors emphasize the importance of social work participation as new health care systems are in the design phase. They identify varied, expanded, and rewarding responsibilities that may be carried out by social workers in current health care settings and those to be developed in the future.

Advancing Social Work Practice in Health Care

Gary Rosenberg, PhD

Social work has been reasonably optimistic regarding our contribution to the well-being of the clients we serve, somewhat less optimistic regarding our contribution to the achievement of desired social utilities, and cyclically either optimistic or pessimistic regarding our contribution to the social policies affecting population groups, neighborhood groups, regions, and the nation.

Historically, social work's contribution to health care has been characterized by an emphasis on social health and on those aspects of social health care that affect patients, families, and populations at risk. From the time that Ida M. Cannon was invited by Richard Cabot to begin an organized social work effort at the Massachusetts General Hospital, social work's contribution to social health care has been recognized with uneven enthusiasm and appreciated by only a fair sampling of physicians, administrators, and client groups. Perhaps it is the characteristically dual focus of social work, which some authors have called "cause and function" and others have labeled "personal services and social policies," that has made social work unique. Our major strength is in placing both individual *and* population needs and problems into a social context and in looking for remedies to these ills not only in the individual and his environment, but in the social policies that affect them.

At the time of writing, Dr. Rosenberg was Director, Department of Social Work Services, The Mount Sinai Hospital and Associate Professor, Department of Community Medicine (Social Work), Mount Sinai School of Medicine, CUNY, and Vice-President, Human Resources, Mount Sinai Medical Medical Center, New York, NY
Reprinted from *Social Work in Health Care*, Volume 8(3), Summer 1983.

Social work has suffered as a profession when we have paid more attention to one or the other of these two foci: to either the social policies/social action aspect of our mission or to the social treatment aspects of our mission. We have done best when we have kept a reasonably balanced perspective on both.

This unique strength of ours has also been problematic. Our dual focus has exposed social work to criticisms from within and without, criticisms that have affected our growth and made the professions hesitant to lay claim to the major contributions we have made. Some social workers specialize in social administration, social policy, community organization — that is, in the larger social policies and social constructs. Other social workers specialize in individual, family, and group treatment approaches. Each group keeps a cautious eye on the other. Yet it is in the blending of the specialists and the generalists — with a uniquely wide-angled focus on the individual, the social environment, the family, and the social policies that affect all of them — that has made social work's contribution significant in the past and also bodes well for its future.

This chapter is optimistic, hopeful, and imbedded in the mission and goals of organized social welfare in the United States. It takes the position that social work in health care will make major contributions along this wide spectrum; in the refinement of a social health perspective; in the provision of services; in the development of treatment modalities and treatment techniques; and in the management of social health services. Social work will contribute in these major ways to the delivery of services to individuals, families, groups, and populations; and it also will continue to contribute as it has in the past to the formation, development, and implementation of social and economic policies affecting these groups.

The series of papers in this book provide us with a set of directions for social work in health care in the present and in the future. They codify the contributions that social work has made up to now and also suggest avenues for increasing the efficacy of social work practice in health. It is helpful to place these contributions in perspective and to review what other colleagues in social work previously have attempted to predict about the future of social work in health care.

In 1974 Neil Bracht offered an overview of trends that were carried over into the 1980s. He suggested that cost control incentives would dominate third-party financing of health care. He predicted correctly increasing conflict between nurses and social workers around the boundaries between the two professions. He suggested that the 1980s would be dominated by the political issue of whether our nation would move to a system of health care or settle for a system of a medical care. He thought that techniques of educational and behavioral change would be primary modes for clinical intervention. He noted also that the predominance of one-to-one clinical intervention by social workers in health and mental health settings had left a short supply of them trained for managing, coordinating, and planning the functions of the emerging health care system (Bracht, 1974).

Highlighting other issues for the future, Caputi (1978), Dinerman (1979), and Dana, Banta, and Deuschle (1974) called attention to our need to gear up for changing family patterns and life-styles, for the increasing numbers of chronically ill and other population groups at high social risk, for accountability structures, and for the study and development of models of interprofessional behaviors.

Lurie predicted an expansion of social work functions in the arenas of ambulatory care, admissions, discharge planning, and emergency room care. He forecasted that by virtue of their training and skills, social workers would be used for liaison, mediation, and the development of programs consistent with community needs. Lurie warned that the direct practice of social work would be influenced by external regulations. He saw as a danger that we might be viewed as allied with the establishment if our functions were corrupted and became institutionally self-serving; that we could become alien to the disadvantaged community we have historically served. He sees social work as part of the caring system, helping patients and families resolve difficulties caused by new technologies in health care. He suggested that social workers would practice as a component of a personal care services system. He thinks that it is likely that our services will be more highly valued when they affect the work productivity of the individual. Lurie identified two future roles for social work: (1) helping health care networks protect confidentiality, and (2) resolving the issues or problems of middle management for the health field at large (Lurie, 1977).

Rehr also ventured a look at the future of social work in health care. As services and financing for services became available to segments of the population that formerly had had limited access, social work experienced increased demand for its services. This was particularly true of the elderly and the poor. Rehr suggested that the health care system may have reached its ultimate size but not the ultimate in quality. She saw the future challenge for social work in what she calls the "challenge of the four P's, the policymakers, the planners, the professionals, and the public," and suggests that this challenge is to put together a rational, pluralistic, multilevel system of social health provision. Within that structure, social work will carry major responsibility in facilitating a broad range of continuous, comprehensive, and coordinated inpatient and outpatient care. She further elucidated a task for social work: to assist in making health care comprehensive, i.e., to piece the fragments together into a pattern of overall resources. Social workers will need to be skilled in dealing with motivation and coping capacities and trained to view the individual and his environment in relation to one another. She suggested further that a large component of our clientele will be the elderly and those with chronic diseases; both groups require a wide range of social supports. Rehr suggested that we will assist in looking at causes in medical care and that social work is competent to contribute to social diagnosis and social medical care. She identified a role for us in fee-for-service social therapy and health education and self-help groups, both in organizing these and in serving as advisors to them. She thought social work will be actively involved in whatever health planning efforts permeate the system. She also suggested that we need to continue to contribute to accountability systems and to efforts to quantify the outcome of our services (Rehr, 1977).

Regensburg pointed out that while professions educate their members for future practice, we cannot accurately predict the ramifications of this practice since it cannot be known what technologies, knowledge, and truths will be available and since we will not know what changes in society will affect the future of social work. Regensburg suggested that the future roles of social work will be shaped by various developments in the profession of social work; by successful nurturing of social workers' currently unrealized potentials; by advancement towards socially desirable goals for health care agreed upon by coalitions and multi-professional groups; by priorities established by governmental bodies in a democratic society for the education, allocation, and recompense of manpower needed in the health care field; and by other unforeseen ways in which political and professional powers influence the form, functions, and substance of health care (Regensburg, 1978).

Harold Lewis raised five persistent issues shaping the professional practice of social work. These are relevant not only to the past views of social work, but to future ones as well:

1. What roles are to be carried by the various parties to the services transaction: the worker, the client, the agency?
2. How should the services be supported: by philanthropic grants, client fees, public taxes?
3. Who should control the helping process: the worker, the client, or the agency?
4. Whose objectives should be worked on and whose goals pursued?
5. To whom is the service and program responsible: the client, the agency, the community, the profession, or the worker?

He anticipated changes in our nation's definition of what constitutes appropriate health care, and expected radical changes in the meaning of these questions and the weight attached to each of these issues (Lewis, 1981).

Nacman suggested that the future direction of social work take place in the academic *health* center rather than the medical school. This new title recognizes the array of different health practitioners who contribute to the care of the patient. He further noted that in order to survive, social workers need to learn how power is distributed within their organizations and their surrounding communities, and how to develop and systematically apply power. Nacman identified a future role for social work in assisting other health care employees in the resolution of organizational and administrative problems that are crucial to fellow health care professionals. He reinforced the need for social work to locate itself both in and out of the health care sector in the hospital and the community and to attempt to set up linkages between them (Nacman, 1975, 1980).

Coulton perceived the future of social work practice in health care concentrating on the degree of "persons/environment fit," which includes physical dimensions, psychosocial dimensions, behavioral dimensions, and economic dimensions. Some of the roles and functions identified by Coulton include giving health information; providing social and emotional support; modifying behavior; engaging in decision-making counseling; helping people obtain resources such as home care, nursing homes, medical equipment, and barrier-free housing; assisting in applications for financial assistance; dealing with the environment of the health care organization by modifying scheduling practices; providing crisis services for evenings and weekends; and modifying restrictive organizational practices. Other work in environmental contexts includes assisting families to adapt to illness, helping to reduce family conflict, and building social relationships, including the use of self-help groups. Coulton also placed strong emphasis on collecting data, organizing pressure groups, providing testimony, contributing funds for lobbying, and supporting professional coalitions for changes in health care policy (Coulton, 1979).

Morris and Anderson urged that social work in health care take on the role of coordinator, manager, and implementor of health care plans for the elderly and chronically ill. They saw social work filling a vacuum in overseeing the multiplicity of presently uncoordinated services needed for the ongoing management of patients who require a designated overseer to direct and coordinate the details of complex care plans (Morris and Anderson, 1975).

Carol Meyer has raised some persistent issues that also affect the future of social work. She states, "It is hard for social workers who are rooted in social reform to confront the reality that fundamental change affecting . . . social conditions will occur politically and not through their professional practice. Effectiveness must derive from harder work than caring, and must come from a mastery of knowledge and skill." She noted that Yarmolinsky provides us with three phenomena that will affect professional behavior in the future: (1) the increasing dissemination of knowledge once held exclusively by professionals; (2) the looming presence of bureaucracies, which stand between the professional and the client; and (3) the democratization of everything, including participation of the client and the public in defining problems as well as their participation in the internal debates of professions themselves. Meyer suggested that the future task for social work is to decide on its *domain* of experience: what it can do and what it can teach; and that it arrive at a consensus regarding these issues (Meyer, 1981).

Two key concepts pervading these predictions of social work in the future health care system emerge as: (1) the role of social work in social health, its definition, provision of services, policies, and the treatment of social health problems; and (2) the social work contribution to the management of the social health system and to the policies governing its organization, structure, control, and accountability.

THE CONTEXT OF FUTURE PRACTICE

Since the social context of practice will influence the future of social work, it can be expected that future social work practice in health care will take place in an environment of declining resources, a condition that will spark an active struggle among health care professionals for economic support from a shrinking health care dollar, as well as persistent attempts to narrow health insurance and contain the cost of health care. Our present model, the one that is most familiar to most social workers, is that of working within the health care settings of hospitals and clinics. This model will continue. Though we will flirt with ideas of community-based social work along the lines of the English model, social work will continue to be characterized and marred by a lack of organized effort coupled with constant struggles as we attempt to find the integrating force for organized social work effort. Market conditions will push social work to concentrate on improved technology of service delivery, cost efficiency, cost effectiveness, and quantifying of the benefits accruing from social work services. This will be coupled by a humanistic, caring perspective of social workers in health care, which will underpin their struggle to maintain the fight for the adequate provision of social health services.

Technological innovation will occur in the area of utilization of behavioral treatment for groups as an effective modality of care in the growing self-help movement. Technical innovation will also come out of the reawakening interest of social workers in general reform and social action. Targets for reform will include the health care system and social policies affecting the health care system; and there will be greater emphasis again on the rights of individuals to self-determination and choice in health care. Much of this resurgence of reform and social action at the practice level will have been fostered by the conservative economic environment of the early 1980s.

While the shape of our practice may change, our social work value system will remain intact. The reforming trend in the profession will help us concentrate on rights, entitlements, and class issues in social health. Once again, social work will do a balancing act between organizational loyalties, loyalties to social reform, and loyalties to the clients it serves.

THE PRACTICE OF SOCIAL WORK

Many issues and concepts will be prominent in the near future of the health social work profession. Social workers will be more concerned with the promotion of health and the preventive concepts surrounding health promotion than at present. Social work will move into a frame of reference that promotes increasing utilization of social epidemiology problem-approaches as well as those of health maintenance and health promotion. Our research will be population-focused and will add to our underlying knowledge base of social epidemiology. Social workers in the community center field will become more interested in health promotion and health preservation. Health education will be an area where social workers will increase their activities, along with nurses and physicians.

Social work's concern for improved services to our patients will continue to put us at the forefront of the consumer movement. Our focus on self-care, consumerism, advocacy, and population approaches to care will place social work in the role of mediating between existing health institutions and population and consumer groups. Social work will focus on consumer satisfaction and consumer needs and help develop new instruments that will rely heavily on epidemiology and survey research, as we did during the birth of our profession, to help health organizations market health promotion and disease prevention in the community.

Retaining the biopsychosocial frame of reference, our research will use randomized clinical trials and move us towards further development of the underlying knowledge base of epidemiology as well as towards innovations in direct practice based on their results. The results of these findings in the field will be applied not only in schools of social work, but in widespread continuing education efforts as we seek to strengthen our knowledge base.

Social work will continue to develop more sophisticated case-finding mechanisms, which identify people at risk, families at risk, and populations at risk. We will expand our work more and more in the areas of occupational health and occupational medicine, and into industry, identifying and treating the social health factors that affect productivity. The pioneering work of leading health care social workers in mechanisms for screening and case-finding of populations at risk will serve as a base for such future expanded efforts in this area (Berkman, Rehr, and Rosenberg, 1980; Clark, 1980).

Social work will struggle with financial support both for its professional input and for health care generally. The next two decades will see continuing argument regarding fee-for-service, market strategies, and insuring entitlements in the general funding base for health care organizations (per diem reimbursement). We believe that social work services should be offered to wider ranges of the population; this need will become increasingly urgent as the United States population continues to age. Social work will have a healthy internal dialogue regarding the place of professional competition in the marketplace. Competition will be linked to different technologies and there will be many value arguments about cost benefits that will have underlying implications for social work funding in health care settings.

It was suggested in 1964 that "in the next decade, medical and public health facilities such as outpatient clinics, nursing homes, and homes for the chronically ill aged are likely to turn increasingly to the profession of social work to fill administrative positions" (Light and Brown, 1964). Some health care organizations note certain advantages in selecting social workers as administrators:

1. Social workers represent well a service-oriented philosophy in which patients' needs receive primary consideration;
2. Social workers are able to create a reasonably permissive atmosphere in which individual differences are accepted;
3. Social workers' special skills in assessing personalities can be applied strategically to selection of staff in order to reduce the likelihood of employing disturbed individuals who might undermine programs;
4. Social workers as administrators convey to other professional staff that there are individuals in a policy-making position who understand and value clinical practice;
5. Social workers are particularly skilled in listening to employees and understanding the content of their communications. (Light and Brown, 1964)

In the near future, social work will not only encompass functions of clinical administration but also functions of program planning and project administration; in short, social workers will assume major positions in human resource management. Social workers have become more and more sophisticated in financial management, human resource management, and in the general principles of business management. They bring to these roles the special skills of social work in an integration that is unique. Further, social workers have become expert in managing social work agencies and bring with them special, valuable experience in the management of human resources and in problem-focused management. It is becoming clearer that the clinical base of social work provides an excellent basic framework for their additional education in management. This combination provides a unique perspective and ability to administer clinical health and social programs. Support for this effort will come not only from continuing social work education efforts, but from a proliferation of joint degrees: MSW/MBA; MSW/MPH.

There will be conflict as social workers will be hard put to face the value dilemmas in working for for-profit health care organizations. On the other hand, out of the conflict will come interesting new sets of organizational forms of health service delivery, many of them community- and industry-based. United States industry will be looking for social workers to help administer health and mental health benefit packages as well as to provide health promotion packages for employees. Additionally, social workers who currently leave positions under social agency auspices to move into businesses and industries in the private sector will have more opportunity to assume management positions and to utilize their skills in both the profit as well as nonprofit organizations.

Social work will face ethical dilemmas, which will inevitably continue, regarding client needs, client desires, client interests, personal interests, and the interest of the organizations where social workers practice. In the short run, in a shrinking economy, social work autonomy will be threatened by the desire of other professions to control psychosocial care. In the long run, collegial collaborative relationships will emerge, which will support a major social work contribution to social health care and which will provide support for the social work practice base. Although social work will struggle with the instrumentalities of collaborative practice and although it is one of the few professions that addresses the collaborative nature of practice, we shall probably miss the opportunity to present definitive research and knowledge in this area.

Social work will continue to be guided in its work by the knowledge of individuals, by knowledge of developmental psychology, and by knowledge of individual life cycles, family life cycles, and the life cycles of groups and populations. Even though our knowledge base will come from a biopsychosocial frame of reference, we will continue to hold to a pluralistic perspective, which will be tested in relation to the identification of problem needs and the services we will continue to provide. This social science base will help social work integrate and modify its clinical practice knowledge base.

As new strategies of interventive techniques are developed, they will be delivered by an organized social work profession with its skills, value, and ethics as well as the key notion of a person within an environment. These mean that we will target and intervene not only in personal and family resources, but in the set of societal resources designed to assist in the social health care of people. The practicing social worker will once again become more attuned to resources and resource development. Computerized information will provide data about resource supports so that we will be able to gather rapid documentation about gaps and lack in resources and their concomitant social, economic, and human costs.

Clearly, the future will require an updated educational system and will probably exacerbate the stresses between the fields of practice and the schools of social work regarding the duration of schooling and the curriculum content. Social work will begin to expand doctoral level education and it may well be that rather than the master's, the doctorate in social work will be seen as the terminal social work degree.

While we move towards better research models and clearer explanations about both what we do and the effects of our intervention, social work will continue to experience conflict between those who believe that scientific findings exist only in randomized clinical trials or experimental research and those who take other perspectives. According to Lewis Thomas (1981):

> Science is thought to be a process of pure reductionism, taking the meaning out of mystery, explaining everything away, concentrating all our energies on measuring things and counting them up. It is not like this at all. The scientific method is guess work, the making up of stories. The difference between this and other imaginative works of the human mind is that science is then obliged to find out whether the guesses are correct and the stories are true. Curiosity drives the enterprise and the open acknowledgement of ignorance. The greatest single achievement of science in this most scientifically productive century is the discovery that we are profoundly ignorant. We know very little about nature and we understand even less.

Social workers in health care settings will continue to see large numbers of elderly sick and those with ongoing chronic disorders — the sick for whom social and physical rehabilitation is possible and those for whom it is not. All these patients require ongoing health and social services and not only periodic, episodic intervention related to crises. Care needs to be continuous and available with an emphasis upon self-care and resource coordination. As this population continues to be buffeted by the changing economic and social climate in this country, the ongoing services they need are best offered by social workers, who have always been advocates for them and served them. The skills social workers have developed out of this long-term commitment meet the needs of this population in a specific and unique way that is hard for other professions to reproduce.

Social work has proven itself to be a unique profession that uses a constellation of hybrid and eclectic knowledge. Our ability to borrow from many others that which is useful to our clients has helped us forge a pragmatic social work approach that is versatile and flexible in each of its three-pronged foci: clinical practice, the formation of social policy, and the management of the social health professions.

Social work will continue to debate the major social policy issues, and the organized profession of social work will continue to move into a political action framework to advocate a more expansive set of entitlements consistent with our underlying values. For those individuals entering the social work profession in health care, the next few decades will be an exciting, stimulating, and difficult time. Social work can meet the challenges ahead and make major contributions toward the provision of social health services, the development of social health policies, and the management of the social health organization.

REFERENCES

Barbara Berkman, Helen Rehr, and Gary Rosenberg. "A Social Work Department Develops and Tests a Screening Mechanism to Identify High Social Work Risk Situations." *Social Work in Health Care*, Vol. 5, No. 4, Summer 1980, pp. 373-385.

Neil F. Bracht, "Health Care: The Largest Human Service System." *Social Work*, Vol. 19, No. 5, Sept. 1974, pp. 532-542.

Marie Caputi. "Social Work in Health Care: Past and Future." *Health and Social Work*, Vol. 3, No. 1, February 1978, pp. 8-29.

Eleanor Clark. *High Social Risk Screening: An Audio Tape.* Society of Hospital Social Work Directors, Denver, Colorado, 1980. John Recording Company, Jackson, Mississippi.

Claudia Coulton. "A Study of Person Environment Fit Among the Chronically Ill." *Social Work in Health Care*, Vol. 5, No. 1, Fall 1979, pp. 5-18.

Bess Dana, H. David Banta, and Kurt W. Deuschle. "An Agenda for the Future of Interprofessionalism." In Helen Rehr (ed.), *Medicine and Social Work.* New York: Prodist, 1974, pp. 77-88.

Miriam Dinerman. "In Sickness and in Health: The Future of Social Work Roles." *Health and Social Work*, Vol. 4, No. 2, May 1979, pp. 5-23.

Harold Lewis. "The Emergence of Social Work as a Profession in Health Care: Significant Influences and Persistent Issues." In Helen Rehr (Ed.), Milestones in Social Work and Medicine. New York: Prodist, 1982.

Harold L. Light and Howard J. Brown. "The Social Worker as Lay Administrator of a Medical Facility." *Social Casework*, June 1964, unpaged.

Abraham Lurie. "Social Work in Health Care: The Next 10 Years." *Social Work in Health Care*, Vol. 2, No. 4, Summer 1977, pp. 419-428.

Carol Meyer, "Social Work Purpose: Status by Choice or Coercion." *Social Work*, Vol. 26, No. 1, January 1981, pp. 69-77.

Robert Morris and Delwin Anderson, "Personal Care Services: An Identity for Social Work." *Social Service Review*, Vol. 49, No. 2, June 1975, pp. 157-161.

Martin Nacman. "Reflections of a Social Work Administrator on the Opportunities of Crisis." *Social Work in Health Care*, Vol. 6, No. 1, Fall 1980, pp. 11-21.

Martin Nacman. "A Systems Approach to the Provision of Social Work Services in Health Settings." *Social Work in Health Care*, Vol. 1, No. 1, Fall 1975, pp. 47-53.

Jeanette Regensburg. *Towards Education for Health Professions*, New York: Harper and Row, 1978.

Helen Rehr, "Social Work Looks to the Future of Health." In *Successful Social Living for Sensory Deprived Persons*. Proceedings of the 70th Anniversary Symposium of Massachusetts Eye and Ear Infirmary, November 3, 1977, pp. 98-106.

Lewis Thomas. "How Should Humans Pay Their Way." *The New York Times*, August 24, 1981, p. 19.

Rape Crisis Intervention in the Emergency Room: A New Challenge for Social Work

Maria I. Vera, MSW, ACSW

SUMMARY. The emerging role of the social worker in the context of rape crisis programs housed in hospital emergency rooms is examined. A brief review of the psychological impact of rape on its victims is offered as a background for delineating this role. The emergency room setting is analyzed in terms of the advantages and disadvantages it presents for this type of crisis intervention. Significant issues of care for the social worker in this setting are discussed, and an outline of tasks for this role is proposed.

INTRODUCTION

In recent years new roles for social workers have emerged in the context of rape treatment programs. Promoted by groups of various orientations throughout the country and designed to meet the special needs of victims of rape, all these programs derive from a recent major reorientation in the conception of the crime of rape. In the past rape was thought to be a sexual crime which the victim had somehow invited. Today, thanks to the initial impetus of feminist writers (Greer, 1971; Brownmiller, 1975) and the accumulating social, psychological, and clinical findings (Sutherland & Scherl,

At the time of writing Mrs. Vera was Instructor of Social Work, Department of Psychiatry, College of Medicine, University of Florida, Gainesville, FL 32601. The author wishes to thank Hernan Vera, George Barnard, and Eve Cech for their valuable comments in the preparation of this manuscript.
Reprinted from *Social Work in Health Care*, Volume 6(3), Spring 1981.

1970; Burgess & Holmstrom, 1974, 1976, 1979; Symonds, 1975, 1976; McCombie, 1975; Groth, Burgess, & Holstrom, 1977), rape is regarded as a primarily violent crime.

This redefinition of the crime of rape has been translated into reforms in legislation, in rules for admissible evidence, and in police procedures. In addition there has been a heightened consciousness about sexual assault in the community and an abundance of ongoing research. The purpose of this paper is to examine the emerging role of the social worker in the context of rape crisis programs housed in hospital emergency rooms. However, the hospital emergency room is not the exclusive setting of rape crisis programs. Community mental health centers, women's clinics, crisis centers, police and prosecutorial agencies, and community groups have established an array of programs specializing in the care of rape victims. In these settings social workers are being called to act as advocates, liaison persons, counselors, educators, and coordinators. Nonetheless, the hospital emergency room has been gaining increasing acceptance as the most appropriate place to develop rape crisis programs.

In delineating the role of the social worker in the emergency room, the following section briefly examines the psychological impact of rape on its victims. Then, a series of features of the emergency room setting are discussed. The last section addresses the issues of care that are necessary for this emerging role for social workers. This paper concentrates on issues of care for adult female victims. While crisis interventions with children and adult males who have been raped are very similar to those with female victims, they also present a number of distinct problems which would lead us far afield in this analysis.

THE PSYCHOLOGICAL IMPACT
OF SEXUAL ASSAULT

Rape shares with other crimes of violence an element which is crucial to the understanding of the life crisis it triggers in the victim: terrorization. As Symonds (1976) puts it, terrorization is the common denominator to all violent crime, and "it is employed by the criminal to insure the immediate compliance of the victim." However, while in crimes of violence, such as muggings, there is little or no interaction between criminal and victim, rape involves a rather prolonged contact between the criminal and his victim. In those crimes of violence which involve a similar prolonged interaction, such as kidnapping and hostage taking, victims are used as a lever to obtain something from another victim. In rape, however, the woman is demeaned in her bodily integrity and often forced to enact utter submission. Thus, the victims' responses to rape are similar in many ways to those of victims of other crimes of violence, but they are also unique.

Symonds (1975, 1976), in his studies of victims of violent crimes, notes that the first response to unexpected violence is shock, numbness, and disbelief, followed by either fright or anger. This fright is particularly notable in victims of sexual assault, who often reach a state of panic when the assailant threatens their lives with a weapon, by physical force, or verbally. In this state of panic, there is a high distortion of perception and judgement, and learned behavior gives way to adaptive responses directed at the immediate preservation of life.

In most instances the anger which the attack provokes in the victim is drowned by terror and manifests itself in the victim's behavior as passive verbal or physical resistance. Some women attempt to introduce anticipatory guilt in the rapist, others try to make him face his "mental sickness"; some say they are pregnant or that they are about to vomit, while still others try to placate the rapist by telling him that he is a nice person. The following vignette illustrates one of the patterns of response. Karen is a 26-year-old graduate student. She related the following about her rape a few days after its occurrence.

> When he caught up with me he was wearing a handkerchief over his face. Grabbing my arm he said, "Come with me, I have a knife and I will kill you if you don't." My arm hurt, I couldn't believe this, I had read it so many times. I said, "I don't think you have a knife, what do you want me to go with you for?" He seemed amused, and said, "Don't play tricks with me, I can be very mean, and don't scream, walk faster." When we got to the place, we had the weirdest of conversa-

tions. He told me about his father beating him every day, his realizing that what he was doing was a horrible, despicable, inhuman thing—by the words he used he could have been a college kid. I told him that I had friends who could help him, that he seemed to be bright, intelligent, and attractive, that if he let me go I wouldn't tell, why didn't we go across the street to talk about it over a cup of coffee. I am sure now that he did not have a knife, but I was so numb then, that I did everything he asked. I didn't even remember I had a brown belt in judo until I got home. I didn't feel anything except anger at the bastard. I remembered every detail of his appearance, the place, everything. The police were really surprised. After they left I collapsed . . . If it hadn't been for my black eye and multiple bruises, I would have thought the whole thing happened to someone else.

Although some victims resist actively by kicking, scratching, screaming, and biting, these acts of active resistance are seldom successful in stopping the attack. Statistically, however, in a majority of cases they do not appear to endanger the victims physically (Symonds, 1976).

Symonds (1976) calls the paradoxical responses to violence "traumatic psychological infantilism." In his view this phenomenon accounts for a number of confusing patterns of responses observed in some victims, such as the feeling of complete helplessness, cooperative and friendly behavior, and at times gratitude toward the criminal for sparing their lives. In my clinical observations, these responses constitute the core of the experience of rape. Each victim I have talked to has related that the overwhelming feeling during the assault was fear for her life. The reaction to unexpected violence must be kept in mind to understand the victim's rather common and apparently absurd expressions of guilt for not having resisted and for thus having cooperated in her own victimization. A "profound primal terror" (Symonds, 1976) is responsible for this apparently cooperative behavior and for the utterly submissive attitudes which most victims cannot recognize as part of their identities. For example, Michelle, a 29-year-old professional, after having been victimized 3 months earlier, said:

When he left, I just laid there not daring to move in fear he would return, and too grateful for being alive to call the police. I kept on asking myself, over and over, why did he have to do it to me, and if I would have been able to help him if I had tried harder to understand his conversation.

Yet, Michelle had been beaten, rough-handled, and repeatedly threatened with death. Her assailant had told her that he knew that what he was doing was wrong, but that he could not help himself. Throughout the assault, Michelle had been forced to repeat how much she had enjoyed and admired her assailant's sexual prowess.

In interviewing rape victims, Burgess and Holmstrom (1974b) have characterized a clinically identifiable "rape trauma syndrome," which is "an acute stress reaction to a life threatening situation." This syndrome is usually a two-phase reaction. The first acute phase of this process is characterized by feelings of shame, anger, fear, and self-blame, as well as by disorganization in the different spheres of the woman's life. Somatic reactions, some secondary to the physical trauma, such as soreness and bruising, others manifestations of psychological discomfort, such as sleep and eating disturbances, are characteristic of the period immediately following the assault. The long-term "reorganizational phase" can start a few days or a few weeks after the attack. This period is characterized by changes in life style and changes in residence and telephone numbers. Many victims develop phobic reactions, such as fear of indoors, fear of outdoors, fear of crowds, generalized mistrust, and sexual fears. Nonorgasmic sex and flashbacks of the assault are also common complaints.

My own clinical observations tell me that the rape trauma syndrome is more than a disorganization of life rhythms. Some victims are unable to resume daily routines such as work and child care activities for days, and at times for weeks and even months. Other victims' daily lives are apparently undisturbed. More crucially, though, women who have been raped are faced with a debacle in their existential horizons. The basic reference points of social life acquired throughout the process of psychosocial development, suddenly appear to be in disarray. If one follows Erikson's (1963) ideas, it appears that victims are launched into a radical reappraisal of the basic parameters of their existence following the rape. The sense of trust, autonomy, and initiative, which this author sees as the achievements of the early ages of development, are called into question. For example, Michelle had to cope with a generalized fear of other persons, of not knowing whom to trust or distrust. Another woman, a corporate executive who was raped in a hotel room, had to resign from her well-paying and rewarding position because she was unable to assess the safety of places other than her home for many months. Because rape triggers a life crisis, professionals assisting rape victims in their recovery must address the task of restoring the women's existential horizons. Furthermore, this assistance must reflect the developmental stage in which victimization occurs, and this stage of development should be taken as the indispensable base on which new meanings and new purposes are built.

THE RAPE VICTIM
AND THE PROFESSIONALS
IN THE EMERGENCY ROOM

The hospital emergency room has been considered "an excellent and appropriate place to develop rape crisis programs" (Bassuk, Saviz, McCombie, & Pell, 1975). The advantages of the setting appear to be numerous. First, the centralization and coordination of services to victims can be achieved using established hospital structures. Second, emergency rooms have professional staff available around the clock.[1] Third, because of the legal ramifications of sexual assault, these professionals can be called upon to testify if the case goes to court.

While a hospital setting for rape crisis intervention offers these advantages, emergency rooms present major shortcomings in that they are designed to treat patients with serious medical or surgical problems; the emotional needs of victims tend to be given a lower priority. And yet, "The rape victim has few medical problems

---

1. This does not mean that emergency rooms are always staffed to meet the psychological needs of rape victims. For a description and discussion of programs which have attempted to address the total needs of victims of rape on a 24-hour basis, see McCombie et al. (1976), Hicks and Platt (1976), and Hunt (1977).

... but for the most part the injury is to the psyche rather than to the body" (Hayman, Lanza, & Noel, 1973). In addition, the social care required by rape victims adds to an already heavy load of patients, and the prospect of a court appearance, no matter how committed the professional and how humanitarian his or her orientation, adds an unwelcome burden to the victim-staff interaction.

Victims of sexual assault bring a wide range of needs to the emergency room. In Burgess' and Holstrom's (1974a) study, these requests for care ranged from seeking medical, police, or psychological intervention to seeking emotional reassurance. The arrival of a rape victim in the emergency ward mobilizes an array of professionals who will attend to the immediate medical, legal, and psychological needs precipitated by the assault. Each of these professionals, the nurse, physician, social worker, and police officer, has a specific set of tasks to perform. Rape treatment centers, responding to the urgings of the medical profession (Committee on Evolving Trends in Society Affecting Life, 1975), have established guidelines for the interview and the examination of alleged victims of rape. These guidelines have been incorporated into protocols, which vary greatly from hospital to hospital. However, some basic responsibilities of the physician and the nurse are usually specified to assure the admissibility of the gathered evidence for legal purposes. The nurse usually does a brief initial interview, collects certain specimens, and prepares the victim for a physical examination. The physician performs a complete physical examination to document the presence or absence of physical trauma and also collects other evidence as specified in the medico-legal protocol. Members of the police force interview the victim to gather information on the circumstances of the assault and other relevant facts which might lead to the arrest and conviction of the assailant. The social worker assesses the emotional state of the victim and provides guidance, support, and information of various kinds. This enumeration of tasks and personnel does not reflect a hierarchy of importance, nor an order of urgency in which these professionals must intervene.

The mobilization of professionals presents two problems which must be underscored, because on their successful resolution hinges the difference between the effective service of the rape victim's needs and her further victimization. The first issue is the setting; the medico-legal concerns can easily overwhelm the emotional needs of the rape victim. Although few rape victims who come into the emergency room in the acute phase of rape show signs of urgently serious physical trauma, nearly every rape victim has been seriously psychologically injured. Emotional trauma is not as visible as physical trauma and often is not recognized as urgent in the emergency room.

In fact, victims in the emergency room exhibit a wide variety of response patterns. Few of us would doubt the urgency of attending to the emotional needs of a woman showing evident signs of distress — shortness of breath, weeping, and screaming. Nonetheless, this is only one pattern of expression, and a not too frequent type of response. Some victims appear composed and serene, others are in a state of shock, while still others appear loquacious and humorous. These responses are poor signs of the degree of emotional trauma experienced. As described in the previous section, terrorization makes the individuals draw on adaptive behavioral mechanisms. For example, Michelle, the victim in our second vignette, appeared calm, cooperative, composed, and self-reliant in the emergency room. Nonetheless, this victim had to face a devastating psychological impact, which literally incapacitated her for over 6 months despite psychiatric intervention.

The second problem derives from the fact that the tasks of the professionals who intervene are independent, goal-oriented processes which do not necessarily complement, and can even conflict with, each other. In this way, as Evrard (1971) has suggested, the victim seems to be at the center of a crossroads, where her well-being appears in conflict with the goals of those attempting to assist her. For example, one particularly hectic night, I was waiting for the physician to finish a physical examination of a victim, when a group of police officers arrived and politely told me that they were going to step in first, explaining that they had a criminal at large and that in addition it was important that they obtain her first recollections, which would be the most accurate. A potential conflict was defused in this instance because I was able to talk to the young woman for a while; with her consent I invited the police officers in, once an atmosphere of trust was established. In another instance, a hurried physician walked in while I was with a woman, requesting to perform a pelvic examination right away because he had to attend to a delivery. The fright this request provoked in the victim was so evident that the physician backed off and decided to return later, when the woman was in a more composed mood.

These conflicts are by no means exclusively centered around the social worker, nor are they as easily resolved as these examples might suggest. This is why there is an urgent need to go beyond the establishment of protocols that define the different professional tasks into a true coordination of efforts. This coordination should establish clear priorities and make the emotional state of the victim the crucial concern. The successful resolution of these efforts is essential to the delivery of care services to rape victims.

THE SOCIAL WORKER AND RAPE CRISIS: ISSUES OF CARE

Since the emergency room is, for most victims, the first contact with a world which can be considered "safe," its staff is among the first with whom the victim interacts after an assault and their attitudes represent the societal response to the victim. The treatment in the emergency room of a woman who has been sexually assaulted cannot be considered as merely an expedient step towards the resolving of medico-legal dilemmas; rather, it should be regarded as a crucial step towards recovery from a traumatic event.

It is for these reasons that the assessment of the victim's emotional state is an essential first step in this time of crisis. A major function of this psychological assessment is to reconcile the intervention of the emergency room staff with the major presenting problem of the victim. This emotional assessment should guide the sequence and timing of the intervention of each professional.

The issue is not whether some tasks should or should not be performed, but rather how and when they ought to be performed. The following case illustrates this point. Janie, an 18-year-old married woman in her fifth month of pregnancy, was brought to the emergency room by a social agency worker after having been raped by a man who worked with her husband. She was terrified by the prospect of a pelvic examination which could, in her mind, harm the baby. She was even more terrified of the suspected reaction of her husband to the attack and of the publicity it could receive if the police were notified. The prospect of reporting the assault to the police was frightening to her, and she expressed fear that her husband would disapprove of it.

Her arrival at the emergency room occurred close to a personnel shift change. In spite of Janie's reluctance, one of the staff members, acting in haste, proceeded to arrange for an immediate physical examination. In this case, after an initial assessment, the social worker had to act as an advocate for the victim and call to the attention of the medical staff the inadvisability of the course of action already set in motion. Eventually, the victim's fears and doubts were addressed, and she willingly agreed to a physical examination and then went through an interview with the police officer. By regaining control over her own body, she initiated her process of recovery.

An obstacle to the performance of this advocacy task is the fact that social work has not been a primary discipline in emergency room settings. Thus, in a very real sense, social workers are outsiders stepping into an established network of interactions, working relations, hierarchical rights, duties, and responsibilities. In this situation the social worker may have been perceived as challenging the established authority; yet the social worker's task is to harmonize the skills and services offered by a number of professionals around the goal of securing the well-being of the woman victimized by rape. This task is even more significant since physicians and other primary care professionals often do not possess the skills to handle the psychological factor of patient care (Brochstein, Adams, Tristan, & Cheney, 1979).

In order to achieve this harmony, the social worker needs to become familiar with the inner workings of the emergency room setting. The social worker should draw upon a theoretical systems framework, which today is an integral part of every social worker's training. In my experience, the particular skills which are derived from this theoretical framework represent a welcome addition to the emergency room, because rape victims have long presented special challenges to the health professional of other disciplines in this setting.

The social worker's role is not so much that of a gatekeeper or that of a coach, but rather that of an interpreter who must convey the needs of the victim to the staff. This interpretation is particularly crucial in those situations where victims display verbal and emotional nonassertive styles, but it is by no means restricted to them. To some extent, all rape victims arriving in the emergency room are confused and filled with doubts. And perhaps the social worker's role in the emergency room is to assist the victim in regaining control over her own body, her interactions, and the course of events in which she will need to participate. For example, it is customary for a victim who has undergone a medico-legal protocol to give up her clothing to the police for evidence. Other routine procedures to which a woman usually finds it difficult to submit are the pelvic examination and an interview with the police. These acts of "submission" need to be interpreted so that the victim does not experience and regard them as additional acts of victimization.

The earlier statements describing the emergency room as the first "safe" contact for the victim following an assault are particularly relevant here. The role of the social worker involves support, guidance, and advocacy. These constitute the areas towards which the special skills of the professional social worker are directed. The supportive role is anchored in the presentation of the social worker as a person with special knowledge and experience; it entails fostering the expression of emotions and doubts. The social worker should allow the victim to tell her story, while providing reassurance of the appropriateness of feelings. In this area the social worker must be prepared to face a series of paradoxes. As said before, terrorization brings about a distortion of perception and a shattering of basic parameters in the victim's life. The victim often seems in a kind of limbo and expresses utter confusion, not only about external events, but also about her own thoughts and feelings. The following statement by Susan, who was raped in her apartment, illustrates her ambivalence towards the assailant:

> I know I should want him behind bars, but I am so lucky to be alive that I am grateful to God that He did not allow him to kill me. Part of me wishes the police to catch up with him, but I don't know what I would do then. This doesn't make sense to you, does it?

Closely tied to the supportive role is one of guidance. The task here can be summarized as the familiarization of the victim with what lies ahead. For the overwhelming majority of victims, rape is the first encounter with violence. Most victims, save those cases presenting physical injuries, do not understand why they are in the emergency room and what procedures are called for. Information on these procedures, their purpose, and most importantly on her option to submit or not to submit to them brings about a significant decrease in fears and apprehension.

Guidance, of course, is not limited to providing information about what is to be expected in the emergency room. At this critical phase, victims express a number of doubts and misgivings. "Whom should I tell about this? If I talk to the police, will they put my name in the paper? Where can I stay now, after this I can't return to my apartment," are only some of the frequent questions. In other instances, potentially adverse reactions of parents, husbands, friends, and colleagues are feared. In addition to addressing these doubts, guidance should include making the victim aware of what feelings, somatic reactions, fears, and apprehensions she can expect later.

Last but not least, the role of providing guidance requires giving information concerning medical, legal, and other community resources which specialize in attending to the needs of rape victims. A most crucial resource is the availability of further counseling. In my clinical experience, the interaction of the social worker with the victim in the emergency room creates a special type of bond, which later greatly facilitates the seeking of further counseling by the victim. In this respect, the social worker's role differs markedly from those of the other professionals in the emergency room. While these professionals complete their care in the emergency room, the social worker's role extends into the future.

Advocacy has already been defined in the context of interpreting and communicating the victim's needs in the emergency room. A number of other tasks fall between support and guidance. One such instance is when the social worker is called upon to enlist other services and resources on behalf of the victim. Other situations require social workers to approach family members and friends to assist them in coping with the trauma, which is bound to touch them in multiple ways.

This enumeration of tasks is by no means exhaustive. It has been offered as an outline from which to map out a new and challenging area of practice which draws upon social workers' knowledge, skills, and values.

REFERENCES

Bassuk, E., Savitz, R., McCombie, S., & Pell, S. Organizing a rape crisis program in a general hospital. *Journal of the American Medical Women Association*, 1975, *30*, 486-490.

Brochstein, J., Adams, G., Tristan, M., & Cheney, C. Social work and primary health care: An integrative approach. *Social Work in Health Care*, 1979, *5*, 71-81.

Brownmiller, S. *Against our will*. New York: Bantam Books, 1975.

Burgess, A., & Holmstrom, L. Crisis and counseling requests of rape victims. *Nursing Research*, 1974, *23*, 196-202. (a)

Burgess, A., & Holmstrom, L. Rape trauma syndrome. *American Journal of Psychiatry*, 1974, *131*, 981-986. (b)

Burgess, A., & Holmstrom, L. Coping behavior of the rape victim. *American Journal of Psychiatry*, 1976, *133*, 413-421.

Burgess, A., & Holmstrom, L. *Rape: Crisis and recovery*. Bowie: Robert J. Brady Co., 1979.

California Medical Association, Committee on Evolving Trends in Society Affecting Life. Guidelines for the interview and examination of alleged rape victims. *The Western Medical Journal of Medicine*, 1975, *123*, 420-422.

Erikson, E. *Childhood and society*. New York: W.W. Norton, 1963.

Evrard, J. Rape: The medical, social and legal implications. *American Journal of Obstetrics and Gynecology*, 1971, *111*, 197-199.

Greer, G. *The female eunuch*. New York: Bantam Books, 1971.

Groth, A., Burgess, A., & Holmstrom, L. Rape: Power, anger and sexuality. *American Journal of Psychiatry*, 1977, *134*, 1239-1243.

Hayman, C., Lanza, C., & Noel, E. What to do for victims of rape. *Medical Times*, 1973, *101*, 47-51.

Hicks, D., & Platt, C. Medical treatment for the victim: The development of a rape treatment center. In M. Walker & S. Brodsky, *Sexual assault*. Lexington: Lexington Books, 1976.

Hunt, G. Rape: An organized approach to evaluation and treatment. *American Family Physician*, 1977, *15*, 154-158.

McCombie, S. *Characteristics of rape victims seen in crisis intervention*. Unpublished master's thesis, Smith College School of Social Work, 1975.

McCombie, S., Bassuk, E., Savitz, R., & Pell, S. Development of a medical center rape crisis intervention program. *American Journal of Psychiatry*, 1976, *133*, 418-421.

Sutherland, S., & Scherl, D. Patterns of response among victims of rape. *American Journal of Orthopsychiatry*, 1970, *40*, 503-511.

Symonds, M. Victims of violence: Psychological effects and after effects. *American Journal of Psychoanalysis*, 1975, *35*, 19-26.

Symonds, M. The rape victim: Psychological patterns of response. *American Journal of Psychoanalysis*, 1976, *36*, 27-34.

The Ecology
of Social Work Departments:
Empirical Findings
and Strategy Implications

Bruce S. Jansson, PhD
June Simmons, MSW, LCSW

SUMMARY. Despite the fact that social work departments are dependent upon hospitals for resources and support, little research has been conducted to analyze organizational factors that promote or impede their development. The researchers hypothesized that departments are most likely to expand in hospital settings with missions that are supportive of clinical, preventive, and community-oriented services; that stress innovation; and that emphasize hospital-funded services and programs. Further, it was hypothesized that social work services would be most likely to expand in settings where hospital administrators perceive them to be relevant to practical needs of the institution. Findings from a survey of 50 nonprofit hospitals in Los Angeles County in 1980 confirm these hypotheses and suggest that social workers need to use knowledge of the organizational context to develop high-level support for their departments.

Relatively few researchers have addressed the question, "why are some hospital social work departments relatively large, while

At the time of writing Dr. Jansson was an Associate Professor in the School of Social Work, University of Southern California, Montgomery Ross Fisher Building, Los Angeles, CA 90089-0411. Ms. Simmons was Director of Patient Services with the Huntington Memorial Hospital, 100 E. Congress Drive, Pasadena, CA 91105.

The authors acknowledge the collaboration of Candyce Berger in the design and implementation of this study as well as eight graduate students in a research practicum (Jan Alperin, Cindy Bockelman, Sarah Cress, Frank Fiorillo, Elizabeth Kautto, Ginny Kent, Brenda Parks, Barbara Victorian).

Reprinted from *Social Work in Health Care*, Volume 11(2), Winter 1985-86.

others are barely able to survive?" This is an important research question because social workers cannot address psychosocial problems of patients if they are unable to obtain funds from their host institutions in the first instance. While few social workers would suggest that expansion of their services should always be favored, many departments are so restricted in size that they cannot address a range of patient and institutional needs.

At least two lines of inquiry can be used to address this question. First, program, political, and administrative strategies of social workers can be analyzed to determine which appear to promote departmental growth. Some theorists speculate, for example, that various political strategies, including the use of assertiveness, increase the likelihood that social workers will obtain favorable responses to requests for additional resources (Jansson and Simmons, 1984).

Second, characteristics of the hospitals can be examined as they discourage or promote the growth of social work departments. This knowledge can help social workers as they develop strategies to obtain funding for their departments by alerting them to obstacles to expansion and by helping them to utilize institutional factors that promote the growth of their units.

This second line of inquiry becomes even more important as the hospital and funding context of social work departments becomes more complex and turbulent with the development of diagnostic and review groups (DRG's), highly competitive relationships between hospitals, and policies that emphasize efficiency in health care. With these kinds of developments, the growth of social work departments could increasingly hinge upon the ability of their staff to analyze their hospital settings and to adapt their program and political strategy to institutional realities.

Various facets of the organizational context, then, were used as independent variables in this study as they were hypothesized to be associated with the size of social work departments, i.e., the dependent variable. While many factors may be associated with wide disparities in the size of social work departments in hospitals, including the political and program skills of their directors and staff, the researchers reasoned that the organizational context itself may influence the extent social work departments expand. Some social work departments may expand more rapidly than others because they exist in a setting that is more favorable to them, though expansion is unlikely even in these settings if social workers do not develop programs that are assessed favorably by administrators and physicians. This article focuses, then, upon the organizational context as it is associated with the size of social work departments rather than upon program and political skills of social workers within those departments. A fuller understanding of departmental size will eventually require linking both organizational and departmental factors together as they jointly influence the growth of social work departments.

REVIEW OF LITERATURE

In this study, the researchers explored a range of organizational literature to develop hypotheses about kinds of organizational factors that might promote the development of social work in hospitals.

When investigating the organizational context of social work departments in hospitals, researchers encounter a predicament. The hospital context is described by an infinite number of factors including formal characteristics of the hospital such as its size and age, decisionmaking processes within it, patterns of staffing, and the nature of its clientele. To devise a focus for this exploratory study, the researchers examined existing hospital and organizational literature to find an initial list of independent variables.

Six hypotheses were tested. First, some organizational theorists contend that departments or units in bureaucracies are most likely to flourish when the mission or objectives of the bureaucracy is supportive to the activities and technology of departmental staff (Thompson and McEwen, 1958; Pfouts and McDaniel, 1977; Rosenberg and Weissman, 1981; Hickson, 1971). It was hypothesized that social work units are most likely to expand, then, in hospitals whose top officials favor clinical services, community services, and preventive services.

Second, it was hypothesized that social work services are most likely to expand in hospitals that are relatively innovative, since social work represents a departure from the typical diagnostic and surgical services of hospitals (Hage and Aiken, 1970; Roemer and Friedman, 1971; Russell, 1979).

Third, it was hypothesized that social work departments would be most likely to expand in hospitals that possess strong central leadership. In this line of reasoning, hospitals with weak central administrative staffs are less likely to emphasize hospital-funded services and programs like social work (Roemer and Friedman, 1971; Bracht, 1978). Indeed, some theorists contend that hospital-funded services are most likely to expand when hospitals have a relatively large number of physicians who are directly salaried to the hospital, since these hospitals are likely to have a tradition of developing and funding hospital-based services (Roemer and Friedman, 1971).

Fourth, the researchers hypothesized that social work departments would be most likely to expand in hospitals whose administrators perceived social work units to be relevant to a range of practical needs of the hospital. A number of theorists have contended that top officials of bureaucracies assess units and departments not only as they are relevant to the mission or goals of the hospital, but as they facilitate the daily tasks and challenges of the institution (Hickson, 1971; Rosenberg and Weissman, 1981; Schreiber, 1981). In the case of hospitals, these practical needs include discharge planning, patient resistance to medical procedures, public relations issues, personal problems of hospital staff, and conflict between departments. Fifth, the researchers hypothesized that the nature of the patient populations of hospitals might be associated with the size of social work departments. Some research suggests, for example, that hospitals whose patient populations include relatively large numbers of children are likely to have relatively large departments since this group clearly needs supportive services (Pfouts and McDaniel, 1977). Finally, the researchers hypothesized that the knowledge of and orientations toward social work services of top officials in the hospital would be associated with the size of departments (Wattenberg, Orr, and O'Rourke, 1977; Carrigan, 1978).

After presenting the findings of the study, a four-stage process of strategy development is discussed to allow social work staff to use knowledge of the hospital context to develop strategy to obtain resources and support for their departments.

SURVEY METHODOLOGY

It was decided to interview both the hospital administrator and the social work director in each of the 75 nonprofit hospitals that exist in Los Angeles County to obtain information both about the social work departments and hospitals. Hospitals were dropped from the sample when appointments could not be scheduled with both respondents; the final sample of 50 hospitals represented two-thirds of all nonprofit hospitals in Los Angeles County. Data was collected in 1980. Since data was not obtained from hospitals that were deleted from the sample, it was not possible to discern whether they differed from hospitals that remained within the sample; attrition seemed largely to be associated with unwillingness of specific administrators to participate in an interview. Interviews were used rather than questionnaires both to decrease sample attrition and to improve the validity and reliability of data. The interviewers, who were participants in a graduate research practicum, were generally impressed by the candor and cooperation of the interviewees.

The interview schedules were developed through intensive consultations between eight students in a graduate research practicum, an academic researcher, the director of a social work department, and a doctoral student with extensive practice experience in hospital settings. It was pretested with a director of a social work department. The graduate students and the doctoral student conducted the interviews with both social work directors and hospital administrators.

Because this is a regional study, findings need to be applied to hospitals in other regions with caution. The data was collected in 1980 before very recent policy developments such as DRG's, but, as we shall note subsequently, these recent policy developments could make the institutional context even more crucial to the expansion of social work departments.

The study was prompted by a surprising absence of empirical studies of relationships between the hospital context and the size of social work departments (Gentry, Veney, Kaluzny, and Sprague, 1973; Pfouts and McDaniel, 1977; Schlesinger and Woloch, 1982). While a number of researchers have analyzed attitudes of top hospital administrators and staff toward social work and toward social work programs and roles, they have seldom examined whether these factors influence the ability of social workers to obtain resources for their departments.

MAJOR FINDINGS

The gamma statistic was used to measure associations between departmental size and hospital characteristics (Weiss, 1968). Departmental size was measured by determining the ratio of social workers to the number of hospital beds and ranged from a ratio of one social worker per five beds to one social worker per 261 beds. The mean ratio was one social worker per 53 beds. The social work units were then divided into three categories representing relatively small (58 or more beds per social worker), moderate-sized (30 through 57 beds per social worker) and large departments (fewer than 30 beds per social worker). This classification was used in cross-tabulation with various institutional variables. The various findings of this study are summarized in Table 3 at the conclusion of this article.

HOSPITAL MISSION

The term "mission" refers to program and institutional objectives that are shared by hospital staff (Perrow, 1970; Thompson and McEwen, 1958). It was hypothesized that the nature of the mission of the hospital influences the growth of social work departments (Nacman, 1975; Pfouts and McDaniel, 1977; Rosenberg and Weissman, 1981). Hospital decision makers who believe their hospitals should address social and psychological causes and consequences of illness, for example, may be more likely to give resources to social work departments than decision makers who do not believe these factors to be important.

The social work directors were asked to rate the relative importance attached to various objectives in their hospitals by key decision makers (see Table 1 where the objectives are listed in order of

TABLE 1
SOCIAL WORK RANKINGS OF THE IMPORTANCE GIVEN
VARIOUS GOALS BY HOSPITAL DECISION MAKERS

Mission-Goals	Importance very important or important		somewhat important		relatively unimportant or unimportant		Totals	
	%	n	%	n	%	n	%[1]	n[2]
1-A Accountability to funding sources	92	(44)	8	(4)	--	--	100	(48)
1-B Hospital growth	89	(42)	9	(4)	2	1	100	(47)
1-C Improvement of present programs and services	90	(43)	8	(4)	2	(1)	100	(48)
1-D Obtaining within the hosp. as much advanced technology as possible	89	(41)	7	(3)	4	(2)	100	(48)
1-E Minimizing Costs per clients	85	(41)	10	(5)	4	(2)	99	(48)
1-F Providing out-patient services	81	(38)	15	(7)	4	(2)	100	(47)
1-G Development of new client programs/services	81	(39)	10	(5)	8	(4)	99	(48)
1-H Increasing staff morale	73	(35)	21	(10)	6	(3)	100	(48)
1-I Providing medical & other health professional edu.	66	(31)	30	(14)	4	(2)	100	(47)
1-J Servicing low income clientele	56	(27)	19	(9)	25	(12)	100	(48)
1-K Helping patients with social or personal prob. as they influence pers. health	56	(27)	33	(16)	10	(5)	99	(48)
1-L Providing preventive medical services	52	(25)	21	(10)	27	(13)	100	(48)
1-M Developing linkages with executive in agencies to whom patients are referred after discharge	44	(21)	35	(17)	21	(10)	100	(48)
1-N Fostering research	28	(13)	30	(14)	43	(20)	101	(47)

1. Precentages may not equal 100% due to rounding.
2. When n does not equal 50, it is because of nonresponses.

their perceived importance). They responded that hospital decision makers emphasized improvement of present programs and services, minimizing costs per client, accountability to funding sources, and obtaining new technology, but they attached considerably less emphasis to helping patients with social or personal problems, preventive services, and developing linkages with agencies to whom patients are referred after discharge. Thus, 44 (92 percent) of the respondents believed their hospital's decision makers attached importance to accountability to funding sources (item 1-A, Table 1) when compared to 27 (56 percent) of the respondents who were perceived to attach importance to "helping patients with social or personal problems as they influence personal health."

A number of associations were found between hospital mission and the size of social work departments. Each hospital was given a "mission complexity" score that was based on the total number of mission objectives that were ranked as relatively important; a hospital received a relatively high score when its social work director responded that decision makers believed a number of them to be important. The association between mission complexity of hospitals and the size of social work departments suggests that social workers are more able to obtain resources in hospitals that have a variety of service and program interests (gamma = .325; p < .05.) This finding may bode well for social work departments in the next decade, since many hospitals appear to be diversifying services, hence enriching their mission, to enable them to compete in the turbulent health environment of contemporary America (Goldsmith, 1981; Brody, 1976).

The researchers wanted to determine as well whether the size of social work departments is associated with the importance that hospital decision makers attach to specific mission objectives. The social work directors were asked to choose the six objectives that are listed in Table 1 that are most important in their hospital and then to rank them from one (most important) to six (least important). In specific hospitals, then, the relative importance of a specific objective could be gauged by considering in tandem the relative importance given to it by decision makers and whether and where it was listed in the list of the six most important objectives.

The researchers used this data to ascertain whether large social work departments were more likely to exist in hospitals where key decision makers placed relatively considerable emphasis upon "helping patients with social or personal problems as they influence personal health" (item 1-K, Table 1) and "developing linkages with executives in agencies to whom patients are referred after discharge" (item 1-M, Table 1). An index was constructed that aggregated data for each hospital regarding these two objectives. An association was discovered between departmental size and the extent these objectives are stressed by key decision makers, a finding that suggests that social work departments are more likely to expand when influential decision makers specifically favor these objectives that are clearly germane to social work services (gamma = .347, p < .05). In similar fashion, a "community services" index was formed by summing data on objectives 1-F and 1-L in Table 1, i.e., objectives concerning outpatient services and preventive medical services. Here, too, an association was found between departmental size and the extent these objectives are favored by influential decision makers (gamma = .434; p < .01). Perhaps social work is perceived to be a "boundary-spanning" profession that links the hospital and its environment through discharge planning and other services, so hospital officials who favor development of community services are more likely than other officials to allocate resources to social work departments. This finding may be auspicious for social work departments in an era when hospitals increasingly have to broaden services to include an array of community-based and preventive services to remain competitive with other providers who are diversifying into services like home health care and community-based clinics.

Low income patients constituted a relatively small portion of the patient load of hospitals in this survey as reflected by the fact that, on average, only 14 percent of hospitals' revenues derived from Medicaid reimbursements. Hospitals whose decision makers were reported to attach importance to serving low income patients were, however, more likely to have large social work departments (gamma = .335; p < .05). Social workers may be perceived as particularly relevant to social and service issues that are encountered by this population, though this finding must be interpreted with caution because of the relatively small proportion of low income persons in the patient populations of hospitals in this survey.

ORGANIZATIONAL TASKS AND CHARACTERISTICS

The researchers hypothesized that relatively innovative hospitals would provide a relatively favorable environment for social work services, since social work services represent a departure from traditional medical services (Russell, 1979). The social work directors were asked to indicate the extent their hospitals develop new programs; hospitals reported to develop them frequently were more likely to have large social work departments than other hospitals (gamma = .341; p < .05). Perhaps "innovativeness" reflects openness to new approaches to health care that includes counseling, community, and other services that are provided by social workers. Or perhaps social workers are emboldened to request resources in settings where influential decision makers prize development of new programs.

The researchers hypothesized that older hospitals would tend to have larger social work departments than newer hospitals both because they are likely to have more financial and program security than newly established hospitals and because social workers will have had more opportunities in them to demonstrate the utility of their services (Neiman and Hoops, 1977). Because of recent population growth in California, the sample in this survey included many older as well as newer hospitals; roughly 60 percent of the hospitals had existed for more than 25 years. Size of social work departments was directly associated with the age of the hospital (gamma = .436; p < .05).

It was also hypothesized that social work departments would be more likely to expand in those settings where a relatively large number of patients are children or elderly persons, since the need for counseling, follow-up, and family-related services is widely accepted in professional literature for these populations (Pfouts and McDaniel, 1977). The researchers also speculated that social work would be perceived as a profession that possesses skills that are particularly germane to the needs of these populations. No significant association was discovered between these patient characteristics and the size of social work departments. Hospital decision makers may not be aware of the kinds of services that these groups need or may not believe that social workers are specifically needed to address their needs.

CHARACTERISTICS OF HOSPITAL ADMINISTRATION

Since social work departments are hospital-based programs that are usually funded from the central budgets of hospitals, the researchers hypothesized that large departments would tend to exist in hospitals with strong central leadership. The hospital administrators were asked to indicate the extent a variety of officials (including physicians, the board of trustees, and themselves) influenced major decisions in their hospital concerning general policies, budgetary choices, and the adoption of new programs. By pooling data regarding these various kinds of decisions, hospitals were identified where central administrators were reported to be relatively influential in the decision making process. Large social work departments were more likely to exist in hospitals where hospital administrators rated themselves as possessing considerable influence over these various decisions (gamma = .315, p < .05). This findings suggests that social workers may find it more easy to obtain resources in settings where central and powerful administrative allies can be found. The size of social work departments is also associated with the number of physicians who are salaried to the hospital, a finding that appears to support the contention of some theorists that social work departments are more likely to expand in those hospitals that emphasize hospital-based services and staff (gamma = .386; p < .05) (Bracht, 1978, p. 167; Roemer and Friedman, pp. 277-301).

ORIENTATIONS OF HOSPITAL ADMINISTRATORS

The researchers hypothesized that social work departments are more likely to expand in hospitals where officials perceive them to be relevant to practical needs of the hospital (Rosenberg and Weissman, 1981, pp. 14-15; Schreiber, 1981). Hospital administrators were given a list of 11 practical problems that confront most hospitals including general personnel problems, conflict between departments, hostile patients, adverse public relations, and patient discharge issues (see Table 2). Administrators were asked both to rank the extent the social work department currently addresses these issues and the extent they believe the departments should provide less, the same, or more effort to addressing them. Each administrator was given a total score based on aggregate responses; an administrator who obtained a high score not only believed the social work unit already addressed many of these issues, but wanted them to increase their effort.

Administrators in hospitals with large social work departments were more likely than others to obtain high scores on this index

TABLE 2

HOSPITAL ADMINISTORS' RANKING OF THE IMPORTANCE
OF SOCIAL WORK IN ADDRESSING PRACTICAL HOSPITAL PROBLEMS

Hospital Problems	Importance							
	very important or important		somewhat important		relatively unimportant or unimportant		Totals	
	%	n	%	n	%	n	%	n
2-A Patient discharge problems	78	(38)	10	(5)	12	(6)	100	(49)
2-B Social/personal needs of patients	75	(36)	17	(8)	8	(4)	100	(48)
2-C Collecting fees from patients	65	(32)	27	(13)	8	(4)	100	(49)
2-D Hostile or "acting out" patients	60	(29)	23	(11)	17	(8)	100	(48)
2-E Utilization review difficulties	49	(24)	18	(9)	32	(16)	99	(49)
2-F Patient resistance to medical procedures	31	(15)	31	(15)	38	(18)	100	(48)
2-G General personnel problems	26	(13)	33	(16)	41	(20)	100	(49)
2-H Public relation problems	20	(10)	31	(15)	49	(24)	100	(49)
2-I Inappropriate use of hospital by many patient	15	(7)	43	(20)	43	(20)	101	(47)
2-J Conflict between departments	13	(6)	15	(7)	73	(35)	101	(48)
2-K Malpractice problems	13	(6)	17	(8)	71	(33)	101	(47)

1. Where percentages do not equal 100%, this is due to rounding

2. Where n does not equal 50, this is due to nonresponses

(gamma = .305; p = .05). This finding suggests that large departments are more likely to exist in settings where they are both perceived to address a range of practical problems and where the top administrator also believes this performance should be expanded even further. As social work departments are perceived to be relevant to a range of practical needs of the hospital, hospital administrators may be more willing to support expansion of them. They may also be more likely to believe that major reductions in the funding of social work could jeopardize the institution, since some of its practical needs would no longer be addressed by hospital staff. Put differently, hospital administrators may psychologically "own" budget decisions about social work units that are perceived to address institutional needs rather than perceiving such decisions to be unimportant to the broader institution. This finding suggests that social workers need to reconsider before focusing their programs largely or exclusively upon clinical counseling services, since administrators may place equal or greater importance upon the provision of services that address practical needs of the hospital.

A number of theorists and researchers have analyzed general attitudes or orientations of hospital administrators toward social work (Caputi, 1978; Nacman, 1975; Schoenfeld, 1975; Schlesinger and Woloch, 1982; Wattenberg, Orr, and O'Rouke, 1977; Carrigan, 1978). It was hypothesized in this survey that social work departments would be most likely to expand in hospitals where top administrators (1) believed that social workers should expand various clinical, planning, and community roles, and (2) had considerable knowledge of the content and location of social work services in their hospitals. A number of questions were developed that probed the knowledge and attitudes of administrators, but no association was discovered between these attitudinal and knowledge variables and the size of social work departments. While further research is needed, these non-findings suggest that abstract or general orientations toward social work may not be as important to the expansion of social work departments as perceptions of the relevance of social work to practical needs of hospitals.

INSTITUTIONAL RELEVANCE AND SOCIAL WORK DEPARTMENTS

Findings discussed to this point suggest that the concept of "institutional relevance" is useful when analyzing the relationship between social work departments and their host hospitals. Social work departments appear most likely to expand in settings where a mission exists that includes a variety of goals that are consonant with social work services such as helping patients with social or personal problems, provision of community services, and assisting low income consumers. Social workers may be more able in such settings to market their services to top decision makers. Social workers may also be able to obtain favorable responses to requests for resources in those settings where they are perceived to be relevant to practical needs of the hospital such as those presented in Table 2. Departments may be particularly well situated that are relevant both to the broad mission of the hospital and to its practical needs.

Findings from this survey suggest as well that a number of other factors, in addition to the relevance of social work departments to institutional priorities and needs, influence the growth of social work departments. Social work departments appear most likely to expand in relatively older hospitals, in innovative hospitals, and in hospitals with relatively strong central administrations.

Further research is needed to develop a measure of the "favorability" of hospitals to social work services. Findings from this survey, which are summarized in Table 3, provide a starting point for further inquiry. The findings suggest that it may be possible in future studies to identify combinations of variables that suggest that a specific hospital provides a relatively favorable or unfavorable setting for social work services.

Formidable obstacles confront researchers who undertake this kind of research. It is often difficult to distinguish between cause and effect in survey research. Social work departments may be more likely to expand when administrators perceive them to be relevant to practical needs of their institutions, but their size may, in turn, make them more visible to officials who are therefore more likely to perceive them to be relevant to institutional needs. Researchers must also contend with methodological issues. It would be desirable to obtain information about the mission and other characteristics of hospitals from many kinds of officials and staff within them, but this strategy is difficult to implement in light of feasibility considerations, particularly when interviews rather than mailed questionnaires are used. As a broader range of officials are interviewed, it is more difficult to obtain data from a large sample of hospitals because of cost realities.

TABLE 3

FACTORS THAT INFLUENCE THE
FAVORABILITY OF HOSPITALS TO SOCIAL WORK SERVICES

A.   Hospital mission variables

    1.   complexity of mission (g = .325; p< .05)

    2.   extent mission is consonant with social work objectives (g = .347; p< .05)

    3.   extent mission emphasizes community services (g = .434; p< .01)

    4.   extent mission emphasize service to low income patients (g = .335; p< .05)

B.   Hospital tasks and characteristics

    1.   extent hospital develops new program (g = .341 p< .05)

    2.   age of hospital (g = .436; p< .05)

C.   Characteristics of hospital administration

    1.   extent hospital administrator influences hospital policies and decisions (g = .315; p< .05)

    2.   number of physicians salaried to the hospital (g = .386; p< .05)

D.   Orientations of hospital administrators

    1.   extent hospital administrator both believes the social work department addresses practical needs of the hospital and desires more of these programs (g = .305; p< .05)

LINKING HOSPITAL CHARACTERISTICS TO EXPANSION STRATEGIES

What are some implications for social workers of relationships between hospital characteristics and the size of social work departments? A four-stage process of strategy development may help social workers to explicitly develop strategies that increase the relevance of their departments to hospitals.

First, an inventory can be made of mission and institutional factors that appear to facilitate or impede the expansion of social work services (Rosenberg and Weissman, 1981, p. 14). These factors should include mission-objectives of the hospital (see Table 1) and practical needs of the hospital (see Table 2). Staff in the social work unit should also examine the extent key officials believe social work is relevant to these various mission-objectives and practical needs. Contextual factors can also be identified including the relative innovativeness of the hospital and the capabilities and interests of its central administration. This inventory allows initial identification of strategic opportunities.

Second, strategy can be devised that allows a department to capitalize on these opportunities. If institutional objectives that are consonant with social work objectives are given priority by influential decision makers, programs should be developed and publicized that address them. Findings from this study suggest that social work departments are most likely to expand in hospitals where top officials favor preventive services, outpatient services, helping patients with special and personal services as they influence personal health, and developing linkages with executives in agencies where patients are referred after discharge. In similar fashion, programs should be devised that are relevant to those specific concrete problems that are important to hospital decision makers.

Third, public relations strategy should be developed that makes decision makers aware of the relevance of social work both to specific mission-objectives and to practical needs of the hospital. A distinction should be made between internal communication within the department and communication with officials who are external to the department. Clinical language and perspectives can be emphasized in internal communications, while communication with external officials should focus upon the relevance of social work services to the objectives and needs of the hospital. Terms and concepts should be used that can be understood even by those persons who possess scant knowledge of clinical services; both empirical and anecdotal information should be used that documents to external officials the relevance of social work to specific mission-objectives and institutional needs of the hospital.

Fourth, social workers should develop strategy that takes into account the increasing importance of the central administration of hospitals (Starr, 1982, pp. 425-427). Hospital administrators are likely to become more powerful than in prior eras when physicians tended to dominate hospital policy and program decisions, since many administrative decisions are needed to help hospitals survive in the wake of recent policy changes and increasing competition between health care institutions. Social workers need increasingly to aspire to become partners in high-level administrative and policy decisions in hospitals. By proactively seeking planning assignments and by initiating program proposals, they can increase their visibility and credibility among key decision makers.

Finally, findings from this survey suggest an ongoing reform agenda for social workers. To this point, we have discussed factors that appear to influence the growth of social work departments. But social workers need to try to shape institutions so they provide a more favorable setting for social work services. In some cases, institutional relevance can be enhanced only by changing the institution itself so that the definitions of "relevance" of its officials and staff include broader perspectives. Thus, social workers need to try to enrich the missions of their hospitals so they place more emphasis upon prevention, community services, and assistance to low income consumers, as well as provision of services that help patients resolve psychosocial problems that frequently cause or accompany illness. As social workers succeed in this difficult task, findings from this survey suggest that they may also promote expansion of their departments.

REFERENCES

Bracht, N. *Social Work in Health Care: A Guide to Professional Practice*. New York: The Haworth Press, 1978.

Brody, S.S. Common Ground: Social Work in Health Care. *Health and Social Work*, February 1976, *1*, 16-31.

Caputi, M.A. Social Work in Health Care: Past and Future. *Social Work in Health Care*, February 1978, *3*, 8-29.

Carrigan, Z.H. Social Workers in Medical Settings: Who Defines Us? *Social Work in Health Care*, Winter 1978, *4*, 149-165.

Gentry, J.T., Veney, J.E., Kaluzny, A.D., and Sprague, J.B. Promoting the Adoption of Socialwork Services by Hospitals and Health Departments. *American Journal of Public Health*, February 1973, *63*, 117-126.

Goldsmith, Jeff. *Can Hospitals Survive?* Homewood, Ill.: Dow Jones-Irwin, 1981.

Hage, J. and Aiken, M. *Social Change in Complex Organizations*. New York: Random House, 1970.

Hickson, D.J. et al. A Strategic Contingencies Theory of Organizational Power. *Administrative Science Quarterly*, 1971, 216-219.

Jansson, B.S. and Simmons, J. Building Department or Unit Power within Human Service Organizations. *Administration in Social Work*, Fall 1984, *8*, 41-56.

Lurie, A., and Hirsch, S. Establishing a Hospital Social Service Department. *Social Work*, April 1959, *4*, 86-93.

Nacman, M. A Systems Approach to the Provision of Social Work Service in Health Settings: Part I. *Social Work in Health Care*, Fall 1975, *1*, 47-53.

Nacman, M. A Systems Framework to the Provision of Social Work Services in Health Settings, Part 2. *Social Work in Health Care*, Winter 1975, *1*, 133-145.

Nieman, D.A. and Hoops, Alan. Can Private Hospitals Afford Private Social Services? *Social Work in Health Care*, Winter 1977, *3*, 175-185.

Perrow, C. *Organizational Analysis: A Sociological View*. Belmont, CA.: Wadsworth Publishing Co., 1970.

Pfouts, J.H. and McDaniel, B. Medical Handmaidens or Professional Colleagues: A Survey of Social Work Practice in the Pediatrics Departments of Twenty-eight Teaching Hospitals. *Social Work in Health Care*, Spring 1975, *1*, 133-145.

Roemer, M.J. and Friedman, J.W. *Doctors in Hospitals*. Baltimore: Johns Hopkins Press, 1971.

Rosenberg, G. and Weissman, A. Marketing Social Service in Health Care Facilities. *Health and Social Work*, August 1981, *6*, 13-21.

Russell, L.B. *Technology in Hospitals: Medical Advances and their Diffusion*. Washington, D.C.: Brookings Institution, 1979.

Schlesinger, E. and Woloch, I. Hospital Social Work Roles and Decision Making. *Social Work in Health Care*, Fall 1982, *8*, 59-70.

Schoenfeld, H. Opportunities for Leadership for Social Work in Hospitals: An Administrator's Expectations. *Social Work in Health Care*, Fall 1975, *1*, 93-97.

Schreiber, H. Discharge Planning: Key to the Future of Hospital Social Work. *Health and Social Work*, May 1981, *6*, 48-53.

Starr, P. *The Social Transformation of American Medicine*. New York: Basic Books, 1982.

Thompson, J. and McEwen, W. Organizational Goals and Environment: Goal Setting as an Interactive Process. *American Sociological Review*. February 1958, *23*, 23-30.

Wattenberg, S.H., Orr, M.M., O'Rouke, T.W. Comparisons of Opinions of Social Work Administrators and Hospital Administrators Toward Leadership Tasks. *Social Work in Health Care*, Spring 1977, *2*, 285-293.

Weiss, R. *Statistics in Social Research*. New York: John Wiley and Sons, 1968.

An Expanded Social Work Role in a University Hospital-Based Group Practice: Service Provider, Physician Educator and Organizational Consultant

Sylvia S. Clarke, MSW
Linda Neuwirth, MSW
Richard H. Bernstein, MD

SUMMARY. This paper reports the development of social work role and functions in a primary medical group practice which was established to replace the general medical clinics of a large urban voluntary teaching hospital in an academic medical center. It traces the shaping and implementation of a role which is functionally integral to the care, teaching and research goals of the practice; is operationalized into its service delivery system; and utilizes a full range of sophisticated social work skills. Along with physicians and nurse practitioners, the social work is a principal provider of patient care, as well as physician educator and organizational consultant who contributes to coordinated, comprehensive and resource conservative care. Implications for other settings are noted.

INTRODUCTION

The recent literature on the contributions of social work to the practice of primary care medicine describes a diversity of models which reflect the various organizational and philosophical attributes

At the time of writing Mrs. Clarke was a consultant, and Mrs. Neuwirth was a social work supervisor, Department of Social Work Services; Dr. Bernstein was Medical Director, Internal Medicine Associates; all at The Mount Sinai Hospital and Medical Center, One Gustave L. Levy Place, New York, NY 10029.
Reprinted from *Social Work in Health Care*, Volume 11(4), Summer 1986.

under which they operate (Clare and Carney, 1982; Coleman, Lebowitz and Anderson, 1976; Coleman, Patrick, Eagle and Hermalin, 1979; Demby, 1980; Ell and Morrison, 1981; Hookey, 1977, 1978; Korpela, 1973; Mechanic, 1980; Miller, 1983).

Adding yet another dimension, this paper reports on the role and functions of social work in an innovative primary care medical group practice which replaced the general medical clinic in a large, urban, voluntary teaching hospital in an academic medical center. It traces how the social worker became a major provider of service, an educator of faculty and residents, as well as a consultant in organizational development within this general internal medical group. The model described is replicable in other primary care settings, especially where there is a conviction that modification of the doctor-centered model of medical practice is feasible and desirable.

IMPETUS FOR CHANGE AND MODEL BUILDING

The impetus for this program, which was eventually named the Internal Medicine Associates of Mount Sinai Medical Center of New York City (IMA), arose formally in 1977 when the Medical Center President appointed a multi-departmental committee to explore the feasibility of establishing group practices to replace the traditional clinic structure in the primary care specialties. The Department of Medicine was particularly interested in piloting this experiment to improve patient care in the general medical clinic (GMC). There was also discontent among the voluntary attendings and residents who staffed the clinic about the quality of care and quality of education there, and concern on the part of the Hospital about the lack of sound administrative controls in this 20,000 visit per year clinic.

Within 16 months, the committee developed a blueprint for change in the GMC (Bosch and Fisher, 1981). The usual pace of institutional innovation was accelerated when the Robert Wood Johnson Foundation selected the site as one of the 15 to receive $800,000 over a 3 year period to develop and evaluate the conversion of a traditional GMC to a teaching hospital primary care group practice.

The underlying principles of the IMA model were to transplant into institutional soil the positive features of private group practice, with the added missions of serving the medically needy in a comprehensive way, of training residents and other health professionals, and of providing an environment for research. The special tasks of primary care (Alpert and Charney, 1975) including accessibility, continuity, and coordination of specialty care and hospital needs, were seen as paramount features of the new model.

Organizationally, all staff, including physicians, nurses, social workers, administrative and clerical staff, report to the Medical Director, who reports to the Division Chief of General Internal Medicine (and in turn to the Department Chairman and the Dean). This contrasts with many other hospital-based primary care practices in which the traditional vertical reporting is along departmental lines (Delbanco and Parker, 1978; Grossman, 1982). In the case of social work, there is a dual reporting channel: to the Medical Director for operational duties and to the Director of Social Work Services for professional affairs. All decisions about hiring or dismissing social workers are made jointly.

The Clinical Teams

Continuity and accessibility needs are accomplished by physicians (group practices medical attendings on the full-time staff, although not necessarily working full-time at IMA), nurse practitioners and social workers organized as teams to provide consistent patient-provider relationships over a period of time. The principal provider, who at different stages in the patient's treatment may be a physician, nurse or social worker, coordinates the health care services the patient receives at the practice, during hospitalization and from consultants who are used with discrimination to avoid fragmented care. There is a comprehensive approach to patient care with each discipline contributing to the bio-psychosocial framework. Team members use a functional definition of illness: how an individual functions in his life, how his illness affects this functioning and vice versa.

Including house staff physicians required a structure to support this thrust. The 84 traditional medical house staff are subdivided among the medical faculty. With the residents away on rotations to affiliates and having only the traditional half-day per week during the weeks they are assigned clinical sessions at IMA, coordinated

904 SOCIAL WORK IN HEALTH CARE: A HANDBOOK FOR PRACTICE

patient care requires a team-approach in which 3 residents (a triplet consisting of a PGY-1, -2, and -3) cross cover each other and, in the event none are available for acute problems and hospitalizations, the faculty-preceptor for the triplet is responsible for providing care temporarily until the primary resident returns.

Because we serve a large Spanish-speaking population, almost all of our staff are bilingual in Spanish and English.

EXPANDING SERVICE ROLE OF SOCIAL WORKER: IMPLEMENTING THE BIO-PSYCHOSOCIAL MODEL

The majority of referrals to social workers in the former general medical clinics were for "concrete" services and patient advocacy within the bureaucracy of community agencies and governmental entitlement programs. Although such services are crucial for many patients served in medical clinics of urban centers, they do not deal with the host of other complex psychosocial problems interrelated with illness. Concerned that help for these problems was rarely provided in the GMC setting, the social work supervisor and the IMA medical director and faculty shared the hope of imbedding the bio-psychosocial framework (Engel, 1977) in the everyday practice of IMA. This was considered to be especially critical because such a large proportion of individuals with emotional problems seek help via the medical doorway (Borus, 1972; Hankins and Oktay, 1979; Noble, 1976; Regier, Goldberg and Taube, 1978; Report to the President, 1978).

A wide range of intertwined medical, social and psychological problems was anticipated in the 5,500 adult patients who were transferred from the GMC to the practice over the first four years. The program needed a structure for reliable identification of and screening for psychosocial problems.

Identifying Patients' Psychosocial Problems

A principal vehicle for integrating the medical and psychosocial dimensions has been the jointly developed, comprehensive, self-administered, bilingual questionnaire which has been routinely administered to all patients since the practice began in September of 1980. It includes the elements found in traditional medical histories as well as several sections and items which represent screening for psychosocial and sexual problems couched in simple, everyday language (Appendix I). This closed-ended part of the medical history is reviewed for positive responses by all primary clinical providers later in the first patient appointment. In addition, there is an initial open-ended section of the medical interview which focuses on the collection of basic demographic variables as well as a global question about environmental stressors. The traditional chief complaint and present illness section of the history follows this "getting to know you as a person" section of the patient profile.

While these questions are superficial, they triggered a flood of referrals for the evaluation of previously unrecognized psychosocial problems. With essentially the same population and the same medical residents, the epidemiology of psychosocial need for social work services virtually inverted from 80% "concrete" to 80% psychotherapeutic. This prompted the delegation of most of the work related to clerical functions, such as application forms for support services, to two medical assistants on the nursing staff. In addition, the demand for social work evaluation and treatment rose to the point where currently 20% of all practice patients are referred for an evaluation by a social worker. The number of clinical social workers to meet this demand (and the average of 7 follow-up visits per referral) reached 3.5 full-time equivalents before the waiting period for the first visit was reduced to less than 2 weeks. (The remaining .5 time of one of the 4 social workers is devoted to supervisory and management activities.)

The referring clinician (faculty, resident or nurse practitioner) provides information on a referral slip about the reason for the referral. Because of the high rate of "no shows" among physician initiated first visits (50%), the patient is encouraged to make his own appointment. This tests his motivation and encourages his participation. For urgent problems where the patient has not made an appointment, the social worker makes outreach efforts to engage the patient by telephone. During each of the 10 half-day clinical sessions each week, one of the 4 social workers is on call for emergency evaluation and crisis intervention, which may include referring the patient to the Psychiatric Emergency Room. Of course, the patient can be referred to the social worker at any point in his treatment.

Social Work Clinical Role

Developing the social workers' clinical role followed naturally from the primary care goal of minimizing specialty referrals and therefore reducing the fragmentation of care. Generally, IMA patients are referred to a psychiatrist or psychologist only after first being evaluated by a social worker, unless such patients already have an established relationship with a non-IMA provider for management of their emotional problem. Medical and psychosocial evaluation by the clinicians and social workers are sufficient to handle the majority of psychophysiologic or somatopsychic problems. Just as the primary care physician can treat the majority of patients' medical problems and use specialists selectively, so the social worker is able to make judgments in the initial evaluation about (1) whether social work will treat the patient, (2) whether referral to a psychiatrist is needed for medication concurrent with social work treatment, (3) whether psychiatric treatment is the primary need and (4) whether psychiatric hospitalization is indicated. The ready availability of a part-time liaison psychiatrist in IMA for medication, consultation or further evaluation has worked well in maintaining role clarity and avoiding the unnecessary use of psychiatric resources.

The Psychosocial Evaluation

Each patient referred to the social worker receives a formal evaluation consisting of: (1) a psychosocial assessment of the etiology of their problem following one or several 45 minute interviews, a review of their medical record, and, if necessary, a discussion with their primary clinician; (2) DSM-3 diagnosis; and (3) a treatment plan often including a formal contract with the patient clarifying mutual expectations and goals.

Treatment Priorities

The psychosocial evaluation serves as the triage instrument to categorize patients' problems and to determine which patients are best served by the group practice social workers. Highest priority is given to those patients whose psychosocial problems precipitate, perpetuate or exacerbate their illness or to those whose psychosocial disturbances are intertwined with their medical problems. Patients followed in IMA are those whose social and emotional problems (a) derive from their illness; (b) exacerbate their medical problems, as in "non-compliance" with prescribed care or in psychosomatic overlay; (c) predispose them to illness, as in obesity or alcoholism, and (d) derive from life crises such as bereavement or divorce. Here intervention may forestall or avoid fixing patterns of somatization of depression.

Patients whose problems are primarily psychiatric and who do not need ongoing medical care are referred to other treatment sources, with social work acting as liaison for motivation, connection and coordination. Exceptions are patients with somataform disorders who are better treated by the practice in order to contain and decrease utilization of physician time. Examples are patients convinced they have cardiac disease because of tachycardia secondary to panic disorder or patients whose headaches are precipitated by psychological stress but who are certain the cause is a brain tumor. The social worker is the main provider of treatment of patients who express psychological distress somatically. Matching provider skill and patient needs results in effective as well as fiscally sound use of expensive professional resources.

Social Work Treatment

Patients' broad range of behavioral, affective, interpersonal, social and environmental problems, along with provider interdependence, require sophisticated social work capabilities in the spectrum of individual, family and group treatment of modalities.

Individual and Family Treatment

Brief treatment of patients and families matches the rapid pace of the service. However, treatment methods and duration vary to meet the needs of the patient population. Social work goals are realistically and functionally formulated. Long term treatment by the social worker is the required course for some patients, just as the efforts of the physician over an extended period of time may be required to stabilize diabetic or labile hypertensive patients.

The functional rubric that shapes all social work treatment is the relationship between patients' inner and outer stresses and their physical disease and illness. The following vignettes illustrate this.

It was essential that a 55-year-old hypertensive patient receive ongoing treatment for anxiety attacks secondary to complicated bereavement which developed after her mother's death from a myocardial infarction. With each such attack, which usually occurred at 4:00 in the morning, she would telephone and wake one of the on-call physicians. The patient's need and physicians' capacity to help did not match. The social worker engaged the patient in treatment. After a year of intensive work, the anxiety attacks remitted with the resolution of her grief reaction.

A 38-year-old woman with labile hypertension profited from a brief period of weekly sessions. Why her blood pressure was so hard to control eluded the nurse practitioner, her primary provider. The patient was suffering from depression caused by a recent separation from her husband and by her daughter's decision to marry and leave home. Treatment focused on helping her resolve the conflicts associated with the loss of these attachments. As the depression lifted, so did her self-esteem. She lost 20 pounds and her blood pressure dropped. Treatment ended with her decision to enter nursing school.

A 68-year-old woman followed medically for several chronic diseases also carried a psychiatric diagnosis of major depression. This was related to a conflictual, intertwined relationship with her dominating and controlling older sister, and to the death several years before of her son by an overdose of narcotics. She had originally presented with symptoms of dementia which turned out to be pseudo-dementia, that is, the decrease in her intellectual abilities were secondary to her depression. Once this lifted through treatment, she no longer showed cognitive deficits. This patient might have been lost in many other settings on the basis that at 68 a "little senility" was natural, and having a sister who talks all the time is not the worst fate. In this practice, the physicians and nurse practitioners are attuned to the relationship between patient's psychosocial stress and mental status so that the exploration of this connection becomes a basic component of care.

Group Treatment

The group method is the treatment of choice for certain patients. Groups are formed by identifying those clusters of patients who have similar problems which are better solved by group than individual intervention.

The wide range of group purpose and composition applicable in health care settings, such as support, education, socialization, problem-solving, psychotherapy, etc. (Northen, 1983), are subject to the priorities dictated by the functional imperatives of the practice: (a) the interconnectedness of patients' psychosocial problems and their illness; and (b) the need to utilize each discipline's expertise appropriately.

Patients with somataform illness have always had high priority for in-house social work treatment. Their psychological disturbances often translate into symptoms that enlist physician and nurse concern though the problems are more responsive to social work than to medical and nursing methods. Timely identification of such patients and matching them with an appropriate treatment modality has proved to be good treatment and also cost effective as it prevents overuse and misuse of medical/nursing visits.

In one instance, a socialization support group for elderly, isolated, depressed women with multiple medical problems had the effect of reducing somatization and overutilization of visits to the practice. Treated individually at first, these 7 women ranging in age from 60 to 84, were all widowed or divorced, with few family and social ties and limited financial resources. Half were wheelchair bound and the others disabled to the extent that the only way they could leave their homes was via ambulette to visit the hospital. These visits to the hospital provided their only contact with the outside world. They had a high rate of walk-in, unscheduled visits to the practice and the Emergency Room. Physicians were troubled that these patients were asking to be seen more often than was medically indicated. Social workers, too, were being deluged with these patients who returned repeatedly without appointments or explicitly stated need.

To receive needed attention they were having to emphasize their physical symptoms, reinforcing their sense of ill health. The costly medical commodity was being misdirected. Time was going into individual treatment of needs, which were palliated, not resolved. It appeared that group social work treatment would be effective for these women, and would be an economical, conserving use of the social worker.

Patients met weekly for 2 years and moved classically through the steps of developing and experiencing a mutual aid process for sharing common concerns and ways of handling them. As group bonds cohesed and strengthened, as the climate became more risk free and their trust in each other deepened, they moved from re-peated recountings of their symptoms and illnesses to levels of dis-cussion which touched and tapped the deeper concerns of their de-pression, anxiety, and isolation. New ways of mastering these emerged, particularly by the self-help network they formed through their increasingly intimate and candid relationships with each other. As their self-esteem grew and as they became psychologically more self-confident and less isolated, their somatization and physical complaints decreased. This phenomenon was documented con-cretely by the decrease in their visits to the primary medical and nursing providers and to the Emergency Room, and by their prefer-ence for the help of the group to that of the social worker individ-ually. Their pattern of overdependence on the practice staff was broken.

Shared Responsibility for Needed Environmental Supports

Many of our patients have chronic long term illness and disability and need a host of aids to enable them to live in the community: practical needs for homemaker, transportation, visiting nurse, home health aides and appliances. In settings which operate primarily from a biological frame of reference, these are usually seen as so-cial needs and become the exclusive domain of social work despite the fact that a medical prescription is needed to procure them and that most of the information needed is medical. In this setting, these needs were redefined and conceptually reframed as health care needs. Responsibility for helping patients obtain these needed aids became the concern of all disciplines since their lack adversely affected patients' medical progress. Requests and forms are now coordinated by medical assistants (nursing aides). Physicians complete the medical data needed, recognizing that their patients' ability to maintain their health status would be jeopardized if they could not travel to the practice offices or did not receive the prescribed wheelchair. Thus, the physician learns directly about patients' life problems. Social workers avoid "taking over" physicians' responsibility for forms primarily medical in nature, knowing this interferes with first hand physician learning.

The drain of social work time, common in ambulatory care settings where the social worker takes over responsibility for monitoring these requests and forms, is recouped for functions which appropriately tap social work skill base.

Where patients have problems with welfare, Medicaid and other agencies which grant these requests, the social worker steps in as the enabler to help them resolve their difficulties.

EXPANDING THE EDUCATIONAL ROLE OF THE SOCIAL WORKER

Team Meetings

Because a team approach does not emerge full blown from its design on the drawing board, ongoing structures are needed to operationalize primary care principles into daily practice (Lee, 1980; Nason, 1983).

Luncheon meetings have been developed and are held weekly with all faculty providers, nurse practitioners, nurses, social workers, and a liaison psychiatrist. Patients who are particularly difficult to manage are discussed. These are usually patients whose behavioral problems are so challenging that the primary clinician and primary social worker need to ask for the advice of others and to develop a multi-disciplinary plan of action. Presentations at the team meetings are selected by the social work supervisor in advance and usually are the focus of an academic discussion about the generic management issue underlying the case in addition to providing specific suggestions for the presenters. Discussions are generally lead by the primary social worker and amplified by the liaison psychiatrist. The goal is to enhance the faculty's skill in diagnoses and treatment of all illnesses whose symptoms are not justifiable solely on an organic basis. They, in turn, transmit their knowledge and skill to the house staff. As internist role models for the residents, the faculty demonstrate that they view social workers as colleagues possessing special skills, and virtually all residents eventually refer a portion of their patients to the social work staff for psychosocial evaluations.

Intramural Consultations and Faculty Support of the Expanded Service Role

Much of the teaching of the clinical staff comes through the process of referring patients and reading the psychosocial evaluations and follow-up notes of the social workers that are sent to the referring clinician (Nason, 1974) before being placed in the IMA medical record.

Over time, the faculty has come to better appreciate the expanded service role of the social workers. Residents who are frustrated and "turned off" by the somatizing, hostile, or non-compliant patient are instructed about the importance of viewing such behavior as requiring further evaluation, usually by the social worker (Monson and Smith, 1983). Over the course of several years, the residents gradually have become a major referral source for the social workers.

The Education of Students in the Health Professions

Social workers are also teachers to medical students in their "Introduction to Medicine" course in the first year. The concepts of primary care, team practice, and the expanded social work role is introduced at this stage of training and reinforced during student electives such as the Community Medicine clerkships in the third year.

A final area of education has been in the placement of social work students in IMA for graduate education in MSW programs.

RESEARCH ROLE FOR SOCIAL WORKERS

The least developed social worker role has been that of research. This is largely because IMA social workers primarily have had service and teaching roles and have not had time allocated specifically for research activities. The epidemiology of psychosocial needs of a population previously served by a traditional GMC, and research "to discover when and with whom treatment of psychosocial problems is most essential and productive" are among the fertile areas for research (Coulton, 1983). Funds for such studies are currently being sought.

EXPANDING SOCIAL WORKER ROLE AS ADMINISTRATIVE AND ORGANIZATIONAL CONSULTANT

The Management Group

The need for multi-disciplinary input in operational decision making was appreciated soon after IMA was established. A management group was constituted which consisted of the medical director, administrator, office manager, a faculty representative, nursing supervisor, and social work supervisor. IMA's missions and goals were formulated by input from the entire staff since it was initially quite small. Intramural policy was created by the medical director and the other faculty. It was the Management Group's purpose to translate the missions and policies into an efficient and effective organization.

In addition to being a valuable contributor as a representative of the social work unit, it soon became clear that the social work supervisor had skills as a process consultant on group decision making, conflict management, and dealing with difficult personnel issues. These skills continue to be particularly helpful to the medical director and are well appreciated by all members of the management team.

Administrative Back-Up for Difficult Patients

Advanced skills in interpersonal relationships are also useful to the clerical staff and office manager. While maturity and public relation skills are criteria in the selection of staff who work at the reception desk in the office, staff find it difficult to manage successfully a small but vocal minority of patients who approach them with hostility. Again, the social worker on call is used as an important part of the management of such patients. This is another source of social work referrals.

Helping Medical Faculty in Their Role Conflicts

The medical faculty has also come to rely on social workers for help in dealing with certain conflicts in their role as preceptors. This is usually done in the context of team meetings but also may be accomplished in one-on-one talks with a social worker. For example, physicians' difficulties in setting clearly defined expectations for the residents' performance were related to their overidentification with the residents' pressured schedules. All the attendings in this practice are young physicians who are close in time to their own training period and remember well the onus of residents' overburdened schedules. These attendings are also new to the institution and have not as yet achieved significant academic status within the Department of Medicine. They are not always sure of their options should residents' performance fall below the mark, and their contracts with the residents are often vague. Their feelings of helplessness are exacerbated by the fact that the residents' complaints about system failures are often reality-based. The process of sorting out these factors helps them begin to take more constructive actions and to function more comfortably as preceptors.

The social worker helps facilitate communication among Management Group members and pinpoints affective impediments to problem solving in the course of their work together. For example, an early, typical agenda item was the issue of patients who repeatedly "no-show." Several approaches proposed seemed mechanical or punitive; the social worker helped the group members shift off this authoritative stance and adopt the use of contracting and paradoxical strategies which were successful.

With the problem of how to lower absenteeism among support staff, the Management Group was helped to shift from a paternalistic to a collegial framework of helping the secretaries see themselves as professionals vital to the operation of the practice and to own their part of the problem.

Social work skills have become helpful to administrative staff as they deal with supervisory and management problems. As the practice expanded and the number of medical assistants, secretaries, receptionists and medical records staff doubled, job responsibilities were redesigned and this triggered competitive struggles between the founding and the new groups: the "oldtimers" feared they would be replaced. The new staff feared criticism. The ensuing resentment pervaded the practice and decreased morale: the close knit family had been invaded. The social worker helped the manager and administrator develop a series of group meetings with this staff in the course of which these conflicts were aired and resolved.

FINANCIAL VIABILITY

What are the costs of this social work model for primary care? Can it be justified in the climate of escalating health care costs and competition for the health care dollar?

Cost and Benefits

As the cited case situations illustrate, many patients seek medical care for other-than-medical concerns; some overutilize the practice's resources; some make many unscheduled visits; some are unable to follow prescribed medical and nursing regimens.

It can be argued that in a fee-for-service design, the prime factor is that these visits are reimbursable and contribute to financial stability. But in examining the quality of these visits, we find they are longer and take more time than normally scheduled visits and give less patient satisfaction because their underlying psychosocial problems are not addressed or resolved. The patient continues to call and visit physicians and nurses in a repetitive cycle costly to their productivity and unsatisfying to patients. Lengthy unplanned for and planned visits disorganize provider schedules and lower productivity. Frequent telephone calls use up non-reimbursable time (and patience) of physicians, nurses and support staff.

Traditional patterns of patient visits to medical and nursing providers in situations where psychosocial stresses precipitate and perpetuate symptoms represent a costly mismatch of need and resource. The conservation and appropriate allocation of interdisciplinary resources is a financial as well as functional imperative (Nason and Delbanco, 1976). The treatment of choice in these instances is much less costly (Hookey, 1979; Schlesinger, Mumford, Glass, Patrick and Scharfstein, 1983).

The social worker's contributions to the team's patient-care plans, to the development of collaborative skills, to the construction of humanistic and efficient policies and procedures, and to the management of systems and staff is cost effective. Job satisfaction and productivity of all staff in the group practice are positively affected.

Revenue Production

Social work generates income through payments for visits by third party private and public insurance plans and through charges for "self-pay" patients (Twersky and Cole, 1976). This income offsets the major salary costs of social work staff (Rosenberg, 1980). Scheduling each social worker for 1000 patient visits yearly, or in a pattern that includes group visits, produces sufficient income to make social work self-supporting. Thus, a formula is established for adding social workers to the practice as its registered population increases. (The .5 FTE time the supervisory social worker spends in supervisory and management activities is conceptualized as administrative overhead and absorbed in IMA along with other administrative costs.)

Experience with the model over a 4-year period has demonstrated its economic viability both in cost benefit and revenue production.

IMPLICATIONS

This experience demonstrates how the organization and philosophy of a medical care program can enhance social work function and effectiveness as a component in care. The model of the social worker as a principal provider in an interdisciplinary group practice taps the full range of social work skills in direct service, collaboration, education, research, management and consultation. Pinned to a bio-psycho-social frame of reference, this model provides patients with a planned way to identify and treat those of their psychosocial problems which interlock with their medical problems, and contributes to achieving the group practice goals of coordinated, comprehensive, unfragmented, effective and resource-conservative care.

What guidelines can we extract for use in similar programs?

(1) One precondition is some commitment on the part of planners to a bio-psycho-social framework for viewing patients' illnesses. If the ambiance allows for demonstration of the described level of social work contribution, even tentative espousal can be influenced positively.

(2) Effective procedures need to be put in place so that there is reliable and consistent identification of complex psychosocial problems associated with patients' illnesses. These structures will facilitate population-based planning for the delivery of social work services and avoid the reactive rendering of these services, which is all too common when social work staff cannot fulfill their potential contribution if they merely deal with visible symptoms: "The patient has no place to live," "no money" or the dramatic behavior of the "hard to manage" patient. We know that many patients seek help via the medical doorway as it is easier to say "my head aches" than "my heart aches," and many patients cannot identify their problems as emotional. Thus, screening methods are needed to identify these significant patient care issues, and social workers can play a crucial role in helping physicians develop appropriate screening tools.

(3) Because social work functions in this model are not circumscribed, the role is a rewarding one. Ell and Morrison (1981) note that the knowledge and skill base in primary care social work is "unique in its breadth." Implementing the expanded role model requires high social work capability in assessment, diagnosis and in individual, family and group treatment, as well as comfort in assuming a principal, as opposed to ancillary, role in the core functions of direct service, collaboration and teaching. The broad knowledge base and sophisticated clinical skills are needed by all

social work providers as a *sine qua non* for the model's institutionalization and perpetuation. At least one social work provider needs to assume the faculty consultant and management roles described and be equipped to each these skills to other social work staff so that the standard of social work input is consistent. The role also calls for openness to learning from other disciplines and a commitment to organizational goals as well as patient needs.

(4) We have seen the benefits of being active in the early stages of designing the system of care. Seizing such opportunities in an institution assures a timely social work presence in planning and counteracts the tendency of medical care planners to work unilaterally, to bring in social work or nursing "later." Design dictates systems, systems shape budgets, and "later" may be too late as budgets lock in designs. Inclusion of social work in the planning process starts the acculturation of professional interdependence and establishes it as a norm (Dana, 1983). Too, the actual beginning operation can start with explicit expectations for social work role. Though these will need to be renegotiated as the operation develops and changes, the negotiations are from a position of strength. The social worker is party, not plaintiff, to the planning. This permits demonstration over a period of time and facilitates the institutionalization of the model as the practice grows and develops.

We have attempted to extract the underlying principles of a way of working that provides effective care to patients, high professional rewards for the social worker and economic viability. These principles are applicable to a broad range of structures and offer a way of addressing and upgrading the social work role in many health care settings.

REFERENCES

Alpert, J.J. and Charney, E. *The Education of Physicians for Primary Care,* DHEW Pub. No. (HRA) 74-3113, Washington, D.C.: U.S. Government Printing Office, 1975.

Borus, J.F. Neighborhood health centers as providers of primary mental health care. *New England Journal of Medicine,* 1972, 6, 697-722.

Bosch, S.J. and Fisher, E. The role and functions assumed by a department of community medicine in planning a group medical practice. *Health Policy and Education,* 1981, 2, 167-176.

Clare, A.W. and Carney, R.H. *Social Work and Primary Health Care*, London: Academic Press, 1982.

Coleman, J.V., Patrick, D., Eagle, J. and Hermalin, J. Collaboration, consultation and referral in an integrative health and mental health program at an HMO. *Social Work in Health Care*, 1979, *5*(1), 83-98.

Coleman, J.V., Lebowitz, M.L. and Anderson, F.P. Social work in a pediatric primary health care team in a group practice program. *Social Work in Health Care*, 1976, *1*(4), 489-497.

Coulton, C. A social work perspective of research in primary care. *Primary Health Care: More than Medicine*, R.S. Miller, ed. Englewood Cliffs, New Jersey: Prentice-Hall, Inc. 1983, 210-228.

Dana, B. The collaborative process. *Social Work Issues in Health Care*, R.S. Miller and H. Rehr, eds. Englewood Cliffs, New Jersey: Prentice Hall, Inc. 1983, 181-220.

Delbanco, T.L. and Parker, J.N. Primary care in a teaching hospital: history, problems and prospects. Mt. Sinai Journal of Medicine, 1978, *45*, 628-45.

Demby, A. Preventive intervention in an HMO: The social worker's role in a marital separation program. *Social Work in Health Care*, 1980, *5*(4), 351-360.

Ell, K. and Morrison, D.R. Primary Care. *Health and Social Work*, 1981, supplement to *6*(4), 355-435.

Engel, G.L. The need for a new medical model: a challenge for biomedicine, *Science*, 1977, *196*:127-36.

Grossman, J.H. Reorganization of ambulatory care in an academic medical center. *Journal of Ambulatory Care Management*, 1982; *1*:44-50.

Hankins, J. and Oktay, J.S. *Mental Disorders and Primary Medical Care: An Analytic Review of the Literature*, Washington, D.C.: Department of Health, Education and Welfare, ADM, 1979.

Hookey, P. Cost-benefit evaluation in primary health care. *Health and Social Work*, 1979, *4*(3), 151-168.

Hookey, P. Social work participation in primary health care: an overview of current developments in industrialized nations. *Primary Health Care in Industrialized Nations*, C.D. Burrell and C. Sheps, eds. The Annals of the New York Academy of Sciences, 1978, *310*, 212-220.

Hookey, P. The establishment of social work participation in rural primary health care. *Social Work in Health Care*, 1977, *3*(1), 87-99.

Korpela, J.W. Social work assistance in a private pediatric practice. *Social Casework*, 1973, *54*, 538-544.

Lee, S. Interdisciplinary teaming in primary care: a process of evolution and resolution. *Social Work in Health Care*, 1980, *5*(3), 237-244.

Mechanic, D. The management of psychosocial problems in primary medical care: A potential role for social work. *Journal of Human Stress*, 1980, *6*, 16-21.

Miller, R.S. *Primary Health Care: More than Medicine*, Englewood Cliffs, New Jersey: Prentice-Hall, 1983.

Monson, R.A. and Smith, R.G. Somatization disorder in primary care. *New England Journal of Medicine*, June 16, 1983, 1464-5.

Nason, F. Diagnosing the hospital team. *Social Work in Health Care*, 1983, *9*(2), 25-45.

Nason, F. and Delbanco, T.L. Soft services: a major cost effective component in primary medical care. *Social Work in Health Care*, 1981, *6*(3), 13-23.

Nason, F. Problem-oriented chart notes as a method of increasing social work visibility, accountability and impact. Presentation at The Meeting of the American Public Health Association, New Orleans, Louisiana, October 24, 1974.

Noble, J. Comprehensive care and the primary health team. *Primary Care and the Practice of Medicine*, Boston: Little, Brown & Company, 1976.

Northen, H. Social work groups in health settings: Promises and problems. *Social Work in Health Care*, 1983, *8*(3), 107-121.

Regier, D.A., Goldberg, I.D. and Taube, C.A. The defacto U.S. mental health system. Archives of General Psychiatry, 35, 1978.

Report to the President, *The President's Commission on Mental Health*, Vol. 1. Washington, D.C., U.S. Government Printing Office, 1978.

Rosenberg, G. Concepts in the financial management of hospital social work. *Social Work in Health Care*, 1980, *5*(3), 287-297.

Schlesinger, H.J., Mumford, E., Glass, G.V., Patrick, C. and Sharfstein, S. Mental health treatment and medical care utilization in a fee-for-service system: Out-patient mental health treatment following the onset of a chronic disease. *American Journal of Public Health*, 1983, *73*(4), 422-429.

Twersky, R.K. and Cole, W.M. Social work fees in medical care: A review of the literature and report of a survey. *Social Work in Health Care*, 1976, *2*(1), 77-84.

APPENDIX I:
EXCERPTS FROM SELF-ADMINISTERED
PATIENT QUESTIONNAIRE

Past History (Historia Medica Pasada)

Please circle (Y) for YES, (N) for NO and (?) for NOT SURE. (Por favor, ponga un circulo alrededor de (Y) si contesta que SI, alrededor de (N) si contesta que NO, o alrededor de (?) si NO ESTA SEGURO).

	YOURSELF (Usted)			CLOSE RELATIVE (sus Parientes)		
16. Alcohol or Drug Problems (Abuso de alcohol o drogas)	N	?	Y	N	?	Y
17. Nervous Breakdown or Suicide Attempt (Problemas emocionales o intento de suicidio)	N	?	Y	N	?	Y

APPENDIX I (continued)

	YOURSELF (Usted)			CLOSE RELATIVE (sus Parientes)		

LIFE STRESSES (STRESS EN SU VIDA)

26. Any relationships with people – family, spouse, children, workers – that continually upset you?
(Cualquier relacion con otras personas – familia, esposo/a, hijos, companeros de trabajo que lo pone nervioso continuamente?)

| | N | ? | Y | N | ? | Y |

27. Do you often feel:
(Se siente Vd. a menudo):
a. sad, blue, "down in the dumps," tearful?
(triste o con deseo de llorar?)

| | N | ? | Y | N | ? | Y |

b. anxious, nervous, panicky, worrisome?
(ansioso, nervioso, con miedo o muy preocupado?)

| | N | ? | Y | N | ? | Y |

28. Would you like help with items in questions 3 or 4? (Quiere Vd. ayuda con los items 3 o 4?)

| | N | ? | Y | N | ? | Y |

29. Do you have problems with appetite, sleep, sexual life, concentration or memory?
(Tiene problemas con el apetito, el sueno, la vida sexual, la concentracion o la memoria?)

| | N | ? | Y | N | ? | Y |

30. Have you ever considered taking your own life? (Penso alguna vez en quitarse la vida?)

| | N | ? | Y | N | ? | Y |

31. Do you feel you need additional help in solving practical problems in your daily life – money, transportation, home care?
(Necesita ayuda para solucionar problemas practicos de su vida contidiana – dinero, transporte, ayuda casera?)

| | N | ? | Y | N | ? | Y |

Commentary

The literature of the eleven-year span covered by this book reflects a long-standing concern that will certainly endure: how to achieve clarity about and acceptance of social work's role and functions in our nation's health care delivery systems (Kerson, 1981; Germain, 1980; Carrigan, 1978; Berkman and Rehr, 1970). Another prominent, allied concern has been the struggle to achieve a balance between an autonomous professional role for social work congruent with developments in the field along with a more secure position as professional colleagues of other disciplines in the health care system (Lister, 1980; Olsen and Olsen, 1967; and Ullmann and Kassebaum, 1961).

The expansion of social work services to new populations and settings has stimulated explorations of social work's realized and potential contributions in the broad field of health care (Berkman, Rehr, and Rosenberg, 1980; and Davidson, 1978). Complex and expanding roles emerged. This collection of articles offers additional segments of needed knowledge and skill.

REFERENCES

Berkman, Barbara, and Rehr, Helen. "Unanticipated Consequences of the Case-finding System in Hospital Social Services," *Social Work* 15(4), April 1970, pp. 63–68.

Berkman, Barbara; Rehr, Helen; and Rosenberg, Gary. "A Social Work Department Develops and Tests a Screening Mechanism To Identify High Risk Situations," *Social Work in Health Care* 5(4), Summer 1980, pp. 373–385. (See Part 6 of this volume.)

Carrigan, Zoe H. "Social Workers in Medical Settings: Who Defines Us?" *Social Work in Health Care* 4(2), Winter 1978, pp. 149–163.

Davidson, Kay W. "Evolving Social Work Roles in Health Care: The Case of Discharge Planning," *Social Work in Health Care* 4(1), Fall 1978, pp. 43–54. (See Part 2 of this volume.)

Germain, Carel B. "Social Work Identity, Competence and Autonomy: The Ecological Perspective," *Social Work in Health Care 6*(1), Fall 1980, pp. 1–10.

Kerson, Toba Schwaber. *Medical Social Work: The Pre-Professional Paradox.* New York: Irvington, 1981.

Lister, Larry. "Role Expectations of Social Workers and Other Health Professionals," *Health and Social Work 5*(2), May 1980, pp. 41–49.

Olsen, Katherine M., and Olsen, Marvin E. "Role Expectations and Perceptions for Social Workers in Medical Settings," *Social Work 12*(3), July 1967, pp. 70–78.

Ullmann, Alice, and Kassebaum, Gene. "Referral and Services in a Medical Social Work Department," *Social Service Review 35*(3), September 1961, pp. 263–264.

Additional Readings

Axelrod, Terry. "Innovative Roles for Social Workers in Home Care Programs," *Health and Social Work 3*(3), August 1978, pp. 48–66.

Current Issues in Health Care Today: A Challenge to the Profession. Proceedings of the Annual Maternal and Child Health Conference, Columbia University School of Social Work and Affiliate Maternal and Child Health Field Settings, New York, June 1986.

Dinerman, Miriam. "In Sickness and in Health: Future Social Work Roles," *Health and Social Work 4*(2), May 1979, pp. 5–23.

Greene, Gilbert; Kruse, Katherine A., and Arthurs, Ruth S. "Family Practice Social Work: A New Area of Specialization," *Social Work in Health Care 10*(3), Spring 1985, pp. 53–73.

Hallowitz, Emanuel. "Innovations in Hospital Social Work," *Social Work 17*(4), July 1972, pp. 89–97.

Jacobs, P. E., Lurie, A., and McLaughlin, M. "Employee Assistance Programs — A New Role for Hospital-Based Social Work Services," *Social Work in Health Care 5*(3), Spring 1980, pp. 313–317.

Jansson, Bruce S., and Simmons, June. "The Survival of Social Work Units in Host Organizations," *Social Work 31*:5, September-October 1986, pp. 339–343.

Lesser, Joan Granucci, and Casaveno, Victoria Hudes. "Establishing a Hospital's Employee Assistance Program," *Health and Social Work 11*(2), Spring 1986, pp. 126–132.

Reamer, Frederic. "Facing Up to the Challenge of DRGs," *Health and Social Work 10*(2), Spring 1985, pp. 85–94.

Rehr, Helen. "Health Care Social Work Services: Present Concerns and Future Directions," *Social Work in Health Care 10*(1), Fall 1984, pp. 71–83.

Rosenberg, Gary, and Rehr, Helen (Eds.), *Advancing Social Work Practice in the Health Care Field: Emerging Issues and New Perspectives*. New York: The Haworth Press, 1983.

Schoenfeld, Harvey. "Opportunities for Leadership for the Social Worker in Hospitals: An Administrator's Expectations," *Social Work in Health Care 1*(1), Fall 1975, pp. 93–96.

Wax, John. "Power Theory and Institutional Change," *Social Service Review 45*(3), September 1971, pp. 274–288.

_____. "Developing Social Work Power in a Medical Organization," *Social Work 13*(4), October 1968, pp. 62–71.

Wilson, Paul A. "Expanding the Role of Social Workers in Coordination of Health Services," *Health and Social Work 6*(1), February 1981, pp. 57-64.

Index

927